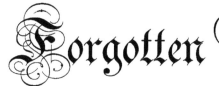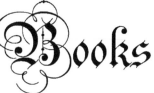

ISBN 978-1-331-06333-9
PIBN 10140007

For support please visit www.forgottenbooks.com

1 MONTH OF
FREE
READING

at
www.ForgottenBooks.com

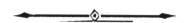

By purchasing this book you are eligible for one month membership to ForgottenBooks.com, giving you unlimited access to our entire collection of over 1,000,000 titles via our web site and mobile apps.

To claim your free month visit:

www.forgottenbooks.com/free140007

TRANSACTIONS

OF THE

clinical

AMERICAN, CLIMATOLOGICAL ASSOCIATION.

FOR THE YEAR 1901.

VOLUME XVII.

"The object of this Association shall be the study of Climatology and Hydrology and of Diseases of the Respiratory and Circulatory Organs."—*Constitution.*

PHILADELPHIA:
PRINTED FOR THE ASSOCIATION.
1901.

Copies may be had of the Secretary.

VOL. XI. contains a complete Index of 11 volumes.

DORNAN, PRINTER.

OFFICERS OF THE ASSOCIATION,
1901.

President.

R. H. BABCOCK, M.D., CHICAGO.

Vice-Presidents.

ALBERT C. PEALE, M.D., WASHINGTON.

S. W. LANGMAID, M.D., BOSTON.

Secretary and Treasurer.

GUY HINSDALE, M.D., PHILADELPHIA.

Council.

JAMES B. WALKER, M.D., PHILADELPHIA.

E. FLETCHER INGALS, M.D., CHICAGO.

E. O. OTIS, M.D., BOSTON.

BEVERLEY ROBINSON, M.D., NEW YORK.

ABRAHAM JACOBI, M.D., NEW YORK.

Representative to the Executive Committee of the Congress of American Physicians and Surgeons for 1901.

FREDERICK I. KNIGHT, M.D., BOSTON.

ROLAND G. CURTIN, M.D., PHILADELPHIA, *Alternate*.

OFFICERS OF THE ASSOCIATION,
1902.

President.

SAMUEL A. FISK, M.D., Denver.

Vice-Presidents.

NORMAN BRIDGE, M.D., Los Angeles.

W. F. R. PHILLIPS, M.D., Weather Bureau, Washington.

Secretary and Treasurer.

GUY HINSDALE, M.D., Philadelphia.

Council.

E. FLETCHER INGALS, M.D., Chicago.

E. O. OTIS, M.D., Boston.

BEVERLEY ROBINSON, M.D., New York.

ABRAHAM JACOBI, M.D., LL.D., New York.

R. H. BABCOCK, M.D., Chicago.

Representatives to the Executive Committee of the Congress of American Physicians and Surgeons.

FREDERICK I. KNIGHT, M.D., Boston.

ROLAND G. CURTIN, M.D., Philadelphia, *Alternate*.

CONTENTS.

LIST OF OFFICERS.

Presidents.

Name.	Year.
A. L Loomis	1884–5.
William Pepper	1886.
Frank Donaldson	1887.
A. L. Loomis	1888.
V. Y. Bowditch	1889.
Charles Denison	1890.
F. I. Knight	1891.
W. E. Ford	1892.
R. G. Curtin	1893.
A. H. Smith	1894.
S. E. Solly	1895.
J. B. Walker	1896.
E. Fletcher Ingals	1897.
E. O. Otis	1898.
Beverley Robinson	1899.
Abraham Jacobi	1900.
Robert H. Babcock	1901.
Samuel A. Fisk	1902.

Vice-Presidents.

F. I. Knight, W. H. Geddings	1884–5.
Frank Donaldson, Beverley Robinson	1886.
V. Y. Bowditch, R. G. Curtin	1887.
A. Y. P. Garnett, J. T. Whittaker	1888.
J. R. Leaming, E. T. Bruen	1889.
A. L. Gihon, H. B. Baker	1890.
E. L. Trudeau, T. S. Hopkins	1891.
E. Fletcher Ingals, Beverley Robinson	1892.
A. H. Smith, E. O. Otis	1893.
I. Hull Platt, E. L. Trudeau	1894.
John H. Musser, G. R. Butler	1895.
Charles E. Quimby, James A. Hart	1896.
S. A. Fisk, John C. Munro	1897.
Beverley Robinson, C. F. McGahan	1898.
James A. Hart, R. C. Newton	1899.
R. H. Babcock, John Winters Brannan	1900.
Albert C. Peale, S. W. Langmaid	1901.
Norman Bridge, W. F. R. Phillips	1902.

Secretaries and Treasurers.

James B. Walker	1884–95.
Guy Hinsdale	1895–1902.

LIST OF MEMBERS.

Honorary Members.

ELECTED

1897. WEBER, SIR HERMANN, 10 Grosvenor Street, W., London, England.

1897. WILLIAMS, CHARLES THEODORE, 2 Upper Brook Street, W., London.

Corresponding Members.

1898. EYRE, G. G., Claremont, Cape Town, South Africa.

1898. GACHE, SAMUEL, 729 Corrientes Street, Buenos Ayres, South America.

1898. LICÉAGA, EDUARDO, 4 San Andres Street, Mexico.

1898. ORVANANOS, DOMINGO, 25 Chavarri Street, Mexico.

1898. SUNDERLAND, SEPTIMUS, 11 Cavendish Place, Cavendish Square, W., London.

1898. WRAGGE, CLEMENT L., Brisbane, Queensland, Australia.

Active Members.

1888. ABBOT, GRIFFITH E., 13½ Street and Pennsylvania Avenue, Washington, D. C.

1897. ALDEN, C. H., Assistant Surgeon-General, U. S. A. (Ret'd.), 33 Washington Park, Newtonville, Mass.

1897. ALTON, CHARLES D., 86 Farmington Avenue, Hartford, Conn.

1898. ANDERS, HOWARD S., 1836 Wallace Street, Philadelphia.

1889. ANDERS, J. M., 1605 Walnut Street, Philadelphia.

1890. ANDERSON, B. P., Colorado Springs, Col.

1900. ARNOLD, HORACE D., 188 Warren Street, Boston.

ELECTED

1893. BABCOCK, R. H., 103 State Street, Chicago.

1885. BAKER, HENRY B., 726 Ottawa Street, Lansing, Mich.

1898. BALDWIN, EDWARD R., Saranac Lake, N. Y.

1901. BARLOW, W. JARVIS, Wilcox Building, Los Angeles, California.

1898. BATTLE, S. WESTRAY, Asheville, N. C.

1885. BELL, A. N., 337 Clinton Street, Brooklyn.

1896. BERGEY, DAVID H., Laboratory of Hygiene, University of Pennsylvania, Philadelphia.

1896. BERNARDY, E. P., 221 South 17th Street, Philadelphia.

1897. BILLINGS, FRANK, 35 22d Street, Chicago.

1897. BLACKADER, ALEXANDER D., 236 Mountain Street, Montreal, Canada.

1895. BOARDMAN, W. S., 57 Hancock Street, Boston.

1897. BONNEY, S. G., 726 14th Street, Denver.

1884. BOSWORTH, F. H., 41 Park Avenue, N. Y.

1885. BOWDITCH, V. Y., 506 Beacon Street, Boston.

1901. BRACKEN, HENRY MARTYN, 1010 Fourth Street, Minneapolis, Minn.

1891. BRANNAN, JOHN W., 11 West 12th Street, N. Y.

1894. BRIDGE, NORMAN, 217 South Broadway, Los Angeles, California.

1897. BROWN, SANGER, Reliance Building, Chicago.

1890. BUCKLEY, J. J., Missoula, Mont.

1896. BULETTE, W. W., Central Block, Pueblo, Col.

1886. BUTLER, G. R., 229 Gates Avenue, Brooklyn.

1896. CAMPBELL, W. A., 424 North Nevada Avenue, Colorado Springs, Col.

1898. CASSELBERRY, W. E., 34 Washington Street, Chicago.

1894. CHAPIN, FREDERICK W., Hot Springs, Va.

1887. CHAPMAN, S. H., New Haven, Conn.

1898. CHAPPELL, WALTER F., 7 East 55th Street, New York.

1898. CLEEMANN, RICHARD A., 2135 Spruce Street, Philadelphia.

1901. COBB, J. O., U. S. Marine Hospital Service, care of Surgeon-General, Washington, D. C.

1894. COLEMAN, THOMAS D., 563 Greene Street, Augusta, Ga.

1901. COLLINS, CHARLES FARNHAM, 50 West 55th Street, New York City.

ELECTED

1891. RANSOM, C. C., 66 West 49th Street, New York (Richfield Springs).

1884. REED, BOARDMAN, 1831 Chestnut Street, Philadelphia.

1885. RICE, C. C., 123 East 19th Street, New York.

1901. RICHARDSON, CHARLES W., 1102 L Street, Washington, D. C.

1893. RISLEY, S. D., 1824 Chestnut Street, Philadelphia.

1899. RIVES, WILLIAM C., 1723 I Street, Washington, D. C.

1884. ROBINSON, BEVERLEY, 42 West 37th Street, New York.

1890. ROBINSON, W. D., 2012 Mt. Vernon Street, Philadelphia.

1892. ROE, JOHN O., 28 North Clinton Street, Rochester, N. Y.

1890. ROGERS, E. J. A., 222 Colfax Avenue, Denver, Col.

1889. RUCK, CARL VON, Asheville, N. C.

1884. SCHAUFFLER, E. W., 1221 Washington Street, Kansas City, Mo.

1901. DE SCHWEINITZ, E. A., 1325 H Street, N. W., Washington, D. C.

1901. SEWALL, HENRY, 23 Eighteenth Avenue, Denver, Col.

1884. SHURLY, E L., 32 Adams Avenue, West Detroit, Mich.

1890. SMITH, A. ALEXANDER, 8 West 47th Street, New York.

1885. SMITH, ANDREW H., 18 East 47th Street, New York.

1887. SMITH, FRANK FREMONT, Palm Beach, Florida, and Bar Harbor, Maine.

1887. SOLLY, S. E., 2 North Cascade Avenue, Colorado Springs, Colorado.

1900. STENGEL, ALFRED, 1811 Spruce Street, Philadelphia.

1898. STUBBERT, J. EDWARD, Liberty, New York.

1901. SWAN, WILL HOWARD, Colorado Springs, Col.

1892. TAYLOR, H. LONGSTREET, 75 Lowry Arcade, St. Paul, Minn.

1896. TAYLOR, J. MADISON, 1504 Pine Street, Philadelphia.

1885. TRUDEAU, E. L., Saranac Lake, N. Y.

1884. TYNDALE, J. HILGARD, 13th and P Streets, Lincoln, Neb.

1884. WALKER, JAMES B., 1617 Green Street, Philadelphia.

1891. WATSON, E. W., 131 North 20th Street, Philadelphia.

1895. WEBER, LEONARD, 25 West 46th Street, New York.

1897. WHITCOMB, H. H., Norristown, Pa.
1898. WHITNEY, HERBERT B., 726 14th Street, Denver, Col.
1898. WILLIAMS, FRANCIS H., 505 Beacon Street, Boston.
1898. WILLIAMS, HAROLD, 528 Beacon Street, Boston.
1885. WILLIAMS, H. F., 197 Gates Avenue, Brooklyn.
1884. WILSON, JAMES C., 1437 Walnut Street, Philadelphia.
1901. WYMAN, WALTER, Surgeon-General, U. S. Marine Hospital Service, Washington, D. C.

Total, 133 active members.

MINUTES.

THE Eighteenth Annual Meeting of the American Climatological Association was called to order at the Cataract House, Niagara Falls, on May 30, 1901. The President, Dr. R. H. Babcock, of Chicago, occupied the chair.

The following members were in attendance during the sessions:

Col. C. H. Alden, Assistant Surg.-Gen., U. S. A., Ret'd.
Dr. Horace D. Arnold, Boston.
Dr. R. H. Babcock, Chicago.
Dr. Edward R. Baldwin, Saranac Lake, N. Y.
Dr. E. P. Bernardy, Philadelphia.
Dr. S. G. Bonney, Denver.
Dr. Vincent Y. Bowditch, Boston.
Dr. John W. Brannan, New York.
Dr. Norman Bridge, Los Angeles, Cal.
Dr. W. A. Campbell, Colorado Springs.
Dr. W. E. Casselberry, Chicago.
Dr. Thomas D. Coleman, Augusta, Ga.
Dr. A. Coolidge, Boston.
Dr. R. G. Curtin, Philadelphia.
Dr. Judson Daland, Philadelphia.
Dr. Carroll E. Edson, Denver.
Dr. H. L. Elsner, Syracuse.
Dr. Samuel A. Fisk, Denver.
Dr. Charles F. Gardiner, Colorado Springs.
Dr. A. C. Getchell, Worcester.
Dr. W. C. Glasgow, St. Louis.
Dr. James A. Hart, Colorado Springs.
Dr. Guy Hinsdale, Philadelphia.
Dr. Arnold C. Klebs, Chicago.
Dr. Frederick I. Knight, Boston.
Dr. C. F. McGahan, Aiken, S. C.
Dr. Charles L. Minor, Asheville, N. C.

Dr. R. C. Newton, Montclair, N. J.

Dr. E. O. Otis, Boston.

Dr. W. F. R. Phillips, Washington, D. C.

Dr. Charles E. Quimby, New York.

Dr. C. C. Ransom, New York.

Dr. Boardman Reed, Philadelphia.

Dr. William C. Rives, Washington, D. C.

Dr. W. D. Robinson, Philadelphia.

Dr. E. L. Shurly, Detroit.

Dr. Frank Fremont Smith, Bar Harbor.

Dr. S. E. Solly, Colorado Springs.

Dr. J. Edward Stubbert, Liberty, N. Y.

Dr. James B. Walker, Philadelphia.

Dr. Herbert B. Whitney, Denver.

Dr. Harold Williams, Boston.

Dr. James C. Wilson, Philadelphia.

Upon motion of Dr. Solly, the minutes of the previous meeting, as printed, were accepted without reading.

The Secretary, Dr. Guy Hinsdale, made the following report:

During the past year the Association has lost by death one active member—Dr. Rufus P. Lincoln, of New York—and one honorary member—Dr. Alfred Stillé, of Philadelphia. Dr. Lincoln was elected to membership in 1890, and died at his home in New York City after an operation for appendicitis. He was a graduate of Amherst College in 1862, and of the Medical Department of Harvard University in 1868. Dr. Lincoln was widely known and highly regarded for his sterling qualities as a gentleman and as a practitioner.

Dr. Alfred Stillé died on September 24, 1900, at his home in Philadelphia, in his eighty-seventh year. He was a man of high attainments and had an international reputation. After graduation from the University of Pennsylvania, in 1836, Dr. Stillé served as Resident Physician in the Philadelphia and Pennsylvania Hospitals; he went to Paris with Dr. George C. Shattuck, of Boston, and came under the teaching and influence of the distinguished Louis. Dr. Stillé read a paper in 1838 in which he presented in tabular form the contrasts and distinctions, clinical and anatomical, between typhus and typhoid fever. In 1848 he wrote the first general pathology published in the English language. He published standard works on therapeutics, and, in conjunction with Professor Maisch, a United States Dispensatory. His publications were numerous, and the effect of his lectures on medicine in the University of Pennsylvania was far reaching.

Dr. Stillé was proud of his honorary membership in this Association. As I personally handed him the annual volume in late years he never failed to speak in appreciation of the work of the Association, the high quality of the papers read at the meetings, and the pleasure it gave him to read the TRANSACTIONS. A fine portrait of Professor Stillé was inserted in the last annual volume.

In June, 1900, by vote of the Council, the attention of members was called to Section 4, Article III., of the Constitution, which provides that "Any member of the Association absent from the meetings, in person or by contributed paper, for three consecutive years, without sufficient cause, may be dropped from the list of members by vote of the Council." It is quite likely that the present large attendance and extensive programme are to be attributed in large measure to this warning.

There have been proposed for membership thirteen names. Descriptive ballots have been printed and forwarded to all members. Notice has also been given of a proposed addition to Article III., Section 1, of the Constitution, "Active members shall not exceed 150." Our present membership is 126.

During the past year the Council held one meeting, June 6, 1900, at Atlantic City. There were present Dr. R. H. Babcock, Dr. E. F. Ingals, Dr. R. G. Curtin, Dr. J. B. Walker, and Dr. Hinsdale. The plans for the present meeting were carefully considered, and it was ordered that a letter be sent to each member relative to time and place of meeting. The result of this was that the vote stood 32 for Colorado and 35 for Niagara Falls. It was accordingly decided to hold the meeting at Niagara Falls.

The publication of our annual volume was delayed by various causes. Several months elapsed before some of the papers were forwarded to the Secretary. The volume finally went to press without one of the papers, in spite of the Secretary's efforts to obtain it.

The previous volume having cost $629, the Secretary made an effort to reduce this heavy drain on our resources. After communicating with our corresponding member, Dr. Septimus Sunderland, one of the editors of the *Journal of Balneology and Climatology*, the organ of the Balneological and Climatological Association, a favorable arrangement was entered into, by which their publishers, Messrs. John Bale, Sons & Danielsson, L'td. of London, would print all the papers of our volume, and by which the editors would utilize some of the papers in their journal. The result was that we secured 300 copies of our TRANSACTIONS at a cost of $220. The preliminary matter was printed in Philadelphia by Mr. Wm. J. Dornan, and the volume illustrated, bound, and distributed for an additional expense of $145, making a total of $365, or $264 less than in the previous year.

The Secretary recommends a renewal of the arrangements for another year.

In accordance with a resolution of the Association, the Secretary forwarded to the Library Exchange of the Association of Medical Librarians, Baltimore, sixty copies of our TRANSACTIONS for 1898, 1899, and 1900. Seventy copies were sent to medical journals and to libraries throughout the world. All our copies for foreign addresses were sent free of charge by the International Bureau of Exchanges of the Smithsonian Institution, to which we are under obligations.

The following is a summary of the expenditures and receipts:

Balance on hand May 1, 1900 .	$102 78	
Received from payment of dues .	600 00	
Received from other sources . .	8 75	
Total		$711 53

Expended:

Reporter's services	$88 52	
Subscription to International Medical Congress	25 00	
TRANSACTIONS for 1900 . . .	365 00	
Miscellaneous printing . . .	55 15	
Other expenses	66 51	
		600 18
Balance on hand May 30, 1901 . .		$111 35

There is due the Association from members $300. Notice has been received from the Secretary of the Congress of American Physicians and Surgeons that a delegate and alternate to the

Executive Committee of the Congress for 1903 should be appointed at this meeting.

A series of communications relative to the choice of a place for holding the next meeting of the Association has been received and submitted to the Council.

On the invitation of Mr. Malcolm Morris, Hon. Secretary-General of the British Congress on Tuberculosis for the Prevention of Consumption, to be held in London July 22–26, 1901, members of this Association are invited to participate. Credentials have been furnished to two of our members—Dr. S. Edwin Solly and Dr. E. O. Otis, who will represent us on that occasion. If any others are anticipating a visit to England at that time, credentials will be furnished on application. The attention of members is called to the great importance and wide scope of this Congress and the distinguished character of its organization.

During the past year the following books have been received :

Transactions of the American Laryngological Association.

Transactions of the Mississippi Valley Medical Association.

Transactions of the Texas Medical Association.

Transactions of the Kentucky State Medical Society.

Bulletin Royal Academy of Medicine of Brussels.

Report of the Weather Bureau, 1898–99, vol. i.

Index Catalogue Library Surgeon-General's Office, U. S. A., vols. i.–vi.

Public Health Reports, 1900–1901.

Climate and Crop Service Reports for Pennsylvania and New Mexico.

Journal of Balneology and Climatology, 1900–1901.

Bulletin of the American Academy of Medicine, 1900–1901.

Dr. Hinsdale presented the Treasurer's account, and it was referred to a committee of two—Drs. Phillips and Elsner—for auditing. The Chairman then appointed the following Nominating Committee: Drs. Walker, Otis, Alden, Solly, and Bonney.

Dr. Walker, referring to the excessive amount of work required of the Secretary-Treasurer and the small sum heretofore paid for such services, moved that $100 be paid to Dr. Hinsdale for such work. The motion was unanimously adopted.

The Secretary announced that through Dr. Quimby the members of the Association were invited to visit the Niagara Falls Power Company's plant, and also to take the trip around the gorge as the guests of Mr. Rankin, First Vice-President of the Company.

Upon motion of Dr. Walker it was decided to accept the invitations as extended, and to make these trips on Friday afternoon, May 31.

It was then decided to hold an evening session, beginning at 8 o'clock. The Secretary read a letter from Dr. Alton, and the subject was referred to the Council for consideration.

Adjournment.

SECOND DAY.

A business meeting was called at 11.15 A.M. The Secretary reported for the Council on the approval of candidates for membership.

The Auditing Committee reported that it had examined the accounts of the Treasurer and found them correct. Upon motion of Dr. Hance the report was accepted.

The Nominating Committee reported through Dr. Walker a choice of the following officers: President, Dr. S. A. Fisk; Vice-Presidents, Dr. Norman Bridge and Dr. W. F. R. Phillips; Secretary and Treasurer, Dr. Guy Hinsdale; Member of the Council, Dr. R. H. Babcock; Representative to the Congress of American Physicians and Surgeons, Dr. F. I. Knight; Alternate, Dr. R. G. Curtin.

Upon motion of Dr. Newton the report was accepted, and the Secretary instructed to cast the ballot electing these gentlemen.

Dr. Newton called for a vote on the amendment to the Constitution limiting the membership to 150; after an extended discussion the amendment was adopted.

Dr. Elsner offered a resolution concerning the State supervision and care of the tuberculous poor:

WHEREAS, The study of tuberculosis has demonstrated the great value of supervision, climatic treatment, and the proper nourishment of the tuberculous; and appreciating the fact that the large number of these are unable, because of circumstances, to take advantage of the necessary treatment, be it

Resolved, therefore, That the American Climatological Association commend State supervision and care of the tuberculous poor, preferably in suitably appointed sanatoria.

The resolution was seconded and adopted, but Dr. Quimby requested to be put on record as opposing the resolution on the basis of the good of the State and the greatest good to the largest number.

The following were elected active members: Dr. W. Jarvis Barlow, Los Angeles; Dr. Henry M. Bracken, Minneapolis; Dr. J. O. Cobb United States Marine Hospital Service; Dr. Charles F. Collins, New York City; Dr. George W. Guthrie, Wilkesbarre, Pa.; Dr. Charles G. Jennings, Detroit; Dr. Charles W. Richardson, Washington; Dr. E. A. de Schweinitz, Washington; Dr. Henry Sewall, Denver; Dr. Will Howard Swan, Colorado Springs; Dr. Walter Wyman, Surgeon-General United States Marine Hospital Service.

On the recommendation of the Council the Association voted to remit the dues of one member and to drop two from the roll.

At the annual dinner, held in the evening, a message of greeting from the American Laryngological Association was read.

SATURDAY, JUNE 1ST—MORNING SESSION.

The meeting was called to order by the President at 9.45 A.M. and the following gentlemen were named as members of the Committee on Nomenclature, in accordance with Dr. Stubbert's paper: Drs. Quimby, Knight, Wilson, Baldwin, Stubbert, and Bowditch.

In accordance with a suggestion of the President, Dr. Fisk moved the appointment of a committee of three to continue the work on Mineral Springs, started by Dr. Hinsdale. The motion was carried, and the Chair appointed Drs. Hinsdale, Peale, and Ransom.

The Council recommended that the next annual meeting be held at Coronado Beach, Cal., and this was adopted; upon motion of Dr. Brannan it was decided to hold this meeting on or about the 1st of June, 1902.

Dr. Newton presented the following amendments to the Constitution providing for the establishment of an associate membership:

To amend Article III., Section 1, by inserting the word "associate" after the word "active."

To amend Article III. by adding the following sections:

Article III., Section 1. This Association shall consist of active, associate, corresponding, and honorary members, the former not to exceed one hundred and fifty, and the latter not to exceed ten.

Sec. 5. Any active member of the Association who shall have

been in good standing for five years may, at his own request, become an associate member.

Sec. 6. Associate members shall be free from the provisions of Section 4, and shall be exempt from the payment of dues. They shall have no vote, but shall enjoy in all other respects the same privileges as active members of this Association.

Sec. 7. The Council may recommend any active member of this Association who shall have failed to comply with the provisions of Section 4 for associate membership, and if the Association shall so vote he shall become an associate member.

The Association passed a vote of thanks to Mr. W. B. Rankin, Vice-President of the Power Development Company, for courtesies extended to the Association ; also to the proprietor of the Cataract House for his efforts to provide for our entertainment.

A vote of thanks was also passed to the retiring officers for their labors in bringing to a successful termination one of the most interesting meetings of the Association.

The Association then adjourned.

GUY HINSDALE,
Secretary.

ADDENDUM.—The President, Dr. S. A. Fisk, subsequently appointed the following committees :

On Programme : Dr. E. R. Baldwin, Saranac Lake, N. Y.; Chairman ; Dr. Vincent Y. Bowditch, 506 Beacon Street, Boston , Carroll E. Edson, McPhee Building, Denver, Col.

On Invitations : Dr. Frederick I. Knight, 195 Beacon Street, Boston, Chairman ; Dr. Roland G. Curtin, 22 South Eighteenth Street, Philadelphia ; Dr. E. Fletcher Ingals, 34 Washington Street, Chicago.

On Transportation : Dr. E. O. Otis, 381 Beacon Street, Boston, Chairman ; Dr. J. B. Walker, 1617 Green Street, Philadelphia ; Dr. John W. Brannan, 11 West Twelfth Street, New York ; Dr. Robert H. Babcock, 100 State Street, Chicago ; Dr. Sherman G. Bonney, 726 Fourteenth Street, Denver ; Dr. W. F. R. Phillips, Washington, D. C.

On Arrangements in California : Dr. Norman Bridge, 217 South Broadway, Los Angeles, Cal., Chairman ; Dr. W. Jarvis Barlow, Los Angeles, Cal. ; Dr. E. J. A. Rogers, 222 Colfax Avenue, Denver, Col.

The President and Secretary members of committees, *ex officio.*

OBITUARY.

WILLIAM H. DALY.

By the death of DR. WILLIAM H. DALY, which occurred at his home, in Pittsburg, June 9, 1901, the medical profession has lost an earnest and able member; the country and the community a loyal, enterprising, and valued citizen; his family and kindred a fond and devoted member, and his intimate associates a genial, large-hearted, and steadfast friend.

Dr. William Hudson Daly was born at Blairsville, Indiana County, Pa., September 11, 1842, and was the son of Thomas and Helen Daly. His father was of Scotch descent, but a native of Ireland; his mother was of an ancient Scottish family. His parents died when he was but seventeen years of age, after which he went to Richmond, Va., where he lived until the outbreak of the Civil War, when he enlisted in the Confederate Army as a private in Company B, 15th Virginia Volunteers, and participated in most of the early battles from Big Bethel to Lee's Mills, where he was taken prisoner by the Federal troops.

Soon after he took the oath of allegiance to the Union cause, went to Philadelphia, under government orders, to take a course in the Jefferson Medical College, during the years 1863 and 1864, and served as medical cadet in the Germantown Hospital. Later he was appointed assistant surgeon in the United States Army, and was assigned to duty in the Army Hospital at White-hall. From that place he was transferred to Savannah, Ga., for service in the general army hospitals, being subsequently appointed post surgeon, and stationed for active service at Hilton Head, S. C.

In 1865 he was stationed at Jacksonville, Florida, and, in company with other medical officers, took charge of the last five thousand prisoners released from Andersonville Prison, and continued to serve actively until the cessation of hostilities and the disbanding of the army.

After the close of the war he continued his medical studies in the University of Michigan and graduated from the medical department in 1866. He then took up the practice of medicine in Pittsburg and continued it until the time of his death. He soon acquired a large practice, attained a leading position among his confrères, and, in recognition of his attainments, was called to numerous important and public positions.

In 1868 he was appointed physician to the Reform School of Pennsylvania, and served in that capacity eight years, until the removal of that institution from Allegheny.

From 1879 until 1887 he served as general surgeon of the Pittsburg and Lake Erie Railroad. He was a senior physician to the Western Pennsylvania Hospital from the time of its organization, and consulting throat surgeon to the Pittsburg Free Dispensary. At the outbreak of the Spanish-American war he was appointed chief surgeon, with the rank of major, of the United States Volunteers, and assigned to duty on the staff of Lieutenant-General Nelson A. Miles. He served through the Puerto Rican campaign, and at its close took charge of one of the largest returning transports.

It was during this campaign that he exposed the fraudulent transaction of the Commissary Department known as the "embalmed beef" scandal, which became the subject of official investigation.

In 1878–1879 he spent a year in Europe, taking special courses and attending the various hospitals of London, Paris, Berlin, and Vienna, studying diseases of the nose, throat, and ear, since which time he made a specialty of and confined his practice mainly to this department, in which he attained eminence both in this country and in Europe.

As an evidence of his interest and high standing in medicine he was elected to active membership in many of the national societies of this country and in some European societies. He was a member of the Allegheny County and State Medical Society of Pennsylvania, the American Medical Association, the Association of Military Surgeons of the United States, the Mississippi Valley Medical Association, the Tri-State Medical Society, the American Social Science Association, and was chairman of the Health Department. He was also a member of the British Medical Association. Of the special societies he was a member of the American Climatological Association, the American Laryngological Association, the American Laryngological, Rhinological, and Otological Society, and was a corresponding member of the British Laryngological, Rhinological, and Otological Society, and of the Société Française d'Otologie et de Laryngologie et de Rhinologie. He was also a member of the Eighth International Medical Congress, held in Copenhagen, Denmark, in 1884, and did signal service at that meeting in upholding the status of laryngology in America in a paper on that subject. He was also a member of the Ninth International Medical Congress, held in Washington in 1887.

Dr. Daly has also been honored by many of the societies to which he belonged. For ten consecutive years he was Recording Secretary of the Allegheny County Medical Society, and was afterward elected President of that body, and also President of the Medical Society of the State of Pennsylvania.

He organized and became the first chairman of the section of Laryngology of the American Medical Association, and was sent three times by that Association as a delegate to the British Medical Association.

In 1887 he was elected chairman of the section of Laryngology of the Ninth International Medical Congress, held in Washington, in August, 1887. He organized this section and carried it through most successfully at a time when, owing to uncalled-for dissensions in the ranks, it had been abandoned by the previous appointees to that position.

In 1896 he was elected President of the American Laryngological Association; in 1897, President of the Laryngological, Rhinological, and Otological Society, and the same year he was elected chairman of the Health Section of the American Social Science Association.

Dr. Daly's contributions to medical literature were numerous and always of a high order, showing marked originality of thought and the positiveness of his convictions. He was among the pioneers of laryngology in this country, and was the first to call attention to the clinical relations between hay fever and nasal disease. He was also interested in many allied and collateral branches of medicine, as shown by his interest in the American Public Health Association ; and it was from clinical observations made by him during his hunting trips of the fact that all persons who avoided drinking the water in malarial districts escaped malarial infection, that led him to believe, long before the plasmodium was found, that malaria was due to a germ and transmitted in the water, and not caused by a contamination of the atmosphere.

Dr. Daly was exceedingly fond of outdoor sports, of hunting, fishing, and travel, and frequently contributed to the press most interesting articles describing his observations and experiences.

It was his custom every year during the hunting season to take trips West or South where game was particularly abundant, and it was on one of these hunting trips that he became acquainted with General Nelson A. Miles, who ever afterward was his steadfast friend. The story of their meeting is a somewhat interesting one. One day while Dr. Daly was in camp in the Big Horn Mountains, during an expedition for elk hunting, a man came tearing over the range asking for a physician to go to a camp many miles away to attend a sick girl. The rider was William F. Cody, better known as Buffalo Bill, and the father of the girl was General Miles. Dr. Daly went and brought the patient safely out of her illness, and the bond of friendship formed between General Miles and himself during the days he remained in the camp was followed by many hunting expeditions together afterward, and continued to the time of his death.

Dr. Daly was a member of the Duquesne Club and also of the Sportsmen's Club of Pittsburg, and an active member and part owner of the Revels Island Rod and Gun Club on the Virginia coast.

Dr. Daly was possessed of a fine physique and commanding presence, which, with great force of character, strong will-power, great determination and perseverance, made him a conspicuous figure wherever he was. He was also possessed of a sturdy manhood, a high sense of honor, and a courageous loyalty to whatever he believed to be his duty and to whatever he regarded as right.

In addition to the high standing of Dr. Daly in the medical profession he enjoyed, together with his estimable wife, a high social position. This followed naturally from his marked social characteristics, for with his friends he was always a hale fellow well met, with ready wit and a great fund of anecdote, which made him a conspicuous central figure in every social gathering.

Dr. Daly was married, June 22, 1869, to Athalia, the eldest daughter of James M. Cooper, a prominent steel manufacturer of Pittsburg, and a member of one of the oldest families. Two children were born to them, but both died during infancy—James Cooper Daly, at the age of four years, in April, 1874, and William Theodore Daly, at the age of eleven months, in 1877.

Dr. Daly was of an affectionate nature, and his home ties were very dear to him. His saddest blow was the death of Mrs. Daly, who had been his constant companion for many years, occurring somewhat suddenly November 22, 1899, at Sioux City, Iowa, where she had gone to accompany Dr. Daly on a hunting trip.

The doctor was very devoted to Mrs. Daly, and in his will, which he had made four months before he died, he left almost his entire fortune, about a quarter of a million dollars, to found a home in Pittsburg for working girls and women as a memorial to be known as "The Athalia Daly Home."   J. O. R.

DR. CARL RUEDI, a corresponding member of this Association, died on June 17, 1901, at Arosa, Switzerland. Dr. Ruedi was formerly an active member, while residing at Denver, and was elected in 1891. He contributed papers entitled "A Comparison of the Winter Health Resorts in the Alps with Some Places in the Rocky Mountains of Colorado," in 1894; "A Peep into the Future with Respect of Pathological Anatomical Researches," in 1895; and participated in the various discussions in previous meetings. He was a man of high scientific attainments, and was widely known and respected.

CONSTITUTION AND BY-LAWS.

CONSTITUTION.

ARTICLE I.—NAME.

THIS Society shall be known as the AMERICAN CLIMATO-LOGICAL ASSOCIATION.

ARTICLE II.—OBJECT.

The object of this Association shall be the study of *Climatology and Hydrology and of Diseases of the Respiratory and Circulatory Organs.*

ARTICLE III.—MEMBERSHIP.

Section 1.—This Association shall consist of *active, corresponding,* and *honorary* members, the former not to exceed one hundred and fifty, and the latter not to exceed ten.

Sec. 2.—Names of candidates for active membership, whose applications have been indorsed by *two* (2) active members, shall be sent to the Secretary at least thirty (30) days before the annual meeting. On approval of the Council, the applicant shall be balloted for at the annual meeting. Three (3) black balls shall be sufficient to reject a candidate. The Council shall have power to nominate active members.

Sec. 3.—The power of nominating honorary and corresponding members shall be vested in the Council. The election shall be conducted in the same manner as that for active members. Honorary members shall enjoy all the privileges of active members, but shall not be allowed to hold any office or cast any vote.

Sec. 4.—Any member of the Association absent from the meetings, in person or by contributed paper, for three (3) consecutive years, without sufficient cause, may be dropped from the list of members by vote of the Council.

ARTICLE IV.—OFFICERS.

Section 1.—The officers of this Association shall consist of a *President*, two *Vice-Presidents*, a *Secretary and Treasurer*, who, with five other members and the delegate and alternate to the Executive Committee of the Congress of American Physicians and Surgeons shall constitute the *Council* of the Association.

Sec. 2.—Nominations. The officers, including the Council, shall be nominated by a committee of five (5) members, which committee shall be nominated by the President at the first session of each annual meeting, and shall report at the business meeting.

Sec. 3.—Elections. The election of officers shall take place at the business meeting. A majority of votes cast shall constitute an election.

Sec. 4.—The President, Vice-Presidents, Secretary and Treasurer shall enter upon their duties at the close of the annual meeting at which they are elected, and shall hold office until the close of the next annual meeting, or until their successors are elected.

Sec. 5.—Members of the Council, other than the President, Vice-Presidents, Secretary and Treasurer, shall hold office for five (5) years.

Sec. 6.— Vacancies. Any vacancy occurring among the officers of the Association during the year may be filled by the Council.

ARTICLE V.—DUTIES OF OFFICERS.

President and Vice-Presidents.

The President and Vice-Presidents shall discharge the duties usually devolving upon such officers. The President shall be *ex-officio* Chairman of the Council.

Secretary and Treasurer.

As Secretary, he shall attend and keep a record of all the meetings of the Association and of the Council, of which latter he shall be *ex-officio* Clerk. At each annual meeting he shall announce the names of all who have ceased to be members since the last report. He shall superintend the publication of the TRANSACTIONS, under the direction of the Council. He shall notify candidates of their election to membership. He shall send a preliminary notification of the annual meeting two (2) months previous thereto, and the programme for the annual meeting at least two (2) weeks previous to its assembly, to all the members of the Association. He shall also send notification of the meetings of the Council to the members thereof. At each annual meeting of the Association he shall read the minutes of the previous meeting and of all the meetings of the Council that have been held during the current year.

As Treasurer, he shall receive all moneys due, and pay all debts therewith. He shall render an account thereof at the annual meeting, at which time an auditing committee shall be appointed to report.

ARTICLE VI.—COUNCIL.

The Council shall meet as often as the interests of the Association may require.

Four (4) members shall constitute a quorum.

It shall have the management of the affairs of the Association, subject to the action of the Association at its annual meetings.

It shall consider the claims of candidates recommended to it for admission to membership.

It shall not have the power to make the Association liable for any debts exceeding in total one hundred dollars ($100), in the course of any one year, unless specially authorized by a vote of the Association.

It shall have the entire control of the publications of the Association, with the power to reject such papers or discussions as it may deem best.

It shall have power to nominate active members at the annual meeting.

The Council shall have power to invite any gentleman, not a member, to read a paper at the annual meeting, on any subject within the scope of the objects of this Association.

The Council shall determine questions by vote, or—if demanded —by ballot, the President having a casting vote.

The Council shall constitute a Board of Trial for all offences against the Constitution and By-Laws, or for unbecoming conduct, and shall have the sole power of moving the expulsion of any member.

The President, or any two members, may call a meeting, notice of which shall be transmitted to every member two (2) weeks previous to the meeting.

ARTICLE VII.—PAPERS.

Section 1.—The titles of all papers to be read at any annual meeting shall be forwarded to the Secretary not later than one (1) month before the first day of the meeting, in order to appear on the printed programme.

Sec. 2.—No paper shall be read before the Association which has already been printed or been read before another body.

ARTICLE VIII.—QUORUM.

A quorum for business purposes shall be ten (10) members.

ARTICLE IX.—AMENDMENTS.

This Constitution may be amended by a four-fifths ($\frac{4}{5}$) vote of all the members present at an annual meeting, provided that notice of the proposed amendment has been printed in the notification of the meeting at which the vote is to be taken.

BY-LAWS.

1. Meetings of the Association shall be held annually.
2. The time and place of the meetings shall be determined by the Council.
3. The dues of active members shall consist of an annual assessment not to exceed five ($5) dollars. The initiation fee shall be ten ($10) dollars. Members in arrears shall not be

entitled to vote. Those in arrears for two (2) years may be dropped from membership by recommendation of the Council.

4. Order of business meeting.

First day :

    Calling the roll of members;

    Minutes of previous meeting;

    Treasurer's report;

    Appointment of auditing committee;

    Appointment of nominating committee;

    Report of Council on recommendations for membership.

Second day—Morning session :

    Report of nominating committee;

    Election of officers;

    Election of members;

    Report of the committee on health resorts;

    Miscellaneous business;

    Adjournment of business meeting.

Any of these By-Laws may be amended, repealed, or suspended by a two-thirds vote of the members present at any meeting.

PRESIDENT'S ADDRESS.

THE LIMITATION OF DRUG THERAPY.*

BY ROBT. H. BABCOCK, M.D.

CHICAGO.

THE purpose for which this Association was established, that is, to promote the study of climatology and hydrology, is a tacit acknowledgment of the great value of the therapeutic agencies residing in nature. Medicine is justly styled the healing art, and therefore, if we would become healers of the sick, as well as diagnosticians, we must endeavour to make a practical application in therapeutics of the truths taught us by pathology, bacteriology, physiological chemistry, &c. We have passed beyond the time when practitioners of medicine were mere empyrical prescribers of nauseous drugs. We have learned that many internal diseases are best managed without medicines, or that if these latter are to be employed at all, it is only in accordance with definite indications, and then only with a view to aiding the natural powers of resistance inherent in the human organism. It is only the tyro or ignorant empyric who fancies he can drive out disease by remedies which at the most only modify symptoms. The fact that we possess two so-called specifics, namely, quinine against malaria and mercury against syphilis, does not at all invalidate the truth of the foregoing remark. Indeed, the very paucity of specific medicinal agencies serves to emphasise the limitation of drugs

* Delivered at the Eighteenth Annual Meeting of the American Climatological Association, at Niagara Falls, May 30, 1901.

in the eradication of those infectious diseases which are the scourge of mankind. We manifest our recognition of this fact every day, and we daily admit our impotence in dealing with these and kindred maladies. We nurse a typhoid fever patient through his attack, often most successfully when we administer no medicine, and then when convalescence sets in we send him into the country or upon a sea voyage that he may avail himself of nature's remedies—fresh air and sunshine. A patient comes to us for treatment because of a bronchitis perchance.. We prescribe appropriate medicines and are or are not successful in bringing about a termination of the process. In many instances we exhaust our therapeutic resources, and at length, discouraged by the continuance of symptoms, the patient takes it into his head to go to a warmer climate, or, in despair over the futility of our efforts, we advise him to go south. Why is this? Because we know that in a suitable climate where he can live out of doors, breathing a balmy air soothing to his irritable respiratory passages, and invigorated by sunshine and plenty of oxygen, away from the dust and germ-laden atmosphere of his home environment, he will get from nature's laboratory what we and our drugs cannot give him. We send gouty and rheumatic sufferers to some resort that they may be benefited by the waters of a natural spring or by a course of baths, while at the same time they may enjoy the invigorating effects of pure air and sunshine; for we know full well that in a way wholly impossible by our medicinal therapeutics these means will modify nutrition and reinforce tissue resistance. These are but a few of the many instances that might be cited in illustration of our dependence upon nature and nature's remedies. Notwithstanding the widespread advertisements of nostrums and the ever-increasing manufacture of pharmaceutical products, all vaunted as unfailing and unequalled, the really intelligent, observing, and conscientious physician grows year by year more impressed with the futility of such medication.

Not many weeks ago I was visited by a representative of

a well-known firm of manufacturing chemists, who, after politely requesting to be excused for trespassing upon my valuable time, proceeded, after the manner of his kind, to enlighten me upon some of the products of their laboratory. In particular he called attention to one of their normal tinctures, echinacea augustifolia, which possessed wonderful curative powers in all conditions attended by the formation of pus. Upon my expressing some astonishment and incredulity regarding such action on the part of a vegetable product he waxed very enthusiastic in its praise, saying it was Black Sampson root and enjoyed great reputation among the American Indians. Indeed, he narrated two very wonderful cases in which its conjoined internal and external use had cured where all other measures had failed. One was a case of purulent discharge from the rectum following an operation, I believe, for piles. Here the medicine had been used as an enema and lotion as well as by the stomach. In the other case a boy had crushed his hand so badly that the surgeon decided an amputation would be necessary. An objection to this operation had been made, and instead, the injured member was dressed with the tincture of Black Sampson root, with the result that the hand was saved in a tolerably serviceable condition. The remedy was also administered internally. As my visitor, a quondam retail druggist, proceeded with his thrilling narrative I sat with my head resting on my hands, and with a scarcely suppressed smile of amusement pondered on the ignorance, or was it the effrontery? of the house that was attempting to retain, nay, to revive, the therapeutics of a century ago. I declined the proffered sample with thanks.

Thirty years ago, when surgeons used to talk about "laudable pus," it might have been in order to attempt to arrest pus formation by means of a vegetable alterative, but in the light of our modern notions of infection such treatment is a manifest absurdity. It seems to me akin to the treatment of acute fibrinous pneumonia by expectorants and tartar emetic, or, if I venture to utter what may sound like heresy, with aconite or veratrum viride.

Not only in suppurative and other infectious processes have we come to realise the futility of the internal administration of ordinary drugs, but as our experience increases in general we find ourselves relying less and less on medicine and insensibly diminishing the number of our remedies in the treatment of disease of all kinds.

We devote more attention to the patient's diet and habits, and more often send him away with good advice than with hastily-written prescriptions. We recommend exercises in the gymnasium, out-door recreation, rest from business and home cares, change of air and scene, the use of water internally and externally; in short, all those various factors and conditions which have been provided by Mother Nature directly and indirectly for the preservation and restoration of health. On the part of the more intelligent lay members of the community, as it seems to me, there is a growing dislike to medicine and medicine givers. This is evinced not only by the frequent remark, " Oh! I'm not much of a hand to take medicine," or by the running after faith healers, mind healers, Christian science healers, and the like, but by the disposition to patronise the numerous instructors in respiratory gymnastics, masseurs, osteopaths, &c., who effect what good they do without the aid of drugs. From the earliest times down to the present, natural springs of one kind and another, health resorts, milk cures, grape cures, and so on, have possessed an unceasing charm for invalids. Some of the attraction, no doubt, lies in novelty, some in the desire to get away from the dreary monotony of medical treatment at home, but in most instances patients are impelled to seek these places and means of cure because of the remarkable benefit there derived by friends and acquaintances; while in a few cases they are sent thither by physicians who have failed in their medicinal management, or anticipate failure.

In this country the distrust of medical men and their

medicines is shown by the great numbers of intelligent people who have turned to Christian Science and mental healing, while from the equally credulous but more ignorant, a Dowie or a Schlatter is able to win thousands of devoted followers who accept faith as the only means of salvation from disease. In Germany the dislike of medical treatment is manifested in a more rational and sensible manner. In various parts of that country there have been established sanatoria where the *natur aertze* subject patients to methods of healing which at first glance seem quite shocking to our notions of propriety. Upon the principle that the more nearly one returns to the ways of primitive man the more surely he will rid himself of the physical evils resulting from modern civilised life, large areas of land are enclosed by high board fences behind which the patients disport themselves in a state of complete nudity. Within separate enclosures men and women without clothing expose their bodies to the action of air and sunshine all day long, working in the earth, playing games, bathing in pools or streams, wallowing in the dirt, and in every other way coming in contact with Mother Nature. They are said to even sleep in the open air with only sufficient protection from the cold night air by a roof, and a modicum of clothing to prevent undue chilling of their bodies. The dietary is extremely simple and is largely vegetarian. It is claimed that thus exposed to wind, rain and sun the skin becomes hardened and glows with the warmth of vigorous circulation, the functions of the several organs become natural, and mere physical existence reaches a degree of enjoyment entirely unknown before. The land is said to be flooded with publications setting forth the wonderful results of such a life for a few weeks or months, and so many thousands flock to these institutions that this *natur heilkunde* has become a serious menace to the prosperity of the rank and file of medical practitioners. The initiative to this method of natural healing seems to have been given, so far as I can learn, by the Kneipp cure. We are wont to

think of this latter as consisting chiefly of morning walks with
bare feet in the grass, wet with the dews of night. This
is, however, but one manifestation of Father Kneipp's teachings.
His method of treatment was founded on the principle that
the body possesses natural power of reaction to cold, and that
if it is subjected to the influence of cold water, great vigour
of body will result. Kneipp cures have been established in our
country, and it will be surprising if the fad for returning to
the nakedness of savages does not invade our land. In these
divers modes of natural healing we see not a mere whim to
try something novel and exciting, but a desire to escape from
bondage to the medical profession, with its time-honoured
adherence to drug therapy, and which, with its conservative
repugnance for whatever smacks of charlatanism, looks askance
upon all such methods. It would be a display of unwarranted
pessimism to assert that a belief in a fad, or any one of the
so-called natural methods of healing is to replace in the popular
mind the well-merited confidence entertained for the art of
medicine. There is, however, a certain feeling of distrust in
many quarters which may be regarded as a reaction against
the heroic dosage of the forepart of the last century. Nor is
this reaction confined to the laity, for among the members of
our own profession it has found expression in the therapeutic
nihilism that still dominates medical thought in Germany.

The wonderful success that has attended the antitoxin
treatment of diphtheria, and the activity shown along the line
of serum therapy, betoken the dawn of a new era in therapeutics ; but as this weapon can be said to be forged only
against those diseases having a definite bacterial origin, there
will still be left that very large class of organic maladies of
a degenerative or sclerotic kind, which are out of reach of sera
and antitoxins, as well as those disorders which seem to depend
upon perversion of function of the chylopoetic viscera and as
yet have no definite pathology. What is to be done with
these ? Indeed, it is for the most part from the sufferers of

these maladies that are recruited the ranks of those runners after new doctrines. Are we to leave them still to the *natur aertze*, faith healers, osteopaths, and the like? We of the medical profession are ourselves largely responsible for the defection of our quondam patients. We have ever looked with suspicion on the methods, however successful and rational from a therapeutic standpoint, of those lay healers; nay, even of those enlightened medical practitioners who have sought to replace pharmaceutical remedies by nature's remedies, and therefore we have practically left the field to ignorant empyrics. This has been shown particularly in our neglect of hydrotherapy. To the shame of the profession be it said that it required the teachings of an ignorant peasant, Priessnitz, to bring us back to the wisdom of the ancients. Although lamentably ignorant of anatomy, physiology, pathology, and the other fundamental branches of medical knowledge which are the just pride of modern medicine, ancient physicians were keen observers, who set us an example in the employment of nature's remedies which we must not find it beneath our dignity to follow. This is eminently true of their use of water. Hippocrates is said to have formulated rules for the use of water in acute and chronic diseases which are still followed by empyrics and even physicians. Asclepiades, a friend of Cicero, achieved great renown as a therapeutist, and mainly through his employment of this agency, although he did not neglect rubbing, exercise, and diet. A disciple of his, Antonius Musa, is said to have restored Cæsar and the poet Horace to health by means of cold baths. Paulus Ægineta, that renowned surgeon and obstetrician of the seventh and eighth centuries A.D., has the merit of having first recommended cold effusions for sunstroke and anuria. During the dark ages, when medicine, like all other arts and sciences, languished under the domination of the priesthood, this potent therapeutic agency was but little employed; certainly not in the form of baths, whether for cleanliness or health. In the seventeenth and eighteenth cen-

turies, on the other hand, there were a number of eminent
physicians who promulgated the therapeutic virtues of water,
both by writings and example. Among these were Floyer in
England, the illustrious Friedrich Hoffman in Germany, besides
Theden, the physician to Frederick the Great, Hahn, Huffland,
and others. Thence the advocacy of water spread to Italy,
France, and again to England. It was employed in fevers,
dysentery, variola and the other exanthemata, in rheumatism,
and other acute and chronic maladies. But as we all know, it
is to Winternitz that we are indebted for a systematic and
scientific knowledge of the physiological effects and rational
application of hydrotherapy. As stated in effect by Baruch,
it has ever been the liberal and enlightened men in our profession who have recognised the value of this remedial agent,
and who have employed it most largely and intelligently. Such
is its potency and almost universal applicability in one form
or another, that although it has passed through many vicissi-
tudes of favour and neglect, water is almost the only remedial
agency that has stood the test of time. Nay more, originating
with the ancients, it stands higher in popular and professional
favour to-day than 2,000 years ago. The same cannot be said
of blood-letting, that other equally ancient means of therapy.

It would be a mistake to think that by hydrotherapy is
meant the internal and external employment of water only
after the manner of the hydropaths. In its broadest sense,
hydrotherapy includes every form in which water can be used,
from the bath and sponging with warm, hot or cold water, to
steam and ice and all modes of administration, internally as
a drink, by lavage and enemata, and externally in ablutions
partial or general, effusions, local or general packs, fomentations, icebags, compresses, bandages, &c. The immense value
of water is shown by the Brand method of treating typhoid
fever, and this alone should suffice to win for it a grateful
appreciation.

By including the study of hydrology among the objects of

our Association, it was the intention of the founders, as I take it, to have us learn to apply this agency therapeutically, whether as pure or medicinal waters. Because of the foregoing consideration, it seems to me greatly to be regretted that as an association intended to investigate and to disseminate facts concerning hydrology, we have allowed this department of therapeutics to remain so comparatively neglected. Thus far we appear to have been contented with holding an occasional meeting at some resort whose springs are its chief attraction, and almost as infrequently with papers upon the benefit of natural waters in some chronic condition of a gouty or rheumatic nature. I therefore heartily commend that portion of the present programme devoted to the clinical aspects of the Spa treatment.

Water in its various forms of administration is so powerful an agency for good in a large number of nervous and other chronic disorders, that a series of contributions upon this subject ought to prove both edifying and interesting. So numerous have been contributions to the subject of tuberculosis, that it has been said, with some show of truth, that we are in danger of becoming a society of tuberculosis rather than of the broader scope originally intended. This is natural, owing to the absorbing interest and universal importance of this class of diseases. Is it not singular that we have not had discussions upon the use of cold in the treatment of pneumonia and pleurisy for instance? To my mind, cold in the form of baths or the icebag is so valuable in these affections, both as an antipyretic and analgesic, and for its tonic effect on the nervous system, that its employment by the rank and file of the profession is altogether too much neglected. Another profitable discussion might be had on the local use of cold in the treatment of pericarditis and endocarditis. There is much diversity of opinion regarding the comparative merits of the icebag and poultices in these affections, and therefore it would be advantageous to have established which is the better; or if both are good, in what cases indications are furnished for one as against the other. The use of normal salt solution falls appropriately under the head of hydrology in its broad sense, and here again is a subject full of possibilities for instructive discussion for our members. I have seen such striking improvement follow the use of alternately hot and cold effusions in a case of acute arthritis consequent upon the injection of antistreptococcus serum, that I am sure we should find instructive a paper on the employment of water in arthritic inflammations, whether rheumatic or not, a plan of treatment which, because employed by Theden more than 150 years ago, is not therefore so old as to merit neglect. These are only a few of the topics belonging to hydrology that might with profit receive consideration at our hands. They would certainly possess the merit of novelty as contrasted with the papers that have composed our programme since I had the privilege of becoming a member of this Association, and therefore they are respectfully suggested for consideration at future meetings.

The remarkable activity of the past thirty years along the lines of bacteriological investigation has culminated in the notion that to some pestiferous microbe is to be attributed every acute infectious disease. The particular micro-organism has not been identified in every instance, but it is confidently expected that the deficiencies of our knowledge in this respect will some day be removed. In the first flush of bacteriological discovery such potency was attributed to these microscopic entities that we thought it was only necessary for pathogenic bacteria to gain access to the human organism to have an infection result. Then it was discovered that they were often carried around in the mouth without disease being necessarily set up; nay further, that under some circumstances they failed to create symptoms of infection even when they gained access by accident or experimentation to the living body. So that we now know there must be some additional factor besides the presence of germs if disease is to follow. This additional factor may be said to be that condition of the tissues which renders them a good soil or medium for the growth of the bacteria. Without entering into the discussion of how it is that the cells of the body are able to resist and even overcome the invading microbes, it may be stated that the likelihood of a resulting infection depends in part upon the degree and vigour of the cell resistance. This varies not only in different individuals, but in the same individual at different times. In other words, the susceptibility of a person to the action of micro-organisms as well as to other causes of disease is greater at one time, less at another. We are not always able to decide whereon this difference in the resistance of an individual depends. We are apt to content ourselves with the vague statement that a person's vitality has become lowered, or that he has lost his powers of resistance, or that he has become "run down." At all events we know that other things being equal he is the most likely to develop disease who habitually violates the recognised laws of health. The dissipated, the intemperate, the unclean, the overworked, the underfed, the anæmic, the infant, the aged, these are the ones who, as a rule, furnish the great contingent of sufferers from tuberculosis, pneumonia and other acute and chronic maladies. How can we best protect these individuals from the evils almost sure to follow their acquired and inherent proneness to disease? Surely not, most certainly, by the administration of medicine. How best can roses be restored to the cheeks and strength to the muscles of the anæmic, flabby child? How can we most surely restore tone to the nervous system and vigour to the circulation of the overworked business and professional man, the devotee of fashion and society, the stoop-shouldered, hollow-cheeked student or clerk; in short, bring back health to any one of that great multitude of victims of modern civilised life? Assuredly not by our long list of so-called hæmatic and nerve tonics. Bunge's researches seem to have proven conclusively that iron is restored to the blood in only minute amounts when it is administered internally. The beneficial effects which seem to follow its use are probably due to its local action within the intestines and not through its absorption, even in the form of the organic preparation now so much in vogue. Therefore, when it is necessary to overcome anæmia it is to be accomplished by the ingestion of foods rich in nucleo-albumens, and by life out of doors where oxygen and sunshine may be had in abundance and the metabolic processes are stimulated. We are of necessity compelled to fall back upon the aid of Mother Nature who has given us pure air and sunshine, mountains and forests, an inexhaustible supply of living water, pools, and springs of medicinal waters for the healing of the multitude. We can find no more striking example of the powerful influence for good of natural remedies, even in organic disease, than in the treatment of circulatory disorders by means of baths after the manner at Bad Nauheim. The use of digitalis in heart disease exemplifies in the highest manner the beneficial effects of medicinal therapy, and it would seem that if any drug were destined to retain its hold on the confidence of the profession, it would be digitalis. And yet it is most significant of the inevitable tendency to abandon medicine, that in this balneological treatment of cardiac affections digitalis is already encountering a formidable rival.

Climatotherapy was employed by the ancients and has ever since been recognised as a most efficient weapon against tuberculosis. Yet it may be said that the profession is being awakened to its possibilities in a manner and to an extent wholly unprecedented. The practitioner is already behind the times who relies upon medicine for the treatment of consumption, and yet the finest climate in the world is of little service to him who is pent up within four walls, while on the other hand, all the benefits of climatic treatment may be enjoyed in an unpropitious climate by him who knows how to make the best of his possibilities.

We Americans are too prone to regard the state of the

weather; as if rain, wind, and sunshine can be hurtful to him who is properly prepared to encounter them.

Let us not as an Association, however, devote our energies too exclusively to the climatology of consumption, ignoring the other natural means of cure in the treatment of diseased conditions in general. Let us broadly preach the gospel that good health means the intelligent daily use of those agencies with which bountiful Nature has supplied us, and which, alas, but too few physicians as well as patients know how to employ intelligently. By instructing people how to make proper use of fresh air, exercise, healthful food and water, we shall not only furnish them with what is better than prescriptions, but we shall guard them against many of those ills to which they now succumb, and thereby rid ourselves of the opprobium of being mere " medicine men."

PUERTO RICO: ITS CLIMATE AND ITS DISEASES.

BY DR. C. H. ALDEN, U.S. Army, Retired.

Late Asst. Surgeon-General.

THE history of Puerto Rico has been comparatively un-eventful. From the discovery of the island by Columbus in 1493, on his second voyage, and its settlement by the Spanish beginning in 1508, it remained continuously under Spanish rule, and although attacks were made by the Dutch, the French, and twice by the English, none of these nations effected more than a temporary lodgment. For more than three centuries the island was governed as a colony under a Captain-General, but the rule was for the most part mild and conciliatory, the revenues were expended within its own borders, and there was, in consequence, no serious revolutionary uprising. In 1870 Puerto Rico was made a Province of Spain and granted representation in the Cortes, and in 1897, in common with Cuba, it was given autonomy. These concessions were, however, more nominal than real. The landing of General Miles' army in July, 1898, and the withdrawal of the Spanish authority a little later, were like an awakening from the torpor of centuries, and were welcomed by the inhabitants as harbingers of progress and prosperity under the "Great Republic." The military control of the United States under Generals Brooke, Henry, and Davis successively, lasted from October, 1898, to May 1, 1900, when the first Civil Governor, Charles H. Allen, of Massachusetts, was inaugurated and a partly representative government established. It was fortunate for the welfare of the people, as we shall see, that the island remained for a considerable period under the exclusive jurisdiction of the military authorities, for through such an agency only could the prompt action and thorough measures, that existing conditions demanded, have been carried out.

Puerto Rico is the smallest of the four larger West Indian islands which are known as the Greater Antilles. It lies about 100 miles south, and 400 miles east of Cuba, having Haiti on the west, and St. Thomas, the Danish island the United States proposes to purchase, on the east. San Juan, the capital, is about 1,000 miles from Havana, the same distance from Key West, the nearest point of the United States, and about 1,500 miles from New York city. The island is about three-fourths the size and of the general shape of the state of Connecticut, forming an irregular parallelogram about one hundred miles long and thirty-six miles wide.

The coast is low with few good harbors, San Juan on the north and Juanica, where General Miles landed, and Ponce on the south, being the most important. Extending along the length of the island from east to west, but nearer the southern coast, is a broken chain of mountains from 2,000 to 3,000 feet high, which trends to the north at the eastern end and there culminates in the peak of El Yunque, 3,600 feet in altitude. From the crest of the mountain ridge the land slopes northward and southward and is deeply cut by streams, giving most of the interior of the island a very broken surface, which becomes more level as it nears the coast. The southern slope is shorter and steeper than the northern with narrower coastal plain. Numerous rivers drain these slopes, but they are short and not navigable, except near their mouths.

Puerto Rico lies within the tropics and has a tropical climate modified by its insular position and physical features. The mean annual temperature of San Juan on the north coast ranges in different years from 78 to 82 degrees Fahrenheit, and the monthly mean from 75 degrees in January to 82 degrees in August, while the highlands in the interior have a mean annual temperature of 72 degrees. The maximum temperature observed on the island is 99 degrees and the minimum 57 degrees. The relative humidity is very high, averaging nearly 80 degrees, and the annual rainfall ranges from 60 inches on the north coast to 100 in the interior elevated region. The south coast is dryer, as the rains are intercepted somewhat by the central range of mountains. Rains begin to increase in April or May, but the rainy season proper extends from August to December. The average number of clear days per month from June, 1899, to May, 1900, was fourteen; of partly cloudy, nine, and of cloudy, seven, December to March having the most clear days and being the best in which to visit the island. The north-east trade winds blow with great regularity, and the sea-breeze by day and the land-breeze by night moderate the temperature. The island is subject to serious storms and to occasional earthquakes. Hurricanes, sometimes of great severity, occur, there being a record from 1493 to 1846 of 127, of which number sixty-eight were in the months of August and September. The great hurricane of August 8, 1899, which caused the death of 2,300 persons, the destruction of many towns and villages, the ruin of crops upon which the food and labour of the poor depended, and resulting in the destitution of 250,000 people, is a matter of recent history. It will be seen later how generously the United States responded to this call upon its humanity.

The climate of Puerto Rico has been called an equable one, but though the annual range of temperature is small as compared with that in higher latitudes, the diurnal variations are very considerable. The records of the Weather Bureau show that during the year ending May, 1900, the greatest daily range of temperature was 45 degrees, occurring in March. In December and February the greatest was 41 degrees, in October, 28 degrees. The chill attendant upon these sometimes sudden changes has to be guarded against.

The island offers the most beautiful and picturesque scenery and all the novel attractions of the tropics to the nervous invalid in search of rest and change. For most other cases it is hardly a favourable health resort. Medical officers serving there have stated that for those from the United States who have been injured or fallen sick, the climate seems to lack recuperative qualities.

The census of 1899, taken under the direction of the United States Government gives some interesting facts about the island, which have a bearing on its health conditions. Its 3,600 square miles of area contain almost 1,000,000 inhabitants (953,243 exactly), being an average of 264 to the square mile. In one department, Aquadilla, with no large towns, it is 415 per square mile. This density of population exceeds that of Cuba seven times, is about equal to that of Massachusetts and New Jersey, and twice that of Pennsylvania. Not only is the population dense but it is evenly distributed throughout the island, being chiefly rural. There are no large cities; the largest, San Juan, on the north coast, has 32,000 inhabitants, the next, Ponce, on the south coast, 28,000, Mayaguez, on the west, 15,000, and Arecibo, in the north-west, 8,000.

About 590,000, or a little more than three-fifths of the entire population, are pure white, and almost entirely of Spanish descent. This proportion of whites exceeds that in the coast states of our country from Virginia to Louisiana inclusive, except in North Carolina. Of the remaining two-fifths, about 304,000 are of mixed blood, and about 60,000 only pure black or negroes. The sexes are reported in nearly equal numbers, with a slight excess of females showing that when the census was taken there had been but little immigration or emigration. This is also shown by the small percentage of foreign-born inhabitants, numbering 14,000 only. More than one-half of the foreign-born came from Spain; the United States contributed but 1,069.

The aborigines of Puerto Rico were a feeble race, not

2

numerous, and under the hardships of enslavement by the Spaniards disappeared entirely it is said, in less than fifty years after the settlement of the island. The present negro population represent the African slaves, imported from time to time to supply the place of the aborigines in the cultivation of the soil. In 1873 slavery was abolished by law, but in order to prevent disastrous results to both planters and negroes the ex-slaves were required to enter into contracts for labour for not less than three years.

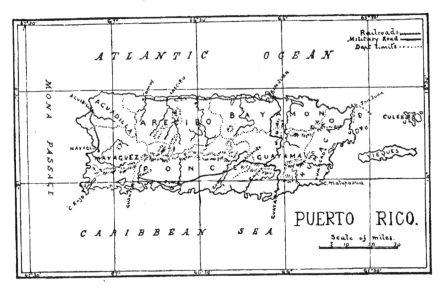

The industries of Puerto Rico are almost exclusively agricultural, those of manufactures, trade, and transportation being of trifling importance. It is an interesting fact, shown by the census, explaining in some degree the greater tranquillity of Puerto Rico as compared with Cuba, that much the larger part, 91 per cent., of the cultivated area is occupied by its owners. In Cuba 43 per cent. only is so occupied. There results consequently in Puerto Rico few large estates and many small farms, agriculture being carried on in a much smaller way than in Cuba. Coffee was formerly the most important crop, 41 per cent. of the cultivated area being devoted to it, but since the destruction of the coffee trees by the recent hurricane, sugar has taken its place. Tobacco is a much less important crop. Bananas and sweet potatoes are extensively cultivated, and these with Indian corn, yams, malangas (a farinaceous root), rice, and other vegetables, and the many native fruits, such as cocoanuts, mangoes, pineapples, oranges, and melons, form the chief subsistence of the people. In the eastern part stock-raising is an industry of some importance.

The lack of means of communication is a great drawback to agriculture. With the exception of the so-called military road constructed by the Spanish government, extending across the island from San Juan to Ponce, and three more short pieces, there is not a good road on the island; even those in the immediate vicinity of the cities are in a poor condition, and during the rainy season all of them, with the exceptions noted, are almost impassable for vehicles. A narrow-gauge railroad was planned some years ago to extend along the coast around the island, but three short detached sections only have been built, about 159 miles in all. Since the United States took possession considerable work has been done on the roads, partly for the purpose of giving employment to the poor.

The degree of illiteracy is high, for leaving out of account children who are less than ten years of age, 22·7 per cent. only of the remaining population are able to read and write.

Owing largely, it is supposed, to the expense attendant upon the celebration of the marriage rites, a large number of persons are living together as man and wife without the sanction of the Church in the, so-called, consentual union, the bonds of which are in general faithfully observed. More than 84,000 of population are sustaining this relation, and consequently the number of illegitimate children is very large, over 148,000. Reports show that over 45 per cent. of the total births are illegitimate, but this is probably under the true ratio.

The houses of the better class are substantially built of stone, usually of one story, roofed with tiles, and have an interior court. In the country the habitations of the poorer people are generally mere huts thatched with palm, and often overcrowded by large families. There are reported to be over 109,000 persons living in families of eleven or more.

It appears from the census statistics that about one-third of the Puerto Rican houses are supplied with rainwater from cisterns, and more than one-half with water directly from streams. About one-seventeenth of the dwellings are supplied with water from aqueducts, these being confined to the four largest cities. One-twentieth only of the houses depend upon wells.

Three-fourths of all the dwellings in Puerto Rico are entirely without any arrangement for the disposal of excreta; in the strictly rural districts nearly four-fifths. In the towns most houses have pits or cesspools, sometimes disinfected with earth, lime, or ashes, and occasionally emptied. Modern water closets are almost unknown, though some have been introduced by the United States military authorities into the buildings occupied by them. Sewers are of course equally rare.

The better class of Puerto Ricans is composed of highly intelligent, refined, and well-educated people, many having been educated abroad; but as a large part of the population is living in poverty and ignorance and amid unsanitary surroundings, the annual death-rate cannot be a low one. It appears from the Spanish records that the death-rate for the eleven years from 1888 to 1898 was a little over 30 per thousand. It is known that these records are imperfect, and it is believed that the true death-rate was considerably larger. In 1899 the death-rate was 41·5 per thousand, being higher than for several years, owing to the deaths from injury and disease, due to the hurricane of that year. The mortality among infants is very great; recent reports show that in the month of July, 1900, out of a total of 4,690 deaths, 1,753 were of children under 5 years of age.

The highest death-rate is from anæmia or "tropical

chlorosis," as it has been called; for the ten years beginning 1890 there was a yearly average of 4,513 deaths from this cause out of a yearly average of 27,915 total deaths. In 1899, the year of the hurricane, there were 8,977 deaths from anæmia out of 39,918 total deaths, a rate of 22·5 per cent. Affecting chiefly the lower classes, it was generally supposed to be due mainly to insufficient and poor food, and, in the low lands, to chronic malarial infection. In 1899, Assistant Surgeon B. K. Ashford, United States army, an alumnus of the Army Medical School, made a special study of this affection, and found in nineteen out of twenty cases in the hospital at Ponce that the diseased condition was due to the presence in the intestine of the ankylostomum duodenale. He seems to have been the first to note this in regard to the Puerto Rican anæmia, though the agency of this parasite in tropical anæmia elsewhere was well known. Dr. Ashford's interesting report on this subject may be found in the *New York Medical Journal* for April 14, 1900. Such cases can no doubt be promptly relieved by anthelmintics and nourishing food, and were it possible to apply these remedies extensively to the population of the island and to prevent the use of contaminated water and food, this disease might be largely abated. Unfortunately most of the people are too ignorant to take the necessary sanitary precautions, and too poor to purchase the needed medicine and food when attacked by the disease.

Intestinal diseases are common, and dysentery is the cause of many deaths. For the ten years beginning with 1900, the annual average deaths from dysentery were 1,183 or 3·83 per cent. of total deaths. During the last three years of that period there was a large increase in the number of deaths from dysentery, there being in 1899, 3,568 deaths or 8·94 per cent. of the total mortality. Lt.-Col. J. Van R. Hoff, formerly Chief Surgeon of Puerto Rico, attributes the large increase in this year partly to the fact that the usual food supply of the poor, bananas, yams, &c., being cut off by the hurricane, the government issued quantities of beans, rice, and codfish which were eaten improperly cooked. Diarrhœal diseases naturally affected largely the troops from the United States, and it is reported that in 1898 there was a ratio of 768 cases per 1,000 of mean strength, with a mortality of 1·41, and in 1899, 543 cases and 2·68 deaths per thousand. The pathology of Puerto Rican dysentery does not seem to have been as fully studied as that in the Phillipines, where it has been ably investigated by Professors Flexner and Barker, and Drs. Strong and Musgrave of the Army, but Col. Hoff considers that it is probably not due to the amœba coli, from the absence of liver abscess.

I have been unable to find reports as to malarial fevers covering an extended period. Col. Hoff states that reports made to the Superior Board of Health for the seven months ending April 30, 1900, give 1,514 deaths from these fevers during that period, being 6·32 per cent. of total deaths, but intimates that the diagnosis was probably incorrect in many cases. The quartan and tertian organisms were found chiefly in the cases examined, the æstivo-autumnal rarely. The troops from the United States suffered severely. In 1898 the admission rate for malarial fever was 77·2 per 1,000 and death-rate 3·86. The admission rate fell in 1899 to 458 with no deaths. Malarial fevers are much less prevalent in Puerto Rico than in Cuba, but chronic malarial infection is believed to be an important factor in lowering the vitality and stamina of its people.

Yellow fever is not endemic in Puerto Rico, though cases have been reported annually for some years. In 1895 it was almost epidemic and caused 360 deaths. The number of deaths in 1897 fell to nine, and in 1899 there were no cases; due, no doubt, to the careful quarantine of our authorities, for there were numerous cases in Cuba in that year.

Typhoid fever gives for the ten years beginning with 1890 an average of 383 deaths annually, or 1·43 per cent. of total deaths with very little annual variation. It is said to have been specially prevalent in the city of San Juan. In 1898 there were numerous cases of typhoid fever among the United States troops, who brought the disease with them from the infected camps they had occupied in this country. From July to December of that year there were among our troops in Puerto Rico 464 cases and 44 deaths, representing an admission rate of 295, and death-rate of 34·6 per thousand.

Among the fevers of Puerto Rico of irregular course and indeterminate origin, it is probable that Malta fever is responsible for many cases, and that it is endemic in Puerto Rico. Assistant Surgeon Walter Cox, of the Army, reported a case in July, 1899, in a member of the Hospital Corps, and there is an interesting report by Professor Musser in the *Philadelphia Medical Journal* for December, 1898, in an officer who contracted the disease in Puerto Rico. These cases were marked by fever of a low type and long-continued course, with intervals of apyrexia, were not influenced by quinine, and did not show the malarial parasite. They did not exhibit the characteristic symptoms of typhoid, nor respond to the Widal test. Neuralgic and rheumatic symptoms were prominent with general glandular hyperplasia. The cases reported showed the presence of the micrococcus melitensis in the blood.

Tuberculosis, presumably almost entirely pulmonary, gave an average of 1,824 deaths yearly for the decennial period referred to, a percentage of 6·78 of total deaths. There is very little annual variation in these rates. Cases are most numerous in the three largest cities where the tenements are crowded. Pulmonary tuberculosis occurred among the United States troops in 1899 at the rate of 5·1 cases per 1,000, with death-rate of·8. Such cases did badly in Puerto Rico and had to be sent back promptly to the United States.

Tetanus is frequent and fatal. For the ten years beginning 1890, there was an annual average of 952 deaths, or 3·57 per cent. of the total deaths. There was but little annual or monthly variation. Col. Hoff states that it is estimated that 90 per cent.

occurs in new-born infants through the filthy dressing of the umbilical cord, a physician being rarely employed as accoucheur among the lower classes.

Venereal diseases, especially syphilis, are very common, and the lower classes are said to be syphilised to a large extent. For the last ten years of the occupation of the island by Spanish troops they had an annual average admission rate from these diseases of 455 per 1,000. The Surgeon General's report shows that the admission rate for United States troops in Puerto Rico in 1899 was 286 per 1,000, being considerably larger than the rate in Cuba or the Philippines, and still larger than that for the United States, which was 127 only. The reports of the British Army show the same disproportion between the cases occurring at home and on foreign service.

The large number of blind in Puerto Rico, some 2,000, or one to every 480 persons, is largely due to the ravages of ophthalmia neonatorum, though smallpox is also a cause. In the United States in 1890 there was one blind to every 1,242 of population.

Puerto Rico is, or has been, no exception to the rule that smallpox is endemic in tropical countries. All classes seem to regard its presence with indifference or take but feeble measures against it. For the ten years prior to 1900 there had been an average of 623 deaths annually, the highest number being 2,362 in 1890, the lowest 11 in 1893. In the fall of 1898 the disease was so general that a quarantine had been declared by other countries against its seaports. The report of the Surgeon-General for 1899 states that from December 15, 1898, to February 11, 1899, 554 cases were reported from sixteen towns and villages. The Chief Surgeon of the Department of Puerto Rico, Lt.-Col. J. Van R. Hoff, who arrived in October, 1898, only, saw at once the importance of taking measures to stamp out the disease, and set about it with promptness and energy. At his instance the Commanding General, on January 27, 1899, ordered the vaccination of the entire population of the island, an immense task, and possible only through military agency. A detailed history of this remarkable achievement would be interesting, but an outline only can be given. Vaccine virus obtained from the United States was unreliable, as it did not keep well in transportation and was too costly in the large quantities needed, and therefore a vaccine farm was established on the island at Coamo Springs, the necessary cattle being generously furnished by a native gentleman, Sr. Simon Moret. The island was divided into five districts, each under a medical officer as Director of Vaccination, with inspectors, vaccinators (generally Puerto Rican physicians), Hospital Corps men as assistants, orderlies, and recorders. The actual vaccinating was performed at each municipality, and the work systematically and rapidly carried out. Col. Hoff states that he is specially indebted for assistance to Majors George G. Groff and Axel Ames, Surgeons U.S.V., Assist. Surg. Reynolds, and A. A. Surg. Leary, U.S.A., Drs. Ames and Reynolds being in charge of the vaccine-producing station. By June 30, 1899, the work was finished. 1,038,000 vaccine points had been produced, and 786,290 persons had been vaccinated at a cost of $28,536, which was paid from the insular funds. The disease rapidly diminished and almost entirely disappeared, as there was but one death from smallpox in 1899 after June, there having been 272 deaths in the six months before that date. The production of virus and vaccination of the unprotected was continued, and though some cases have appeared in the last few months there is no fear of an epidemic.

Cerebro-spinal meningitis is the cause of considerable mortality, there having been 305 deaths annually on the average from 1890 to 1899, a percentage of 1·12 of total deaths.

Leprosy exists in the island, but to the extent of about 100 cases only. Under Spanish rule no attempt had been made to isolate these unfortunates, but recently the authorities have taken steps for their separation from the community and for their proper treatment and care. The tubercular form is the usual one. Elephantiasis, which is ͺquite common, has often been mistaken for leprosy.

It is not to be understood from what has been said that there was no provision under Spanish *régime* for the sanitary and medical supervision of the island. Sanitary laws did exist but they were inadequate and imperfectly executed. There were quarantine officials at the principal seaports, but one quarantine station only, that at San Juan. Puerto Rico was divided into seven Departments and seventy-one municipalities, each one of the latter having its Board of Health, the reports of disease and death being made by the Alcalde to the Secretary of State at San Juan. A royal sub-delegation of medicine and surgery at the capital was charged with the licensing of medical practitioners, though some were also licensed by the Governor-General. Physicians from the medical schools of Spain seldom had the Doctorate degree, but were styled " Licensiados." A few physicians had the degree of Doctor of Medicine from European and American schools. Another class of practitioners were licensed as " Practicantes," these being assistants to the physicians proper or doing the rough work of the profession in the mountains and among the poor. Midwives were also licensed as " Comadrones." Each district had at least one physician to the poor, employed by the Government at a salary of $400 to $500 gold. In 1900 there were but 125 physicians in the whole island, or one to nearly 8,000 of the population. Naturally quackery does not flourish. There are a few pretenders who claim to be the direct representatives of celebrated deceased physicians, and who practice and prescribe in their names. Christian Science is said to have been recently imported.

The advent of the United States authorities found sanitary affairs in a very demoralised state, due partly no doubt to the confusion incident to the change of jurisdiction. The medical departments of our services were not slow to see the necessity for systematic organisation. The Marine Hospital Service at once established efficient quarantine, and · the Commanding General, again at the instance of Lt.-Col. Hoff, the Chief Surgeon, ordered in June, 1899, the establishment of a Superior Board of Health composed of one officer from each of the three services, the Army, Navy, and Marine Hospital, and two native physicians, with Col. Hoff as President and Major George Groff as Secretary. This Board was charged with the supervision of the municipal boards of health and of all the various interests affecting public health, such as the licensing of medical practitioners, dentists, druggists, and nurses ; the collection of vital statistics ; the investigation of the causes of disease and recommendation of preventive measures ; the sanitary inspection of hospitals, schools, and prisons ; the inquiry into the purity of the water supplies, food, drinks, and medicines ; the establishment of a laboratory for their examination ; the supervision of municipal sanitation, of sewers, plumbing, &c. This list gives but the principal duties committed to the Board, which was armed with powers to act efficiently. The Superior Board of Health, organised under the Civil Government, has taken up the work of the Military Board.

Not only did the Medical Department of the Army during the military occupation of the island have in charge the important duties already inadequately sketched, but under the Chief Surgeon, Col. Hoff, as President of the Board of Charities, it was the principal agent of the Government and the people of the United States in relieving the victims of the great hurricane of 1899. The 2,390 deaths and wide-spread destitution and disease which followed that great calamity have been referred to. Col. Hoff reports that an average of 183,000 persons were fed daily from September, 16, 1899, to January 22, 1900, chiefly with food supplied by the Government. About $115,000 was contributed for food and clothing in the United States. It is estimated that the total relief extended reached a cost of over a million dollars with practically no expense for personal service. The island has not yet recovered from the effects of the hurricane, and nothing speaks more eloquently of the sad condition of the poor than their willingness to emigrate in large numbers to Hawaii, as they are now doing. But we may confidently hope that the new Government under the wise leadership of Governor Allen, continuing the good work already begun will ultimately bring about great changes for the better. The sanitary measures instituted under Col. Hoff and Major Groff cannot fail to be important factors in improving the health conditions of the people, in spite of climatic and racial hindrances.

The facts and statistics embodied in this paper have been derived from the official records of the census of 1899, the reports of the Surgeon-General of the Army for 1899 and 1890, of the Chief Surgeon of the Department of Puerto Rico, of the Superior Board of Health of the island, and published letters from medical officers who have been on duty there.

DISCUSSION.

Dr. SHURLEY: May I ask whether the anæmia spoken of was confined to or predominant in either sex?

Dr. ALDEN : No, it occurs in the whole population.

Dr. HAROLD WILLIAMS : I would like to ask if it was a pernicious anæmia or a secondary one?

Dr. ALDEN : It is a secondary anæmia and now that the great prevalence of the intestinal parasite, the ankylostomum duodenale, has been discovered it is supposed to be due to that. Out of twenty cases taken to the hospital at Ponce nineteen were found to have the parasite and the anæmia was relieved when the parasite was destroyed.

Dr. NEWTON : I would like to ask where the parasite comes from, does it come from the drinking water?

Dr. ALDEN : The streams from which most of these families obtain their drinking water were infected and this probably because there is no systematic care of excreta. It also comes, no doubt, from contaminated food.

Dr. F. FREMONT SMITH : Does this disease attack others than natives?

Dr. ALDEN : Yes ; a few cases have been noted among the United States troops.

THE CLIMATOLOGY OF AUGUSTA, GEORGIA.

BY THOMAS D. COLEMAN, M.D.

AUGUSTA, GEORGIA.

———

THE fact that climate tends to eliminate, or reduce to a minimum some forms of disease, and to favour the development of others, cannot be gainsaid. Some diseases thrive more luxuriantly and are associated with localities, just as peculiarities of person and provincialisms of speech characterise a people. Asiatic cholera has usually been focussed at Mecca as its point of origin; the bubonic plague in the far east: yellow fever in the tropics, &c.

Longfellow has said, " As turning the logs will make a dull fire burn, so change of studies a dull brain." I have been told by farmers that sheep will not thrive well if left long in one pasture; of other animals the same is true, and man is no exception to the rule. A change of climate is oft-times beneficial to those in perfect health; it is truer still of those whose bodies are diseased.

If such be the case, and I think it is beyond the possibility of dispute, then it behoves us to make a closer study of climate in relation to disease.

This point may be contested by those who advocate the home treatment of tuberculosis, but, in my judgment, this is simply a compromise measure. I am far from being willing to affirm that tuberculosis is incurable in the locality where it develops, but I am unalterable in my belief that such individuals would stand a better chance of a speedier and more perfect recovery if they sought some region other than that in which the disease developed.

I believe Augusta, Georgia, to be a climate exceedingly well adapted to the cure of tuberculous patients, and yet I should unhesitatingly advise residents of that region developing the disease there, to seek some other climate. These considerations have led me to feel that a short presentation of the advantages and disadvantages of Augusta's climate, may prove profitable to the members of this Association.

In treating of the climatology of this region I shall limit my consideration largely to that portion of Augusta that is known as a health resort, and upon which Augusta should have been built, viz., Summerville. It is not possible to separate the two portions however, or to give the full value of Summerville's climate, inasmuch as the meteorological data are all recorded by the United States Signal Service down in the city proper, 300 feet below the Sand Hills upon whose summit Summerville is located.

Augusta is situated upon the Georgia side of the Savannah River, which along this region separates the States of Georgia and South Carolina. By the river route it is about 231 miles from the Atlantic Ocean, and in an air line about 90 or 100 miles. The city proper has an elevation of 167 feet above the sea level. With its immediate suburbs it has a population of between 50,000 and 60,000 people. It is one of the oldest as well as one of the most beautiful cities in the South; and the third city in industrial importance in the State. A huge canal seven miles in length furnishes water to run its large and numerous cotton mills and other industries. From the number and size of its cotton mills it has been styled the Lowell of the South. It has about eighteen miles of electric railway, (most of which is double tracked), which is modern in construction, equipment, and conduct. It has public schools; a high school for boys, the Richmond Academy; the Tubman High School for girls; a Jesuit College; and the Medical Department of the University of Georgia is located here. Strangers sojourning here may have school facilities for their children if they desire.

There is a modern opera house, a public library, and churches of the more prominent religious denominations. The city proper is quite level, and the streets are wider and more beautiful than those of any city with which I am acquainted. The chief residence street, Greene Street, is 175 feet wide, and throughout its length of several miles there extend four rows of majestic elms and oaks, the majority of which are half a century or more old. Between the central avenue vehicles are not allowed to pass; this being stone curbed and grass plotted is reserved for pedestrians, and as a playground for children.

The city has a water supply that is not excelled by any city in America. This supply comes from the Savannah River, which from its origin in the water-shed of the Blue Ridge Mountains to Augusta has upon its banks neither city, nor villages, nor hamlet. As if for additional precaution it breaks into shoals which extend irregularly for forty or fifty miles above Augusta. This water is taken three miles above the city, carried by mains to reservoirs on the hill-top where it is filtered, and thence delivered to the city mains.

The city has an excellent sewerage system, which in my opinion plays an important part in its healthfulness.

The death-rate for Augusta has decreased from 23·36 per 1,000 inhabitants in 1880 to 17·15 per 1,000 inhabitants in 1899.

Again in the case of the one disease, typhoid fever, the death-rate has diminished from 1 in 41·7 in 1880 to 1 in 133·6 in 1899.

Augusta is easy of access from any of the ten railroads which centre there, and also by the Savannah River, as this is the head of navigation for that stream. Crossing the river at this point is a row of sand hills which, beginning in the region of Chester, S. Carolina, pass down through Aiken,

Augusta, and on into Georgia. On the crest of these hills, 298 to 300 feet above the city level is the village of Summerville located. This has for more than a hundred years been an aristocratic suburb of Augusta, and on account of its healthfulness was early known as Mount Salubrity; it is also perhaps more generally known as the Sand Hills. This suburb is connected with Augusta by fine gravel roads and by an electric line which runs on a fifteen-minute schedule to and from the city, and the borders of the village of Summerville touch the city limits of Augusta. From this elevation one gets a sweep of landscape that is rarely excelled by mountain scenery, the view extending far over the hills of South Carolina and the plateaux and hills of Georgia.

The village of Summerville has churches and schools of its own, and is governed by an intendant and town council. Here is also located the Bon Air Hotel, which stands easily with the first of the winter resorts of the South. This hotel has accommodation for 250 guests, and the demand upon it is so great that a thirty or forty room annex is now in course of construction. Connected with the hotel is an eighteen-hole golf course, said to be the best in the South, and an elegant club-house is to be built upon it the coming year. In addition to the hotel there are numerous boarding-houses on the hill, and many of the private families will take a few boarders.

The chief amusements consist in riding, driving, and bicycling over the splendid gravel roadways which ramify in every direction through Richmond County, and in hunting, fishing, and playing golf.

These hills are covered with pines, elms, oaks, and such grasses as will grow in a sandy soil. Wild flowers are abundant, and the honeysuckle, cherokee roses, and yellow jessamine make the region most attractive in the spring. The soil is very sandy, it being necessary to go down from 80 to 150 feet before striking water, so that the region is always dry. No water accumulates on the surface of the ground, it being like a huge filter; and one can, in a few minutes after the hardest rains, go out and walk for miles without getting the feet wet. Bad drainage is therefore a practical impossibility.

The meteorologic data for this health resort are unfortunately not accessible, and almost the sole data that we have is gotten from the United States Signal Service Station located 300 feet below and in the river valley. I think it is unfortunate that the Government does not locate its bureau at its Arsenal, which is a splendid property located on the summit of the hill. A register was kept there from 1849 to 1869. The observations taken there during that period at sunrise, 9 a.m., 3 p.m., and 9 p.m., show the mean average temperature to be as follows:—January, 46·7 degrees; February, 50·7 degrees; March, 58·8 degrees; April, 65·1 degrees; May, 72·2 degrees; June, 80·9 degrees; August, 79·7 degrees; September, 72·8 degrees; October, 63·5 degrees; November, 53·8 degrees; December, 46·3 degrees.

Mean temperature of spring, 65·3 degrees; summer, 79·9 degrees; autumn, 63·4 degrees; and winter, 47·9 degrees.

Mean number of fair days 238, cloudy days 70. Snow about two days to every three years. Unfortunately no record of the humidity is made. Dr. Kenworthy, in an article on the climatology of Florida has shown that, in an observation extending over from three to five years for the months of November, December, January, February, and March, the mean temperature of Cannes was 50·8 degrees; Augusta, 51·4 degrees; Aiken, 50·3 degrees; Jacksonville, 58·7 degrees. He also pointed out that for these months the mean relative humidity was for Cannes and Mentone, 72·4, Augusta, Georgia, 68·9, and Jacksonville, 68·8 per cent.

The mean relative humidity of Augusta therefore (and it should be borne in mind this for the city in the valley, not the village of Summerville on the hill-top) was 2·5 degrees less than Cannes and Mentone, and one-tenth of a degree more than Jacksonville, Fla.

CLIMATE OF AUGUSTA, GEORGIA, LATITUDE, 32° 28′ N.; LONGITUDE, 81° 54 W.

	Jan.	Feb.	March	April	May	June	July	August	Sept.	Oct.	Nov.	Dec.
Temperature:												
Average or normal for 29 years ...	47	50	56	64	73	79	81	79	75	64	54	48
Average daily range for 20 years ...	18·1°	19·4°	21·4°	22°	21·9°	19·9°	19°	18·3°	18·5°	20·8°	20·7°	19·5°
Mean of warmest for 29 years ...	56	58	62	69	77	83	85	84	79	71	60	57
Mean of coldest for 29 years ...	39	38	50	59	69	74	78	76	70	58	48	38
Highest of maximum for 29 years...	80	84	89	93	100	103	105	105	101	94	85	78
Lowest of minimum for 29 years ...	6	3	22	29	41	46	57	58	41	29	23	7
Average date of last killing frost for 29 years, March 18th.												
Average date of first killing frost for 29 years, November 8th.												
Humidity:												
Average relative for five years ...	74	71	70	66	66	70	76	80	74	74	78	76
Average absolute for 5 years ...	2·457	2·550	3·414	3·936	5·555	7·441	7·980	8·240	6·563	4·372	3·539	2·366
Precipitation:												
Average in inches for 29 years ...	4·35	4·30	4·97	3·48	3·28	4·50	5·52	5·27	3·80	2·42	3·08	3·36
Wind:												
Prevailing direction for 29 years ...	W.	W.	W.	W.	S.E.	S.	S.E.	N.E.	N.E.	N.E.	N.E.	W.
Average velocity in miles per hour...	4·5	7·0	7·0	6·5	5·8	5·4	5·1	5·0	5·2	6·2	5·5	6·0
Weather:												
Average number clear and fair days for 5 years...	20	18	22	23	25	23	23	23	23	25	22	21
Largest number clear days for 5 years	19	23	22	25	28	29	26	26	27	27	25	24
Smallest number clear days for 5 years	16	14	12	22	22	23	19	18	21	21	19	19
Average number cloudy days for 5 years	11	10	9	7	6	7	8	8	7	6	8	10
Largest number cloudy days for 5 years	15	14	19	8	9	7	12	13	9	10	11	12
Smallest number cloudy days for 5 years	12	5	9	5	3	1	5	5	3	4	5	7
Average number rainy days for 29 years	11	10	10	8	8	11	12	13	7	7	8	9
Smallest number rainy days for 5 years	7	2	9	7	3	6	8	10	5	2	5	6
Largest number rainy days for 5 years	13	14	15	11	13	15	13	19	8	8	13	11

The foregoing table for the city of Augusta, located 300 feet below the village of Summerville, extends over a period of twenty-nine years, and is furnished me by the United States Signal Service Office at this place.

In studying this table, even with due allowance made for the advantages of altitude and dryness possessed by Summerville, it will be noted that Augusta is not a tropical climate. The chief advantages would seem to consist in, first, the fact that we have a bracing climate that holds neither the inhospitable rigors of the North nor the debilitating and depressing influences of the far South; second, it is moderately dry, and this can be increased or diminished by getting down into the river valley or further up on the hill-top; third, the absence of sudden and decided atmospheric changes which characterise the regions further north; fourth, the large percentage of sunshiny days which makes it possible to spend most of the time out of doors, a point insisted upon by medical practitioners in the treatment of tuberculosis, and other diseases running a more or less protracted course.

As to those cases which do best in this region, I am limited almost exclusively to my own observations, as the village of Summerville keeps no mortuary records.

Blodgett, in his " Climatology of the United States," shows that the rate of deaths from consumption to total mortality was less in Georgia than in any State in the Union. And Dr. Huntington Richards, in the " Ref. Handbook of the Medical Science," vol. i., page 443, writes: " The following figures deducted by calculation from the statistics of the United States Census for 1880, showing the deaths attributed to consumption which occurred in every 10,000 of population during the census year, are herewith presented to the reader:—Maine, 28·18; Vermont, 24·46; Massachusetts, 29·20; Rhode Island, 24·98; New York, 25·29; New Hampshire, 24·96; New Jersey, 23·25; Connecticut, 22·67; Philadelphia, 18·85; and Georgia, 11·14."

With regard to tuberculosis it is, both in its distribution and destructiveness, the greatest scourge of the human race, and no region, it seems, is suited to all cases. If such a locality existed, it would be the Mecca for such cases, and would doubtless be shunned by the healthy.

It is well known that some authorities advocate the home treatment chiefly because it is the best that can be done under the circumstances; others prefer a mountain climate; still others the arid stretches of New Mexico and Arizona; others again such a mild and equable climate as that shown by Augusta and regions further south.

Tubercular cases with cardiac complications certainly do better here than in mountain regions, and until Arizona and New Mexico have further development it is not practicable except in a few localities to send any but robust cases there, and these may be treated nearer home.

To sum up the climate in and around Augusta (and in this I include Aiken, for I do not believe there is any appreciable difference in these places), is, according to my experience, well adapted for the treatment of tuberculosis, and especially when complicated by heart lesions, of cases of bronchitis and asthma. For the last named class of cases it seems especially adapted. The equable and mild climate make it suitable for those suffering from nephritis with its complications; rheumatic and cardiac cases as a rule do well here; and it is especially well suited as a place of convalescence, and for those who desire to avoid the rigors of the northern winter and its changeable spring seasons.

DISCUSSION.

Dr. BRIDGE: I would like to inquire as to character of the filtration of the drinking water of Augusta and would also like to ask if Dr. Coleman knows any possible explanation, apart from the water supply, for the mortality of the town as compared with such a town as for example Omaha, which has a mortality of not more than 8 or 9 per thousand? Why should

Augusta have a mortality twice as large as that, and why should Chicago have a mortality of only about 14 per thousand ?

Dr. PHILLIPS : Dr. Coleman remarked that it was an unfortunate condition that he had no meteorological record for Summerville. Now I wish to say that there can be no decided difference between the meteorological conditions of Summerville and those of Augusta. An elevation of 300 feet, if one were to go directly up from the earth's surface into the free air, would show a fall in the temperature of one degree. It would thus be seen that Summerville could have a temperature one degree lower, on the average, than Augusta. However, that would be too great an average difference to apply. In the United States Weather Bureau's efforts to reduce the temperature of elevated stations to sea level temperatures it was found that it was only permissible to apply a difference of one degree for every two or three thousand feet of ascent. The Weather Bureau's results were obtained by a most careful comparison of all known statistics of places located near each other and yet at different altitudes. The stations at Pike's Peak and Colorado Springs, and at Mount Washington and a neighbouring town, at lower level, were some of the stations studied. So it is probable that the temperatures of Summerville and Augusta differ only by a fraction of a degree. Inasmuch as humidity is dependent upon temperature, other conditions being equal, the difference in the humidity of these two places can be but slight. I will also just remark that a good many persons in referring to the meteorologic service in this country call it the Signal service. It was a part of that service at one time, but now it is the Weather Bureau and it is best to use the proper term in referring to its reports.

Dr. QUIMBY : Fifteen years ago it was the custom among New York physicians to make very sharp class distinctions, based on the nature of the pathic processes, in the cases to be sent to different localities. It seems to me that the influence of altitude and climate as bearing upon our selection of the proper place for each special case should be distinctly separated. The effect of altitude is primarily purely physical and the results of all others definitely determinable. Moreover, as climatic conditions are often the same at high and low altitudes it may be the dominant factor determining our decision. I should, therefore, like to ask the gentlemen from the several resorts if they make any such distinction between altitude and climatic influences ?

Dr. COLEMAN : In replying to the question about filtration, I wish to state that the Savannah river water has always been considered an extremely pure water. I presume because there are so few cities located on its banks. I know that formerly seamen often used to make special trips to this river for their ship's water supply. It contains a great deal of clay, however, and the filtration is used particularly to get rid of that. I am not familiar with Omaha's death rate, but it strikes me that the figures given are very low. Two conditions contribute to make the death-rate of Augusta higher than it should be and one of these is that 40 per cent. of the population are negroes. As a race they are shiftless and their health is not so well taken care of now as it was before the war.   Their houses are not well built and in winter they huddle together in small ill-ventilated rooms to keep warm.   Their death-rate in tuberculosis, for instance, is twice as high as in the white race, whereas before the war the disease was hardly known among them.   Another is in the large factory element of white people, in many of whom are found the elements of poverty and thriftlessness.   I want to make my apologies to Dr. Phillips for styling his service the United States Signal service.   Without going so deeply into the scientific aspect of the subject as he has, it seemed to me, that in addition to the elevation, the condition of the soil of Augusta proper and proximity to the river might have some effect upon the humidity.   Moisture stands in our lower districts for a long time, whereas on the hill-tops it is impossible for it to remain, and I have often noticed a mist over the low country when the atmosphere was perfectly clear about the hills.

REMARKS ON THE CLIMATIC INFLUENCES OF NEWPORT, RHODE ISLAND.

BY WILLIAM C. RIVES, M.D.

WASHINGTON, D.C.

THE climate of Newport, Rhode Island, taken as a whole, may be described as a cool marine one, of moderate humidity, this latter element becoming excessive in summer. The mean annual temperature (Report of Chief Signal Officer for 1883, War Department) is 50·0 degrees.

Mean temperature of January, 30·7 degrees F.; of July, 70·5 degrees F. Mean annual barometer (corrected for temperature and instrumental error only), 29·964 inches. Mean annual rainfall, 49·97 inches. Mean monthly wind movement, 6847·3 miles.

The temperature and relative humidities of the seasons are as follows:—

	Winter	Spring	Summer	Autumn
Temperature	32·1	45·2	68·2	53·5
Relative humidity	74·7	72·9	77·8	76·9

In 1888 there were 164 clear days.

Newport's climate of course shares in the general features common to marine ones, but is further influenced by two other factors, the direction of the winds and the Gulf Stream. The prevailing winds at Newport are from the south-west, while in the northern part of the State a northerly wind is most frequent. The effect of the Gulf Stream is shown[1] in the temperature of the water—far warmer than is found north of Cape Cod—and by the presence of marine algæ, which, with many of the fishes of Newport, as Dr. Storer* has pointed out, are southern forms.

The comparative equability of the Newport climate—its coolness in summer and mildness in winter—has long attracted the notice of observers, several of whom have called attention to it, among them Surgeons Head and Campbell,† who were stationed for four years at Fort Adams, Newport Harbour, Dr. Fisher,‡ Secretary of the State Board of Health, and especially Dr. Storer, to whose articles I shall presently refer. The climate is not only milder than that of the east coast of New England, but differs considerably from the climate of the Northern' part of the State of Rhode Island, of which that of Providence is fairly representative. The annual temperature of Newport and Providence is about the same, but there is a marked difference in the maxima and minima and the yearly, monthly, and daily ranges. The mean yearly range at Newport is about 87 degrees F. The mean monthly range varies from 44·4 degrees in January to 28·6 degrees in August. Mean daily range about 13·5 degrees. The ranges at Providence are considerably greater.

Although the island of Rhode Island is surrounded by the salt water it is so short a distance from large masses of land that it is obviously somewhat less subject to oceanic influences than Nantucket and Block Island, both of which, as regards each other, possess a nearly identical climate, and have a still smaller monthly and daily range, and somewhat greater humidity than Newport.

A special result of the oceanic influence at Newport becomes apparent when we compare the monthly temperatures at

---

[1] This influence of the Gulf Stream is now questioned.

different seasons; the surrounding waters, which become heated in summer, lose their heat but slowly, so that Newport, which is cooler in summer, begins in September to be warmer than Providence, and the autumnal climate is proportionately warm. In the spring, however, the cold water becomes warm slowly, so that May is a warmer month in Providence, and the springs at Newport are somewhat more backward than in the interior.

The local topographical features of Newport have had much to do with its celebrity as a health resort, and deserve to be regarded in considering its climate. Newport is greatly favoured by nature in being chiefly situated on an irregular high plateau, two and a half miles long by three-quarters of a mile broad, usually from forty to sixty feet high, but attaining an elevation of 100 feet and sloping rapidly to the east and west; less abruptly to the north and south. This high situation well above the water gives good ventilation and admirable facilities for drainage. The old town being mainly on the western slope, unlike most of our seaside resorts, faces west, and is comparatively sheltered from the easterly winds. As it lies along the bay, and the harbour is comparatively land locked, it is not fully exposed to the Atlantic breezes.

The rock underlying the compact part of Newport belongs to the coal measures; it is chiefly of a slaty character and forms the cliffs east of the town. To the south and south-west especially, there are large tracts of rocky land, of varied geological formation, more or less devoid of surface soil. Apart from the easy facilities of drainage, the nature of the soil is not particularly favourable. I am indebted to Captain J. P. Cotton, City Engineer, for the following account:—"A limited area of the thickly settled parts of the town bordering on the tide water is flat and elevated but a few feet above tide. Here the surface drainage is not good and the ground water not far below the surface; its level is, however, nearly constant. The soil is for the most part clayey, underlaid by a gravelly hard pan with clean gravel of varying thickness overlying the rock.

In some sections this clay is so nearly impervious to the passage of water that cisterns have been built without brick walls—plastering with cement on the clay. In excavating for sewers we seldom find much water until the gravel bed is struck. This carries large quantities of water. In the early days of sewer building the sewers were not in favour because they so often drained the wells in their neighbourhood. Bored or drilled wells have been sunk in some sections of the town that give a good supply of water from the gravel; some have been deepened through the gravel into the rock for a greater supply and have lost in the rock the supply from the gravel. Deep wells in the rock have seldom proved satisfactory either in quantity or quality of water; chlorine in excess being often found where no contamination was in evidence." The rock has been known to have been the means of conveying sewage and foul matter considerable distances; in one case nearly 100 feet.

In most of our sea coast watering places the exact situation chosen for a dwelling, provided the sanitary surroundings are good, makes but little difference, but at Newport the climatic conditions vary very greatly with the locality, for the town proper is several miles away from the full influence of the Atlantic, notwithstanding its nearness to the salt water.

Much of the summer life goes on at points remote from the sea; the hotels and boarding houses are, with very few exceptions, at a distance from the shore, and many visitors spend but little time near the water. To get the full effect of the ocean, one must go to the southern and especially the extreme south-western point of the island, which is always cool and comparatively bracing, even when it is intolerably close and relaxing in the town, as it occasionally is. The situations on the cliffs facing east occupy an intermediate position with regard to coolness. The most thickly settled and lowest parts of the town near the harbour are the least healthful, with the exception of the so-called " Point." The very compact portions of the town, however, are not large, and it has the advantage of being spread out over a wide extent of surface, many of the dwellings, even the humbler ones standing in grounds of their own. The sewerage system has been extended during recent years, and sanitary conditions are, with occasional striking exceptions, good, and are improving. No epidemic has been traced to the use of the city water.

During recent years vegetation has much increased, and mosquitoes are more troublesome than formerly, though not so numerous as to be a serious annoyance.

The feature of the Newport climate which most impresses itself upon the visitor in summer, is its humidity. This is greatest in the months of July and August, and heavy fogs abound, particularly in the month of June.

The moisture is so excessive that doors and window-frames swell to an astonishing degree, and articles are very apt to become mouldy. Disinclination for active exertion of both body and mind is a marked effect of the Newport summer climate. It seems even to have had its effect upon the character and temperament of the inhabitants. The actual summer temperature is seldom excessive, and the nights are almost always cool. The highest temperature recorded for Newport by the United States Signal Service was 92 degrees in July 1878; the lowest, 7·8 degrees in January, 1882.

"Thunderstorms," says an observer,§ "rarely pass over the place; they seem to divide about the head of Narragansett Bay, sending one division to follow the eastern shore, while the other passes over the land west of the Bay. In fact the storms seem to avoid the water and follow the land."

Newport's climate has a tendency to cause disorder of the digestive organs, and often produces diarrhœa, especially in a new-comer. In spite of its generally relaxing character, due to the atmospheric moisture, which to those in ordinary health is uncomfortable rather than unhealthful, the coolness of both days and nights and freedom from extremes, are great summer attractions.

The remarkable natural healthfulness of Newport for the average human being is a matter of some pride to the inhabitants, and is generally acknowledged, besides being, in a measure, confirmed by statistics. A climate with constant moderate variations in its principal factors is considered to be the best for the maintenance of health, and this is in the main, the character of the Newport climate. It is, in fact, though far less equable, about as near an approach to the climate of England as we possess in the Eastern United States. It is peculiarly favourable for children. Dr. Rankin, of the Newport Board of Health, called attention‖ to the fact that the excess of the birth-rate over the death-rate in Newport for the five years, 1884 to 1888, was from 17·9 to 15·6 per 1,000, and that the average excess in the whole State of Rhode Island for five years prior to 1886 was only 6·3 per 1,000—a striking confirmation of the truth of this supposition. "Few cities," said Dr. Rankin,¶ "have as low a general death-rate, as low a death-rate from zymotic diseases, as small a percentage of deaths among children under five years of age, and as few deaths from consumption."

A further indication of the healthfulness of Newport, given by Dr. Rankin is that but ten deaths occurred among the 8,000 to 10,000 summer visitors in 1889, and of these but one under five years of age.

Longevity is also very noticeable, and old residents, not only over 80 but over 90 years of age, are by no means infrequent. This, too, when the standard of sanitation and efforts for the prevention of disease are as yet not what they might be.

The average death-rate in Newport for ten years prior to 1888 was 15·9 per 1,000; in the whole State for the same period it was 17·9 per 1,000. In 1890 and 1891 the effects of epidemic influenza were experienced, the death-rate rising to the high figure of 21·5 in the latter year. Since then the death-rate has again decreased; for 1897 it was 16·5 per 1,000. But the population of Newport is so largely increased in summer, that the death-rate, as recorded, is higher than it actually is.

Dr. H. R. Storer, formerly a resident of Boston, who took up his residence at Newport as an invalid, was among those who recognised the comparative equability and mildness of the winter climate, and writing with his well-known ability, brought forward statistics** to show that the ratio of deaths from phthisis in Newport (at that time 12·93 to the total mortality per 1,000; 12·92 to the deaths from known causes; and 1·53 to every 1,000 of the population), was smaller than in most other parts of the country, except the north-western States. "What then," says Dr. Storer, "are the probable reasons of Newport's marked exemption from this scourge." His answer is absence of the two great causes, collective in-door occupation, and soil moisture, and secondly, freedom from cold moisture and from great sudden variableness of climate. It is also possible, he claimed, for a delicate person in Newport to lead comparatively an out-of-door life throughout the year. Dr. Storer also suggests that the dampness and moisture arising from inland waters seem to have a different effect from that rising from the sea, and that a saline marine atmosphere is beneficial.

He says Newport's insularity, which he regarded as producing its climatic conditions, is the chief of the causes of its immunity from phthisis, and while not recommending Newport as having an ideal climate for the consumptive, recommended it for such New England patients as were unable or unwilling to take more distant journeys in search of health. Dr. Storer's views were combated by our fellow member, Dr. J. Hilgard Tyndale,†† who, as an adherent of dryness and altitude, said that "It is a direct and indirect injury to consumptives to seek the moist and unequable climate of Newport, &c. Its oceanic character is a myth, as its stubborn moisture and temperature tables show, which in no wise vary from those of the general character of the whole northern coast." Dr. Tyndale claimed

(with some justice) that equability of temperature may be said
to exist, broadly speaking, where monthly ranges are below
25 degrees F., and the annual range not above from 30 to 40
degrees F. (maximum 80 degrees F., minimum 40 degrees F.).
" Here," said he, " we have for Newport monthly ranges of
32 degrees F, and from that up to 53 degrees F. and an annual
fluctuation of 84 degrees.   In short, not one of the elements of
climate which are suitable for consumptiives." These observations of Dr. Storer and the comments of Dr. Tyndale were
published just before the recognition of the tubercle bacillus as
the exciting cause of phthisis, and we are now able to estimate
them more accurately in the flood of light which has been shed
upon the climatic and hygienic treatment of tuberculosis in recent years.

That Newport has at least relative advantages of winter
climate, however, whatever may be thought of it absolutely,
Dr. Storer has clearly demonstrated, nor can his contention that
the death-rate from phthisis is unusually low be gainsayed,
though it is less exceptional in view of our present more complete statistics, than at first appeared, as we can partly infer by
an examination of the census maps of the mortality from
disease in various parts of the country.   It has been even
more favourable than was stated by Dr. Storer, and has
been as low as 1 · 14 to the thousand of the population and 7 · 93
per thousand of the total mortality.   It compares favourably
even with many inland localities and stands in marked contrast
to the rate of the coast of Massachusetts taken as a whole.   In
that State it is well known that the mortality from phthisis
diminishes strikingly in its ratio to the distance from the sea
coast, as Dr. Abbott‡‡ and others have shown.   Along the
coast of Rhode Island the reverse is the case, a condition
partly to be explained by the general uniformity of climate
over the whole state, without very marked differences in altitude
and dryness.

As far as Newport's climatic conditions are concerned—by

no means the only causes—its comparative exemption from phthisis seems to be due to its comparative mildness and equability, its sheltered yet airy position high above the water, with opportunities for out-of-door life at all seasons, while it possesses those two great factors which it now seems to be admitted are the most essential in choosing a locality : (1) a well drained if not naturally dry soil, and (2) purity of air, a view to which the excellent results of the Massachusetts sanitaria lend strong confirmation.

The best climates, however, it has been well said, for healthful development and for maintenance of health, need not be the best, may even be injurious to delicate or diseased persons. In view of the general opinion that the majority of consumptives do better, other things being equal, the further they are removed from the sea, more evidence than that afforded by the death rate is required to uphold the claims of Newport. Dr. Storer quotes Dr. Rankin as having reported two advanced cases in which the disease had been arrested and material improvement obtained, and many other cases in the earlier stages in which he had perceived very marked improvement, and the Newport Medical Society at that time expressed their endorsement of Dr. Storer's views. These cases, however, were not sufficiently numerous, and unfortunately were not reported in detail. Dr. Storer's opinions we must now consider as having been too favourable.

I cannot myself recollect having observed benefit in phthisis from the Newport climate, and unfavourable views have recently been expressed to me by Newport physicians.

Dr. Henry Ecroyd, of Newport, writes me : " I do not look upon Newport as a good place for consumptives. The spring with its heavy fogs is especially bad for lung cases. Few consumptives fail to decline rapidly here—and at all times too much moisture. Trust my remarks will not discourage any one from coming to Newport, but would consider it a great misfortune if lung troubles should drift to Newport, as we have too many now." Dr. T. A. Kenefick is even more emphatic, and has been struck with the rapid progress of the disease in certain cases, which he attributes to the heavy, moist atmosphere. "Any inland high country place is far more desirable than Newport. I have seen patients come to Newport from inland New England cities in fairly good general condition with only slight physical signs in the lung, and the general wasting took place so rapidly that in a week it was impossible for them to be removed, and shortly after they were carried home dead. I never saw a consumptive improve. I have always recommended immediate removal to a more inland and a high and drier altitude."

Taken absolutely, Newport has a bad winter climate for the consumptive; at the same time as it possesses the qualifications of very pure air, greater mildness, less variability, fewer piercing winds, little if any more moisture at that season, and allows of an out-of-door life with more comfort, I should prefer it to other parts of the New England coast, and with the present improved methods of treatment and cases taken early, should look for better results.

With regard to other diseases there is not much to be said. "I consider Newport," said the late Dr. William F. Hutchinson,§§ one of the very best summer climates for nerve invalids in the world. The heavy sea fogs which are sometimes complained of, are in themselves most active agents in quieting irritable nerves." This statement is too broad, and presupposes patients possessing considerable bodily vigor and powers of reaction.

There is one class of cases which does not do well in Newport in summer. This comprises persons of feeble vitality with imperfect powers of digestion, especially anæmic and dyspeptic girls who need exercise. Newport is too sedative and relaxing for such, and they do much better in the drier and more bracing air of the mountains. As was before said, the climate of Newport tends to derange the digestive organs, especially at the close of summer. In illustration of this, it may be mentioned that of 44 deaths in Newport in 1891, from diarrhœal diseases (nearly three fourths infants under two years of age) thirty-nine occurred in August and September.

No special benefit has been observed from Newport in renal diseases. Dr. H. G. MacKaye, of Newport, considers the climatic influences distinctly unfavourable to them, rheumatic affections are not usually helped. Some asthmatics are favourably affected; others are not. Newport, in spite of the advocacy of Dr. Storer, is not frequented as a winter health resort, although he regards it as the Isle of Wight, or as we might say, the Atlantic City of New England. It has, however, undoubtedly attracted to it persons seeking for a less vigorous winter home. Whether, as it is as yet practically the only really available winter resort close at hand, it may not be advantageously employed for convalescents from acute diseases, and for threatened or very early organic disease in patients from Boston and the neighbouring parts of eastern New England, is a question which its meteorological and local conditions and its satisfactory provision for the hygenic needs and comfort of the sick, would seem to answer in the affirmative, but still requires to be further and more systematically subjected to the test of experience.

REFERENCES.

* " The Mild Winter Climate of Newport, Rhode Island, as the effect of Gulf Stream." *New York Medical Record*, vol. xxiv, 1883, pp. 679-81.

† Circular No. 8. War Department, Surgeon-General Office. A Report on the Hygiene of the United States Army, with Description of Military Posts.

‡ Third Annual Report, State Board of Health of Rhode Island.

§ Annals of Harvard College Observatory, vol. xxi, part ii. New England Meteorological Society, 1891.

‖ Fourth Annual Report of the Board of Health of Newport, Rhode Island.

¶ Fifth Annual Report of the Board of Health of Newport, Rhode Island.

** *The Sanitarian*, vol. xi.

†† *Boston Medical and Surgical Journal*, vol. cviii, 1883.

‡‡ " Climate Cure in Nervous Diseases." *New York Medical Record,* vol. xvii, 1880, pp. 3-6.

§§ " On the Geographical Distribution of certain Causes of Deaths in Massachusetts." (Twenty-third Annual Report, Massachusetts State Board of Health for 1891.)

DISCUSSION.

Dr. HAROLD WILLIAMS : I would like to ask the writer his authority for what he said in regard to the Gulf Stream as modifying the climate of New-port ? The latest authority on the Gulf Stream, so far as I know, is Dr. Peterman's charts, and my impression is that the Stream does not come within 300 miles of Newport, so that it could not affect the temperature of that place in the least.

Dr. RIVES : The temperature is certainly warmer than it is north of Cape Cod, and it seemed to me reasonable to attribute to the Gulf Stream. I am not able to give authority for it.

Dr. NEWTON : Speaking of climate for consumptives, I personally believe we are too prone to lay stress upon dry climates. I believe that if patients stayed out of door in climates like Newport as much as they do in Mexico, it would be better for most of them. We are told, for instance, that in the English navy the number of consumptives has increased greatly since steam war-vessels have come into use and the sailors have been confined in close, steam-heated quarters.

Dr. SOLLY : That is true, but it has also been found that those sailors who develop consumption have to be taken away from the sea for treatment. People may live very well in a damp climate, but when they contract that disease they do not do well in such a climate.

Dr. RIVES : It seems to me that even if Newport is, absolutely speaking, a bad climate for consumptives, it is better than we have at most places along the New England coast. It escapes the east winds of Boston, and its death rate is less.

NANTUCKET AND THE OCEAN CLIMATE.

BY DR. HAROLD WILLIAMS.

BOSTON, MASS.

———————

SOME fifteen years ago, in a paper read by the writer before the Massachusetts Medical Society, entitled " Climatic Treatment of Phthisis," climate, therapeutically considered, was divided into four classes : —

(*a*) Mountain, (*b*) inland, (*c*) sea-board, and (*d*) ocean.

Mountain climate as experienced at altitudes of 6,000 feet or thereabouts, and ocean climate as experienced upon shipboard, represented the extremes of therapeutic climates. Those of other stations were classified as inland or maritime, according as they more nearly resembled the one or the other of these therapeutic extremes.

This classification seems to the writer a good one, and is adopted in the present paper. It is obvious how the climate of the low mountain resorts like the White Mountains, for example, resembles that of higher altitudes, like Denver or Colorado Springs only in degree. In the same way, it is obvious how the climate of the various sea-shore stations resembles that of the ocean itself simply in degree, and it is the object of the present paper to show : —

(1) How the climate of Nantucket resembles more closely that of the ocean itself than does the climate of any of the summer sea-shore resorts of the Atlantic coast, from Old Point Comfort to Grand Manan, with the possible exception of Atlantic City.

(2) To give the Association a brief description of the island itself, following the plan laid down by Dr. E. O. Otis in the *New York Record* of August 25, 1900, and the results of my experience there during twenty years of summer practice.

The ocean climate differs from mountain climate in that it contains:—

(*a*) The maximum amount of oxygen; (*b*) the maximum amount of aqueous vapour; (*c*) the maximum amount of ozone; (*d*) small saline particles—iodine and bromine; (*e*) it presents more regular variations of barometric pressure; (*f*) it presents the minimum diurnal variations of temperature.

Together with mountain air, it possesses the common element of purity. Of these various attributes, the first three are practically common to all sea-board or island resorts. The fourth depends largely upon the direction of the prevailing winds, and, so far as we know, it is not of particular therapeutic importance. This leaves us with the diurnal range of temperature and the purity of the air as the chief points of difference between the various sea-board and island stations. The most characteristic peculiarities of the air of the ocean itself, as compared with the climate of the sea-board or of islands upon the coast, are its freedom from organic impurities, the iodine and bromine it contains, and the minimum of its diurnal range of temperature. Theoretically, and as I believe practically, we should expect the air of islands would most nearly approximate to the air of the sea in these two most important respects. A glance at the map (Department of the Interior, 1898), shows us that between the parallels of latitude 37 and 45 degrees, or from Virginia to Canada, there are but six principal islands available for and frequented by the summer visitor. These islands are Long Island, Block Island, Martha's Vineyard, Nantucket, Isles of Shoals, and Mount Desert. Our glance at the map will also have shown us that of all these islands, Nantucket is situated furthest from the mainland, or furthest out to sea, and we should consequently expect of it that its climate would more nearly resemble that of the ocean than would that of any of the others. The following tables, prepared from the reports of the Weather Bureau for the year 1899, taken at haphazard, would seem to confirm this expectation.

I.

TEMPERATURE CHART FOR MONTH OF JUNE, 1899.

RESORTS—Nantucket		Block Island		Vineyard Haven		Bar Harbour
Maximum temperature	78°	...	83°	...	86°	...	85°
Minimum temperature	63°	...	65°	...	68°	...	59°
Maximum daily range	24°	...	26°	...	29°	...	35°
Minimum daily range	8°	...	9°	...	11°	...	14°
Average daily range for month ...	11·9°	...	13·8°	...	17·3°	...	24·4°

II.

TEMPERATURE CHART FOR MONTH OF JULY, 1899.

RESORTS—Nantucket		Block Island		Vineyard Haven		Bar Harbour
Maximum temperature	80°	...	80°	...	85°	...	88°
Minimum temperature	55°	...	52°	...	59°	...	44°
Maximum daily range	18°	...	22°	...	22°	...	34°
Minimum daily range	5°	...	6°	...	7°	...	12°
Average daily range for month ...	11°	...	11·9°	...	15·2°	...	23·5°

III.

TEMPERATURE CHART FOR MONTH OF AUGUST, 1899.

RESORTS—Nantucket		Block Island		Vineyard Haven		Bar Harbour
Maximum temperature	82°	...	80°	..	84°	...	88°
Minimum temperature	57°	...	49°	...	51°	...	45°
Maximum daily range	18°	...	22°	...	25°	..	32°
Minimum daily range	4°	...	3°	...	6°	...	13°
Average daily range for month ...	10·5°	...	11·2°	...	14·6°	...	23·2°

IV.

TEMPERATURE CHART FOR MONTH OF SEPTEMBER, 1899.

RESORTS—Nantucket		Block Island		Vineyard Haven		Bar Harbour
Maximum temperature	77°	...	79°	...	81°	... No Record.
Minimum temperature	49°	...	48°	...	47°	...	,,
Maximum daily range	19°	...	16°	...	24°	...	,,
Minimum daily range	5°	...	5°	...	6°	...	,,
Average daily range for month ...	10·8°	...	10·4°	...	14°	...	,,

V.

AVERAGE DAILY RANGE FOR THREE SUMMER MONTHS, 1899.

RESORTS—Nantucket		Block Island	Vineyard Haven	Bar Harbour	Atlantic City
Average diurnal range for three months	11·1°	... 12·3°	... 15·7°	... 23·7°	... 11·03°

From these tables it is evident that Nantucket possesses a climate more nearly resembling that of the ocean than the climates of the other islands with which it is compared in the principal attribute of the ocean climate—the smallness of the diurnal range. It is almost exactly the same as that of Atlantic City, which, so far as I know, possesses the most equable climate of any health resort upon the Atlantic coast. It is to be regretted in this context that the Isles of Shoals could not have been included in the comparison, but no record of these islands is kept by the Weather Bureau. My own experience, however, with this group is that the diurnal range is great. Probably it approximates more nearly to that of Mount Desert than to that of the other islands.

In the absence of positive data with respect to relative purity of the air, comparison of Nantucket with other islands or with Atlantic City, is, of course, valueless. It may be said, however, that natural conditions are favourable here in the highest degree to the purity of the atmosphere. The island is sparsely populated; there are no high mountains or hills to interrupt the sweep of the wind, the prevailing direction of the latter is westerly, blowing over miles of ocean before it reaches the island; this would seem to be more highly favourable to its becoming purified and charged with saline particles than would be the case of other islands or stations.

From this brief *résumé* of its climatic peculiarities, it would seem that the climate of Nantucket resembles more nearly that of the ocean, as experienced on shipboard, than does the climate of the other islands of the North Atlantic.

THE ISLAND OF NANTUCKET.

The island of Nantucket (41° 15′ north latitude, 70° west longitude) lies in the Atlantic Ocean twenty-five miles due south of the metacarpal joint of the beckoning finger of Cape Cod. It is of a long-horned crescent shape, and roughly speaking, is fourteen miles long and four miles wide. It is the most easterly of the group sometimes known as the Elizabeth Islands, in which are also included Martha's Vineyard, Naushon, Tuckanuck, and Muskeget. It is almost exactly 100 miles from Boston. Structurally considered, it is a vast mound of sand, gently undulating in surface, and presenting a series of high bluffs to the sea. At various points its surface is dotted by fresh water ponds of varying size. The soil is of a light, porous, sandy nature. Rocks are so rare that it would be easily possible to count those worthy of the name upon the fingers of the hand. There are, practically speaking, no trees. The flora is large and varied. Five hundred varieties of species are described as growing without cultivation. The botanic range is wide; heather grows upon the moors; cactus is to be found freely flowering in the month of July, while in August, a visit to a vast field of hollyhock-like blossoms of the pink hybiscus is a favourite excursion. A large variety of birds pause at the island upon their semi-annual pilgrimages; black duck and quail (the latter protected throughout the entire year), live there the entire year round, and the neighbouring island of Muskeget is a breeding ground upon which thousands of families of seagulls are annually reared.

Nantucket, the chief town, is situated upon the northern side of the island, on Vineyard Sound. The resident population in 1900 was 3,000, though the summer population is, of course, much in excess of these figures. In 1894, 16,306 passengers, not including children exempt from the payment of fares, were brought to the island. At the height of its prosperity, when the whaling industry flourished, the population was

10,000. The town is very old (the oldest house bearing the date 1686). Many of its dwellings and warehouses are built of brick, and the number is surprisingly large in proportion to the present population. A general impression of size and antiquity is given to the town. The streets are, for the most part, paved with stone. Outside the town clay roads extend in many directions, and the State Road, a fine piece of macadamised road, connects the town with Siasconset. At a greater distance from the town the roads consist chiefly of "ruts," and one may drive or ride in almost any direction at will over the moors.

Siasconset, formerly a small fishing village, eight miles and a half from the town of Nantucket, and connected with it by a narrow-gauge railroad, is now an exceedingly popular summer resort. It is situated on the ocean, and is possessed of several hotels and boarding houses,* a casino, and a fine golf course. The surf bathing is excellent.

The following tables, compiled from statistics, prepared for me by Mr. A. W. Crosby, at the Weather Bureau in Boston, show the temperature and the number of pleasant days for the summer months of the years 1897, 1898, 1899, and 1900.

" A. B. C. and D."

Average maximum and minimum temperature; average maximum daily range and average monthly daily range at the Island of Nantucket for the months of June, July, August, and September of the four years 1897, 1898, 1899 and 1900.

	MONTHS—June	July	August	Sept.
Average maximum	$77 \cdot 5^{\circ}$ ...	$80 \cdot 7^{\circ}$ ...	$80 \cdot 2$ ...	81°
Average minimum	$48 \cdot 5^{\circ}$ ...	$55 \cdot 5^{\circ}$ ...	$57 \cdot 7^{\circ}$ ..	$48 \cdot 5^{\circ}$
Average maximum daily range...	20° ...	$18 \cdot 5^{\circ}$ ...	$16 \cdot 7^{\circ}$ ...	$18 \cdot 2^{\circ}$
Average monthly daily range ...	$11 \cdot 27^{\circ}$ ...	$10 \cdot 8^{\circ}$ ...	$10 \cdot 6^{\circ}$ ...	$10 \cdot 6^{\circ}$
Average number of rainy days...	$8 \cdot 7$ ...	$10 \cdot 5$ ...	8 ...	$7 \cdot 2$

It may be of interest to compare these records with those of Boston, New York, and Chicago, during the hottest weather of last summer.

---

* Hotels :—Beach House, Ocean View Hotel. Price of board: Hotels, 10 to 20 dols. per week ; boarding houses, 10 to 12 dols. Rent of cottages from 100 to 500 dols., average 250 dols. Absolute accuracy is not claimed for these data.

	July—14th		15th		16th		17th		18th
Boston	...	81°	...	82°	...	95°	...	95°	...	97°
New York	...	84°	...	94°	...	93°	...	94°	...	94°
Chicago...	...	92°	...	90°	...	85°	...	74°	...	68°
Nantucket	...	78°	...	78°	...	81°	...	76°	...	78°

From the Tables A, B, C, and D, it will be seen that the average number of partly rainy days for the four summer months for the years 1897, 1898, 1899, and 1900, was 8·6 per month. This number represents the number of days during which it rained at some period of the day. The number of days in which an invalid could not exercise out of doors was, of course, very much smaller. In 1894, for the months July, August, and September, there were ninety-two consecutive pleasant days.

The prevailing direction of the wind is westerly. One of the most remarkable meteorological phenomena of the island is the rarity of electric storms. Thunderstorms are exceedingly uncommon, passing north or south of the island. In the twenty summers I have passed at Nantucket I have known the lightning to strike but on three occasions.

The average temperature of the water for the summer of 1894 was 72 degrees. At the bathing beach it is somewhat higher. The cause of this high temperature of the water is a much discussed question. It is believed by some to be due to the proximity of the Gulf Stream, but this theory is not borne out by fact. Any one interested in the matter is referred to Dr. Peterman's charts of the Gulf Stream. The water supply of the town is derived from a large fresh water pond. It is between two and three miles from the town, and is in an isolated position so far as dwelling houses are concerned, the house of the engineer being the only human habitation within the water-shed. It would be difficult to conceive of its ever sustaining dangerous pollution. During the latter part of the season, especially when the weather is exceptionally dry, and the pond is low, the water is at times rendered of objection-

able taste and odour because of the decomposition of weeds.
This year wells were constructed in close proximity to the
pond, and it is expected that in future this defect in the quality
of the water will be remedied.

The sewerage of the town has been greatly improved in
recent years by the construction of a main to the deep waters
of the harbour channel, but the cess-pool system still partially
prevails. The average hourly velocity of the wind, however
(nine miles for the three months of 1894), renders the air free
from the odours usually attendant upon the cess-pool system.
From its isolated position, Nantucket is particularly free from
contagious diseases. During the past ten years (1890 to
1900), there have been forty-four deaths from tuberculosis,
and fourteen from diphtheria, averaging, respectively, 4·4
tuberculosis, and 1·4 diphtheria per year for the ten years in
a population considerably in excess of 4,000, or 10 per 10,000
as compared with 22 per 10,000 in Boston. Last year one case
of questionable typhoid was reported. It was, however, an exceedingly doubtful case, and did not give the Widal reaction.
Contagious diseases when present are for the most part imported to the island, and are generally so managed as to reduce
to a minimum their further dissemination. This is the more
readily accomplished because of the co-operation of an intelligent Board of Health.

· The amusements afforded to the summer visitors are unusually varied. The boating is excellent. Large cat-rig boats, under
the charge of experienced skippers, are provided in abundance.
Those prefering still waters may sail in the land-locked waters
of the inner harbour, eight miles in extent. The more accomplished sailors can pursue their excursions upon the rougher
waters of the sound. A daily trip by sail boat and by launch
is made to Wauwinet, about seven miles up the inner harbour.
Still water for rowing is always found in the waters of the
latter, and excellent light boats can be hired by the hour. It
is particularly safe for women and children because of the shal-

lowness of the water. The fishing is excellent : blue fish abound
in the season ; scup and plaice fish (the latter a species of large
flat-fish) are found in great abundance, as are also the English
turbot. Lobsters, clams, quohogs, and oysters, are also abundant. Perch abound in the fresh water ponds. There is some
shooting. Marsh birds are found throughout the summer ;
plover and snipe are frequently killed during their flights, and
black duck and rabbits are numerous. Driving is very agreeable at Nantucket. The moors are for the most part unfenced
and level, and it is the custom to ride and drive across them
in any and every direction. Excellent carriages are to be had
for one dollar per hour, with special prices to prominent points.
Bicycling is also excellent. The State road is a perfect piece of
road construction ; the clay roads are fair, and there are several
agreeable bicycle paths. Golf is the principal amusement.
The golf course is remarkably fine, and in many respects an
exact counterpart of the Scotch links. The course consists of
eighteen holes, is about 5,500 yards in length, and is over gently
undulating ground, in which neither tree nor stone interferes
with the pastime. Fine views of the sea are to be had from
many of the tees and greens. Afternoon teas and tournaments
are held every week during the season.

From twenty years of summer practice on the island, the
writer feels able to recommend the climate as especially suited
for the extremes of life, for the very old and the very young,
the immunity from contagious diseases and the smallness of the
daily range making it especially suitable for the latter ; those
suffering from functional nervous affections, neurasthenia, insomnia, and neuralgia ; for convalescence from diseases of the
respiratory organs ; for chronic dysentery ; and especially is it
specific for the enterocolitis of children.

Nantucket possesses an excellent public library, a museum
containing many objects of interest, the valuable and interesting
collection of the Historical Society, an old mill, several light-
houses and life saving stations, churches of nearly every denomi-

nation, gas and electrical plants; also an excellent hot water bathing establishment.

There are several hotels, among which may be mentioned the Ocean House, Point Breeze, the Sea Cliff and Springfield House,† prices varying from ten dollars to eighteen dollars per week. There are also a large number of excellent boating houses.‡

Mr. A. T. Mowry, real estate agent, has a list of available cottages for rent, and solicits correspondence upon all mattters pertaining to Nantucket. Cottages vary from 150 dollars to 1,000 dollars; average about 400 dollars. An eminent Boston surgeon and a distinguished oculist from Philadelphia are among the summer residents, and can be called upon for special services.

DISCUSSION.

Dr. SOLLY: I was delighted to hear this paper, which confirms all I knew of Nantucket clinically as well as the climatic parts. I am glad to have the question of the Gulf Stream settled, but it is further off than it ought to be. The equability of the climate of Nantucket in the summer seems to be very commendable and very valuable to many patients. I have sent a great many chronic consumptives to Nantucket in the summer, and they have benefited very much by the change. We have on the Pacific coast an island that approaches it very closely, that is Santa Catalina. The remarks the doctor made about Atlantic City, too, were very interesting, and it is interesting to consider why that place should suffer very little from the land winds that give rise to such wide ranges of temperature. The great difficulty at most seaside resorts is the change from land to sea breezes.

Dr. RIVES: I would like to ask if a few years ago the death-rate of tuberculosis at Nantucket was not the highest in the State?

Dr. WILLIAMS: I am very glad that question has been asked, because thereby hangs a tale. Some years ago the population of Nantucket was 10,000 as compared with 3,000 now. At that time the main industry was

---

† Not intended to be complete.

‡ Mrs. Ayers ; Central House ; Albert Easton ; Mrs. G. G. Fisk ; Miss Folger, Cliff Road ; Holiday Inn ; Island Home House ; Nesbitt House ; Pitman's ; Rest Haven ; Roberts' House ; Mrs. Smith, The Cliff ; Mrs. E. A. Waitt. Prices varying from 8 to 12 dols. per week.

removed from the island and with it migrated the mass of the population. When these people died, however, in various parts of New England—some, possibly, in Newport—their bodies were returned to Nantucket for burial, and the published statistics of the island were not of people *dying* at Nantucket but of the people *buried* there. I wrote a criticism of the Board of Heath at that time, in which I compared the death-rate at Nantucket with that of Gettysburg at the time of the battle, which, of course, was somewhat out of proportion to the population of the town. Our death-rate at Nantucket from tuberculosis is about 4 per 10,000 as compared with 12 at Newport and 20 throughout the State. One reason why I read this paper was that I wanted to call attention to the great importance of the diurnal range of temperature which, it seems to me, has been disregarded too much in the description of the climate of health stations. I regard the diurnal range as one of the most important things to be considered in regard to the climatic conditions of any place. There is another matter, suggested by Dr. Smith's paper, to which I also desire to call the attention of the Society. This is, the subject of the development of typhoid fever in persons returning home from different health resorts, and often unjustly ascribed to the health resort, whereas, in truth, they are acquired in travelling. One or two such cases came to my knowledge with respect to Nantucket last summer. It was impossible, however, that they were acquired there as there were no cases on the island from which such infection could emanate ; and careful inquiry further showed that the incubation stages of the cases in question were too long to render it possible that the cases should have been acquired there. I am sure that the same thing is true of other health resorts, especially of the southern health resorts, and in justice to these stations I desire to impress this matter upon the notice of the Association.

THE CLIMATE OF NEW ENGLAND.

BY GUY HINSDALE, M.D.

PHILADELPHIA.

THE climate of New England is a peculiarly changeable one. This is due not altogether to its diversity of surface, but rather to its situation with reference to storm tracks. Modern meteorology traces with accuracy the paths of storms —cyclonic disturbances—and it is found that the areas of lowest barometric pressure pursue two distinct courses, meeting in New England. Cyclones of the first group come from the Great Lakes, and generally move in a north-easterly direction down the St. Lawrence valley, north of the boundary line, or they may pass more directly east, crossing New England to the Atlantic Ocean. The second group of cyclones comes from the south, and moves in a north-easterly direction along the coast, sometimes within the coast line, and at other times in the Atlantic. These are much more severe than the former, and bring a greater amount of rain and snow, but they are fewer in number.*

It should be understood that cyclones are not to be confounded with tornadoes. The latter have occurred in New England, but are comparatively rare, pass along narrow paths, and are of intense violence. Cyclones, on the other hand, may

---

* See *Investigations of the New England Meteorological Society*, 1889, vol. xxi., part 2, and Appendix, 1888 and 1889.

pass through or near New England as often, on an average, as once in four days the year round ; they affect a wide extent of territory, and are rarely attended, but occasionally, as at Galveston, by loss of life. The term cyclone may thus be applied to any barometric depression in which a distinct centre of low pressure is formed with the isobars approximately circular, and does not involve the idea of extreme violence of the winds. There are no periods of the year when the cyclones cease to move near New England, though they are somewhat less numerous in summer than in winter. April, May, and October are the months of greatest frequency.

The average annual rainfall is from 40 to 50 inches in the interior ; to 50 inches on the coast ; and the amount is subject to a variation of 20 or 30 per cent. in individual years. Rainfall is quite evenly distributed in the different months on the average. This is readily explained as due to the comparative uniformity in the distribution of cyclones throughout the year.

Though New England is a small district, it possesses a diverse topography, and therefore varied climatic conditions.

The characteristics of mountain climate are exemplified in Maine, New Hampshire, and Vermont, and those of the sea-level throughout a long and interesting coast. Maine alone has something like 3,000 miles of shore-line owing to its remarkable indentations and numerous islands.

The New England climate is characterised by (1) its changeableness. During the whole year there are clear days followed soon by cloudy ones ; during the winter and spring there is great variation of high and low temperature. Rain or snow falls in some parts of New England on nine-tenths of the days of the year, and at any given place, occurs once in three or four days. The same conditions prevail but for a few days at a time, and there is rarely what is called settled weather. An exception to this must be made in the climate of the Cape Cod peninsula. Here the conditions are much more uniform, and in the adjoining islands of Nantucket and Martha's

Vineyard the temperature range is remarkably uniform and the winds constant. At these localities a marine climate is experienced. (2) The great ranges of temperature both daily and annual. The large daily ranges 10 to 20 degrees F. on the average from the coast inland, and of 50 degrees in individual instances, are also due to the rapid succession of cyclone and anticyclones. The large annual ranges, 90 to 120 degrees from the coast island, are due to the fact that the climate is essentially continental, for while situated on the coast, the weather conditions are brought to it from the west, and are therefore those of a great continent somewhat tempered by the Atlanic Ocean.

The cold of northern New England is constant, but in Massachusetts and Connecticut it is liable to sudden interrup-tions. Occasional temperatures of 20 degrees below zero (F.) in winter, and of 100 degrees above in summer, are re-corded. The mean average temperature at Boston is about 48 degrees, and is one or more degrees lower in the western counties. Sudden changes are common, and the passage from winter to summer is often rapid. The climate of the south-eastern portion and the two islands is much more equable than that of the interior. The ground often freezes to a depth of three feet, and snow covers the ground to a depth of two feet or more in winter, especially in the western counties. The aver-age annual rainfall is from 40 to 45 inches.† As Charles Dudley Warner says, " New England is the battle ground of the seasons. It is La Vendee. To conquer it is only to begin the fight. When you have completely subdued, what kind of weather have you ? None whatever. It is alternately invaded by the hyperborean legions and the wilting sirens of the tropics." He likens the Gulf Stream to a white knight of the south going up to battle with the giant of the north. The two meet in New England and have it out there. He sarcastically

---

† Report State Board of Health, 1892.

calls New England the "exercise ground of the weather." This may seem rather unfair when all seasons of the year are considered, but one who has spent long winters and springs in Southern New England knows very well the exasperating features of the climate. The prolonged dry, crisp, freezing weather of the north is invigorating; but variable conditions, freezing, thawing, snow melting and freezing again, make nearly half the year dreaded by the healthy, not to speak of its effect on the sick. Warner, speaking from experience, says, " A New Englander is a person who is always just about to be warm and comfortable. That is the stuff of which heroes and martyrs are made ! " It is only too true. New Englanders, as far as they are a hardy race and long-lived, are so in spite of the climate. The fittest have survived from generation to generation. They have been brought up in hardship, and show a resisting power very great when their mortality is compared with that of immigrants from foreign lands.

Dr. E. P. Hurd,‡ of Newburyport, has shown that the foreigners coming to that manufacturing town are much more susceptible to pulmonary phthisis than the native population.

The isothermal lines are roughly parallel with the coast, the mean annual temperature diminishing in a north-westward direction. The difference between the boundaries is about 9 degrees F. for 4 degrees difference in latitude. The daily ranges of temperature are very great at times, especially in winter, and to this may be attributed, in great part, the prevalence of colds and pulmonary diseases in New England. The atmospheric humidity varies for the year from 60 to 90 per cent. in different parts of New England. In Boston there is less humidity in spring and early summer than in the other seasons, while at Block Island this is reversed. May and December are the cloudiest months, and September is the least cloudy; the aver-

---

‡ *Trans. Amer. Climatological Assoc.*, 1889.

age cloudiness is 50 per cent. The number of rainy days each month averages nine to seven.

The general characteristics of New England climate, and a scientific analysis of the weather for the year, are given in the bulletins of the New England Meteorological Society, particularly in the appendices each year. Reports are received from 175 observers, and the records are published and discussed in the Annals of the Harvard College Observatory. The Director of the Society, Prof. W. M. Davis, and the Secretary, Prof. Winslow Upton, have made the valuable reports in connection with these studies.||

A discussion of types of New England weather is found in Prof. Davis's report for the year 1889. Attention is called to certain disturbances of the ordinary diurnal variation of temperature due to the passage of cyclones, particularly in the winter season. Instead of the regular mid-day rise and evening fall there is, at times, a continuous rise of temperature from one day to the

---

THE NEW ENGLAND CLIMATE.—There is a marked difference in the mean temperatures of the ocean on the north and south sides of the Cape Cod peninsula. On the northern side the average summer temperature of the air is 69 degrees, and that of the water 70 degrees lower ; on the south side the average is 67 degrees, with the water but 1 degree cooler. The fauna and flora of the northern waters are semi-arctic in their character, scarcely varying from Massachusetts Bay to the Bay of Fundy, but in Buzzard's Bay the marine life approaches more nearly to that distinguishing the tropics. This decided difference is attributed to the action of the cold Arctic current, which flows along the northern coast, and the Gulf Stream, which washes the southern shore. With regard to the atmospheric temperature, a different condition of affairs prevails ; the towns on the northern coast, swept by the south-west winds which have traversed a heated territory, are hotter during the summer than the more favoured places on the southern shore, which are cooled by breezes which have crossed the expanse of the ocean. The sole exception to the former unfortunate spots is Sandwich, which is kept constantly cool by the indraft of cold air which passes through the funnel-shaped Buzzard's Bay.

|| See Appendices to the Bulletins of the Society for 1888 and 1889 ; "Investigation of the Sea Breeze," by W. M. Davis, L. G. Schultz, and R. de C. Ward ; "Thunderstorms in New England in the Summer of 1885," W. M. Davis.

next through the night, or, conversely, the continuous fall of temperature from one night to the next through the intervening day,
even though that day may have a clear sky with bright sunshine.
Such events are, of course, not confined to New England, but
the position of New England with regard to the two systems of
cyclone tracks renders these peculiar atmospheric changes more
liable to occur here than elsewhere. Thus, on November 27,
1889, the temperature rose at a certain point in New England
continuously from 28 degrees at 1 a.m. until 2 p.m. on the 28th,
when it reached 56 degrees ; again, the temperature rose steadily
from 28 dgrees at 6 a.m., on December 8, 1889, to 60 degrees
at noon on the 9th, both these occurrences being due to brisk
southerly cyclonic winds. On January 20, 1887, the southerly
winds of a strong cyclone from the great lakes carried the temperature upwards through the night to 40 or 50 degrees ; at
Windsor, Vermont, the temperature thus rose 81 degrees in
about forty-two hours. Similar changes occurred on Jan. 23
and 24, 1887, and once more on the 28th and 29th, during the
passage of cyclones to the north. The frequency of such abnormal changes decreases as winter passes away. Examples of
the continuous fall of temperature through the day, the direct
reverse of the preceding cases, are also not uncommon.

While cyclones or areas of low pressure advancing towards
New England produce marked disturbances of the weather, it
must not be forgotten that there is an anticyclone, or area of
high barometer, the direct antithesis of the cyclone. They
are considered by Loomis and Ferrel as the passive products of
adjacent cyclones. These periods of anticyclonic weather are
brief, rarely remaining in New England more than two days in
succession. Areas of low pressure are sure to take their place.
It is during the winter anticyclone that the lowest temperatures
are recorded. The air is clear and relatively still ; its lowest
strata lie very quietly on the earth, especially at night. The
nights are long and the days are short, with weak sunshine.
The air is dry and inspiriting. Such days are of bearable cold

on account of the absence of wind and moisture. Under such,
conditions the lower air becomes extremely cold at night and
thermometers may give readings below zero even near the
Southern coast, and in northern New England as low as — 20
to — 40 degrees F. When comparison is made at these times of
the records in adjacent hill and valley stations, it will be found
that the valleys are much colder than hillsides and·hill tops,
while on peaks, like Mount Washington, the temperature is
relatively moderate. For example, in the early morning of
January 19, 1887, after a quiet clear night, the temperature had
fallen close to zero on the coast, and records of — 40 to — 42
degrees were reported from the interior further north. It was
found that at Waterbury, Connecticut, the records rose in very
regular gradations, from — 25 degrees at the lowest point in
the valley, to 0 degrees 200 feet higher on the hills; at
Lexington, Massachusetts, one thermometer eight feet above
the ground, read — 15 degrees, while another on the same
building, but thirty feet above the ground, read — 7 degrees.

At Mount Washington, at such periods of anticyclones, the
temperature has been observed at + 16 degrees, while in the
neighbouring lowlands it ranged from — 10 degrees to — 24
degrees, a reversal of the usual temperature gradients. This
cold at night in lower strata of air in times of anticyclones, is,
of course, of local production, the cooling of the ground by
radiation through the clear air then prevailing, and secondarily
to the cooling of the quiet lower air chiefly by conduction, and
partly by radiation to the ground.

Such observations are of the greatest practical importance in
the choice of building sites, particularly in mountain regions.
Even for summer occupancy houses should never be at the
bottom of mountain basins. The lowest portion of the valley
first feel the frosts, which, in portions of the White Mountains
and the Adirondacks, may occur even in August, and it is in
these localities that banks of mist are seen in the early morning,
white clouds of fog, which send a chill through those who ven-

ture through them. Lakes lying at the base of mountains are in early autumn mornings almost invariably covered with white clouds, which quickly disappear before the sun. Cold air is like water, it seeks the lowest levels, and thus it is desirable in choosing a location, to seek an eminence or sheltered declivity; such a site is much cooler at mid-day in summer, and warmer at midnight in winter than the lower levels. An example of this variation of temperature between the lower and higher levels is seen in the so-called " ice storms." It is probable that in such cases the air half a mile or more above the earth is warmer than that below, and the rain that is formed aloft as a cyclone approaches is cooled close to the freezing point while falling, and freezes on reaching the ground or any solid object. Thus great damage is done to branches of trees; telegraph wires and other objects are frequently unable to withstand the thick ice which weighs them down.

Cold waves occur when the cyclone is intense, its passage rapid and central over New England, and when an area of very high pressure lies to the north-west. At these periods of cold north-westerly winds in the lowlands the upper currents are strongest and coldest. On Mount Washington at such times the wind may attain a velocity of over 100 miles an hour for several days, and temperatures below — 30 degrees for part of the period. On January 22, 1885, the Mount Washington record showed a minimum of — 50 degrees, the lowest temperature recorded there, and a north-west hurricane of over 100 miles an hour, the total daily movement being 2,140 miles. At such times the observers on the mountain must have wished for the speedy arrival of the quiet anticyclone with its relative warmth, and it is no wonder that this station has been abandoned.

The typical winter of New England lasts well into March, and after a rapidly warming spring, many days of May are almost like summer. The gales of March and its cold waves have always been characteristic, but never so terrific as on

March 11 to 14, 1888, when New England as well as the middle States were buried in the " Great Blizzard."¶

The extraordinary features of this storm were the result of two cyclones moving northerly from Arkansas, the northern centre passing north-easterly beyond the New England boundary, while the southern centre passed up the North Atlantic coast. The southern centre reached the south-eastern coast of Massachusetts on the evening of March 12, then curved westward, and advanced into Connecticut on the 13th. This change in direction was apparently due to the arrival of an area of low temperature from the north-west, and the rapid cooling of air fully saturated caused a great excess of precipitation. This was in the form of snow west of Rhode Island and Central Massachusetts, and rain and snow mixed in the eastern part of southern New England. From over 400 reports of the snowfall, it appears that in the southern part of Vermont and of New Hampshire, west of the Merrimac River, the western half of Massachusetts, nearly the whole of Connecticut, and of New York east of the Hudson River, as far north as Lake George, the average depth of unmelted snow exceeded 30 inches, while in central Connecticut and a large part of eastern New York, the average fall was between 40 and 50 inches. A minimum area of about 20 inches occurred near Hartford, Connecticut. The snow was badly drifted by the wind, and drifts from 30 to 40 feet by actual measurement were reported. The snow caused a complete suspension for several days of railway traffic entering New York City; no trains could pass from New York to Philadelphia until the fourth day, and violent winds exceeding 50 miles per hour prevailed. Boston reported a maximum velocity of 60 miles; New Haven 60; Block

---

¶ For a full account of this " blizzard " from a meteorological standpoint, see *Monthly Weather Review*, U.S. Signal Service, 1888 ; *Nautical Monograph*, No. 5, U.S. Hydrographic Office ; and *American Meteorological Journal*, May, 1888.

Island 70; and Eastport 72 miles per hour. Men were frozen to death in Broadway, New York, and many perished in consequence of exposure. Fortunately nothing like this has ever been known to have occurred before, and it is extremely unlikely that those now living will ever see such an event again. The great blizzard and cold wave of February, 1899, failed to reach New England, but expended itself in the Mississippi Valley, the Southern and South Atlantic States.

REFERENCES.

Winslow Upton, "Investigation of Cyclonic Phenomena in New England," *Amer. Meteor. Journ*, October, November, December, 1886, and January, 1887.

W. R. Dewey, "The Causes of Anticyclonic Cold in Winter," *Amer. Meteor. Journ.*, iii., 1886, 25-32.

"Winter on Mount Washington," *Science*, vii., 1886, 40.

Winslow Upton, "The Distribution of Rainfall in New England, February 10 14, 1886," *Science*, vii., 1886, 254.

Winslow Upton, *Bulletin N.E. Met. Soc.*, No. 41.

Winslow Upton, *Signal Service Monthly Weather Review*, March, 1888.

Winslow Upton, "The Cyclone of January 9, 1886," *Amer. Meteor. Journ.*, iii., 1886, 367-382.

W. M. Davis, "Mountain Meteorology—Appalachia," iv., 1886, 336.

F. V. Pike, "Three Ice Storms," *Amer. Meteor. Journ.*, 1886, pp. 32-39.

H. H. Clayton, "Cause of a Recent Period of Cool Weather in New England," *Science*, vii., 1886, 233.

A. Lawrence Rotch, "The Inversion of the Wind's Diurnal Period at Elevated Stations," *Amer. Meteor. Journ.*, ii., 1885, 29.

A. Lawrence Rotch, "A Connecticut Tornado," *Amer. Meteor. Journ.*, iii., 1886, 310-316.

H. W. Parker, "A Tornado Brood in Hampshire Co., Mass.," *Science*, vii., 1886, pp. 118, 220.

MAINE.

The State of Maine is the most important and the most interesting of the New England States from a climatic standpoint. Its name, the Pine Tree State, characterises it well. The forest stretching throughout the central and northern portions, has been long the source of the heaviest timber of the East. The trees are chiefly coniferous. The soil is sandy. The northern and western portions are mountainous, the range being part of the Appalachian system. Lakes abound,** and the marvellous indentation of its coast line affords innumerable bays and harbours, providing the most delightful seaside resorts, and affording the inhabitants every facility for maritime pursuits. The climate of Maine is therefore not alike throughout the State. While the interior and more remote portions of the State may afford a suitable refuge for the consumptive, and the comparatively dry soil, moderate altitude and pure air from pine forests are an aid to recovery ; the coast has very different properties. Its high latitude, rocky shores, and distance from the Gulf Stream, render the waters cold and the air chilly during the greater portion of the year. The great variability of climate and prevalence of fogs, which increase in density and penetrating qualities as we go further east, render it undesirable for persons with bronchial or pulmonary affections to remain near the sea. A great portion of the population is located near the coast, finding employment in maritime pursuits. The lumber regions are comparatively thinly settled. The death rate from phthisis is large, and in 1898 was 15·44 per 10,000 of population, or in other words, there were 647 persons living to one death from phthisis.

Those who have had experience in Maine unite in condemning the sea coast, and nearly all unite in praising the interior and backwoods as a resort for throat and lung troubles. The sea coast may be suitable, however, for cases of malaria and general and nervous debility. There is no doubt but that the exhilarating sea air, when free from fog, is of the greatest benefit in most cases of convalescence from acute disease, nervous exhaustion, and the debility of age. The air is bracing, and free from the debilitating character so often felt on low sandy coasts, especially during periods of " land breeze."

** Maine has 1,700 lakes, each not less than one mile square, and a greater number of smaller ones. One-fourteenth of its surface is thus covered.

The Maine coast is therefore to be sought only in summer, and particularly in order to avoid extreme heat. Bathing, except on the south-western coast, is safe only for the vigorous. Among the resorts most frequented is Moosehead Lake, surrounded by dense woods, forty miles from Mount Katahdin (elevation 5,385 feet) it is a favourite resort, and affords the best accommodation. The deeper woods of the Aroostook country are accessible from this point, and the salmon fishing of the Restigouche, Metapedia, and the St. John's, may be enjoyed if one can make the necessary arrangements. The right to fish in many of these waters is controlled by private clubs, which, however, are very hospitable to visitors properly introduced. The Rangeley Lakes in Western Maine afford fine trout fishing

Beginning at the eastern extremity of the coast, the resorts are Campobello, Grand Manan, and Mount Desert Islands. This last island is especially attractive, and presents some of the most picturesque scenery on the Atlantic coast. Comprising thirteen mountains and thirteen lakes, as well as a rugged shore line, the scenery is not like that of any other point on the seaboard. There are several harbours. Bar Harbour is the chief resort. Other harbours are North-east Harbour, Southwest Harbour, Seal Harbour, and Somes Sound. The elevation of Green Mountain, Mount Desert, is 1,500 feet. Winter Harbour, opposite Mount Desert and Isleboro, are also desirable summer stations. Castine has a beautiful situation, and is of great historical interest. It is at the head of Penobscot Bay, is more protected than Bar Harbour and is safer for boating. The mean annual temperature is 43·78 degrees. Other resorts are Isleboro, Old Orchard Beach, Biddeford Pool, Kennebunkport, Wells Beach, York Harbour, and Portland.

	Mean y'rly 1883	Temp. 1887	Max.	Min.	Prev. Wind	Rainfall		Mean Cloudiness	Humidity
Eastport ...	40·6°	41°	81·6°	17°	South	53·18		4·9	73
Portland ...	46·4°	44°	89°	8°	West	1883 32″	1887 49″	4·7	66

JULY / AUGUST

Day	JULY 8 a.m.	JULY 2 p.m.	JULY 8 p.m.	JULY Wind 3 p.m.	JULY Weather a.m.	JULY Weather p.m.	AUG Temp 5 a.m.	AUG Temp 8 a.m.	AUG 2 p.m. Temp	AUG 2 p.m. Weather Wind	AUG 8 p.m. Temp	AUG 8 p.m. Weather	AUG 8 p.m. Wind
1							60	72	72	O	66	Clear	S. Mod.
2							—	68	66	S. Str.	62	,,	O
3							54	70	63	S.E.	58	,,	O
4							48	66	67	S.	60	,,	O
5							58	66	65	S.E.	68	,,	O
6							62	72	72	S.	68	Cloudy	O
7							68	64	68	S.E.	64	Rain	O
8							62	76	63	,,	63	Clear	O
9							64	76	78	S.	66	Rain	S.
10							66	76	72	,,	66	Clear	O
11							72	61	91	W.	82	,,	O
12	—	—	64	S. Str.	Cloudy	Rain	70	62	69	S.E.	63	Rain	Lt.
13	65	72	67	W. Lt.	Clear	Clear	56	54	60	O	56	Cloudy	O
14	68	80	68	S.W. Lt.	Cloudy	,,	52	62	65	—	57	,,	Lt.
15	68	72	66	S. Lt.	Clear	,,	60	62	65	S.W.	62	Clear	,,
16	67	70	67	,,	,,	,,	58	67	67	S.	64	,,	O
17	68	85	70	W. Lt.	Cloudy	,,	50	67	72	S.W.	62	,,	S.W. Lt.
18	68	87	74	S.E. Lt.	,,	,,	59	64	78	W.	67	,,	W.
19	74	85	68	S. Lt.	Clear	,,	52	64	71	S.W.	65	,,	,,
20	66	65	62	,,	Rain	Cloudy	48	60	69	S.E.	60	,,	O
21	60	63	64	S. Lt.	Clear	Clear	50	70	67	,,	63	Cloudy	S.E. Lt.
22	70	69	62	,,	,,	,,	56	63	67	S.	62	,,	O
23	67	72	64	S. Str.	,,	Rain	62	75	65	,,	62	,,	O
24	70	74	66	O	Rain	Cloudy	66	73	70	,,	63	Clear	O
25	68	67	66	S. Lt.	Clear	Clear	64	81	72	,,	63	,,	O
26	65	67	63	S. Str.	,,	,,	70	71	83	S.E.	71	,,	Lt.
27	68	67	62	,,	,,	,,	70	68	71	S.	73	,,	O
28	70	67	62	S. Mod.	Cloudy;fog	,,	66	67	72	S.E.	64	Cloudy	Lt.
29	67	68	62		Clear	,,	64	66	71	,,	66	,,	,,
30	62	65	63				60		66		66	,,	—
31	67	68	63								64	,,	
Aver.	67·2	71·7	67·2	—	—	—	60·2	66	69·5	—	64·4	—	—

Records kept at Bar Harbour, Belfast, Cornish, Fairfield, Gardiner, Kent's Hill, Lewiston, and Orono, correspond closely with these figures. Unfortunately no records are available of the climate of the backwoods.

Poland Springs, in South Poland, Maine, are among the most famous in the United States. The waters are diuretic, and are indicated in cases of renal calculus, acute and chronic congestion of the kidneys, acute nephritis, acute and chronic hepatic congestion, and catarrhal inflammation of the mucous membrane lining, the biliary passages, or catarrhal jaundice. The good effects of the water are, doubtless, to be attributed largely to the systematic methods adopted, and large quantities in which the waters are taken. The Rangeley Lakes, in South-western Maine are favourite resorts for sportsmen and for summer camps. The prevalent diseases are typhoid, bilious and rheumatic fevers, in summer and autumn, and diseases of the respiratory tract in the winter and spring.

DISCUSSION.

Dr. PHILLIPS : I would like to ask Mr. Hinsdale how his thermometers were exposed and what instruments he used ?

Dr. HINSDALE : The therometer which I had was not exposed in the way in which the Weather Bureau thermometers are supposed to be. I had two, one on the shady side of the house in the morning, and one on the shady side in the afternoon, so that they were under the conditions which would be experienced by persons sitting in the shady sides of the porch either morning or afternoon ; they were not housed in the shelters with open slats as used by the Weather Bureau. The thermometers were mercurial ones, but I cannot say that they were of a standard make.

Dr. PHILLIPS : We get several thousand thermometers a year, and one half of them have to be thrown away because they are two or three degrees out of the way, and I am afraid that is the kind which most amateur observers get hold of. Most people seem to think it is only necessary to get a thermometer and that any kind of instrument will do for the purpose, but our experience is that with anything but properly made thermometers we have decidedly varying results. The Weather Bureau never gets as high temperatures in the summer and never as low ones in the winter as the local thermometers show. We got some record breakers last summer because it was a phenomenal season, but there were many local instruments that gave much higher readings. It is just as important in climatological work to have a good thermometer as it is in clinical thermometry, and I think this Association should insist that those of its members who essay meteorological work should provide themselves with proper instruments. In regard to the question of cyclones, recent investigations have shown that the cyclone is the product of the anti-cyclone and not the reverse as heretofore has usually been supposed.

Dr. GIBSON : What month does this thermometrical work represent ?

Dr. HINSDALE : From July 13 to August 31.

Dr. GIBSON : They are very similar to the records I took in the Adirondacks for about the same period, and I hope at some future time to report the observations I have made in that region. I would like to ask Dr. Phillips if he regards J. Green's thermometers as accurate.

Dr. PHILLIPS : They are the best made, and almost any instrument he sends out can be relied upon.

Dr. OTIS : It does seem as if some of us New England men should say something about our climate, but the fact is that there is so much of it we do not know where to begin. I will make some remarks about the prevailing winds in our locality, and I suppose it applies to other parts of New England. There is a general error, which I fell into myself, in saying that our prevailing winds are easterly, and almost any Boston man would make that statement ; whereas the Weather Bureau has determined that the prevailing wind is from the north-west. It is a fact that as bad as the easterly winds are, they are not the prevailing winds. The cold easterly wind is so keenly felt, however, that their remembrance abides with us so long that we come to consider them more frequent than they really are.

Dr. QUIMBY : What the Doctor has just said leads me to add that the most frequent winds about Hanover, N.Y., where accurate records have been kept at the observatory for thirty years, are south-westerly.

Dr. SOLLY : When considering the influence of wind upon climate it is very important to separate the night winds from the day winds, as they frequently blow from different directions.

Dr. FISK : For the last dozen years I have spent the summers on the Maine coast near Kennebunkport. I have been careful where I go because of my tubercular tendency, and I wish to say that I have a feeling of assurance along the Maine shore, for my tubercular patients do well along this coast, provided they make a good location. There are places that have local disadvantages, such as fogs, that have to be avoided, but my experience is favourable to the Maine coast in general. I wish to call the Society's attention to Prince Edward's Island in the Gulf of St. Lawrence, where hay fever patients frequently find relief. I would like to ask Dr. Phillips whether he notices that his thermometers are influenced by barometric pressure ?

Dr. PHILLIPS : No, sir, a mercurial thermometer will not, under any circumstances, be influenced by barometric pressure. In the case of clinical thermometers such influences may be due to the patient himself.

I would suggest, in view of some observation of my own, that these changes may be due to certain changes of clothing ; for I found that my temperature would fall half a degree readily upon exposure out of doors, and that this fall remained for an hour or more after going into the house, that the fall would be more pronounced the more the wind blew ; that if the wind blew strongly the fall in temperature occurred more rapidly, and also that there was an evident cooling of the entire body brought about on exposure to low temperature. In other words, the body temperature in health is not constant without certain limits, but varies within these limits with variation in the meteorological movements. Mention has been made concerning the winds of New England. Dr. Otis spoke of the prevailing wind as being from the north-west rather than the east. I think if he analyses the winds of this region he will find that there are two prevailing winds, a south-westerly wind in the summer and a north-westerly wind in the winter. The United States, like all countries on large continents, has a monsoon wind, from the ocean to the interior in the summer and from the interior to the ocean in the winter, with periods of shifting or somewhat variable winds between.

Dr. REED : I would like to ask Dr. Hinsdale whether we are to take his remarks about the contest with the Gulf Stream as a joke? My understanding is that the Gulf Stream makes a divergence about the New Jersey coast and does not come anywhere near the coast of Massachusetts.

Dr. BOWDITCH : It is curious to notice the different effect of the southwest wind upon the coast of Maine and upon the southern shores of Massachusetts. Where it comes across the cold currents of water in Maine it is a delicious tonic, but coming across the warmer waters to Massachusetts it is debilitating. I have lived on the coast of Maine much during the last ten or twelve years, and these differences are very noticeable ; I have seen clothes drying in the thin fogs there, while we know that along the coast of Massachusetts boots and shoes will get mouldy in the closets ; a condition which rarely occurs on the Maine coast.

Dr. HINSDALE : Regarding the Adirondacks, I may say that I also kept records there during July and August for a number of years. The average temperature at Lake Placid, elevation 1860 feet, was nearly identical with what I found at Kennebunkport, Maine ; the record at that hour was usually the maximum. There was, however, a much lower minimum in the mountains than at the shore. The last report of the Weather Bureau shows that in Boston the prevailing wind was east only one month during the whole year, and that happened to be, last year, July. In regard to the day and night winds, the general experience on the sea coast is that the wind dies out about 6 o'clock. There is not as much wind on the coast in the evening as there is inland at a higher elevation. As to the Gulf Stream, my quotation from Charles Dudley Warner was used simply as a figure of speech. The centre of the Gulf Stream is about 300 miles from the Massachusetts coast. It is about 300 miles in breadth at that latitude, and its influence is felt, especially during southerly and south easterly winds.

SOME OBSERVATIONS ON SOUTHERN CALIFORNIA.

BY SAMUEL A. FISK, A.M., M.D.

DENVER, COLORADO.

THE State of California, the second in size in the United States, covering 155,980 square miles of territory, is usually subdivided, for convenience sake, into Northern, Central, and Southern California, each portion having its well-defined characteristics not to be confounded with those of the others, any more than one brother should be taken for another, simply because he bears the family name. In Southern California I spent the months of February, March, and April, of this year, and it is of this portion that I want to say a few words in a chatty way.

By Southern California, is usually meant that portion of the State which lies to the south of the Tehachapi Pass, or, roughly speaking, the seven southern counties of Santa Barbara, Ventura, Los Angeles, Orange, San Diego, Riverside, and most of San Bernardino. On the Atlantic Coast, this would reach from a point somewhat south of Cape Hatteras, about to Charleston. Its boundaries, for vacation purposes, are fairly represented by Santa Barbara to the north, San Diego to the south, Redlands to the east, and Catalina Island to the west. Parallel with the coast, but back from it at varying distances, up to ninety miles or so, is the Coast Range, which cuts the sea-coast off from the desert to the east, and at right angles with this range, and running sometimes to the shore, are numberless spurs, making a series of valleys but sparsely inhabited.

While there are characteristics which these places have in common, and which are not, by any means, to be confounded with those of portions of the State, further north, they, nevertheless differ from each other, for in this region we have sea-shore and mountain, low and high altitude, the ocean fog, and the absence of that fog, so that these conditions must constantly be borne in mind.   Here are the well-known places of San Diego, Coronado, Lakeside, Santa Anna, Orange, Los Angeles, Santa Catalina Island, Santa Barbara, Montecito, the Ojai Valley, Nordhoff, Pasadena, San Bernardino, Redlands, Riverside, Mentone, Cotta, Strawberry Valley, &c., while Montery, Santa Cruz, San Jose, San Francisco, lie further to the north, and are in central, rather than in southern California.

It so happened that our journey was made in a snowstorm, and icicles hung to the car windows, and this emphasized to us the fact, that from first to last, we did not see snow in southern California, except occasionally on the distant mountain peaks. The ice on the tables was manufactured, and most of the houses are supplied with " cool rooms," rather than refrigerators.   On the other hand, but little provision is made for fires.   The hotels have steam here and there, to take the chill off the air when necessary, but coal is brought from a distance at a considerable cost, and a few sticks of cotton wood are harboured almost as an Easterner would cherish hickory.   At times a blazing hearth would be cheering, and is welcomed when met.

The foliage, too, struck me as being so different from that to which we are accustomed.   It was the winter season, and the green trees were of the evergreen variety, cypress, palm, pepper, eucalyptus, rarely a pine.   Live oak, magnolia, orange, lemon, and olive, there were, of course, and the groves of these trees, which are on all sides, in this southern country, I saw none of as we went further north.   The elms, maples, oaks, chestnuts, and spruce, were absent, though I did run across some beeches high up in the canons, and now and then I saw a drooping willow.   The mistletoe, in large clusters, usually on some sycamore, was not an unusual sight.

The bird life was novel and interesting. The mocking-bird, singing away from some thick tree or chimney top, the wild canary, the linnet, the quail, and, most of all, the meadow lark, made music. It seemed odd to have the lark pouring forth his melodious strains from the top of a post on the one side, while the surf was breaking on the beach on which we were walking, and the snipe were scurrying before the incoming wave, and all this in early February, where we could see snow on the distant mountains.

And who can speak of this country and neglect to mention the flowers? One thinks of roses blooming on all hands in the open air in mid-winter in California, but he will not soon forget the luxuriant growth of the gold of Ophir roses, trailing over the very roofs of the cottages, or, with his companion, the Cherokee, making an impenetrable hedge for hundreds of feet, nor the paths bordered by marguerites and calla lilies. And as for the orange groves, with their trees weighted down with fruit, and at the same time white with blossoms, and the air heavy with fragrance, the experience is a never-to-be-forgotten one. As one invariably associates some particular brookside with the trout, or Duluth with the planked white fish, or lower Cape Cod with the broiled blue-fish steak, or Digby, Nova Scotia, with fried herring, and each particular food never tastes so good anywhere else, so one can never, I think, wander amongst a grove of orange trees at will, and pick up from under one of them a Washington navel that has just fallen, so ripe that it is thrown down by the wind, as juicy as any water melon, dripping as it is peeled by the fingers (without a knife), and as sweet as sugar, one cannot have such an experience, I think, and not put a pin in it, to fasten it there, and make it one of the events of his life. He may eat the best oranges the market can produce, surrounded by all the comforts and luxuries of club life, spotless table linen, polished china, silver, steel, and glass, noiseless carpets, attentive servants, but he will still sigh for the hillside, the view, the caroling of birds, the breeze, the perfume, the sunshine, the luscious and juicy fruit, and that orange grove.

This country is full of seeming contradictions, and alongside of this cultivation, may be rough fields or tall growths of cacti, or what looks like unproductive land. Acres upon acres of waving grain, bordered by barren fields, or even by marshy lagoons. Like a pretty girl, she pouts and smiles with the same lips, but she is always beautiful. There are the same reds and browns as in the landscape of Colorado, but it is not so rugged, and the effects of rocks and bowlders is lacking. In fact, were a comparison to be made between two things so alike in some respects, and unlike in others, it might be said that Colorado is stimulating, while California (*i.e.*, the southern portion), is soothing. The soil is porous, and dries rapidly, and dust is on the clothes and shoes, and follows the carriage wheels.

The towns are furnished with abundant water supplies of clear mountain water, and the lay of the land makes fine drainage, which, in many instances, is into the ocean. While dryness is the prevailing impression, I recall a wet and nasty day spent in Los Angeles, in the very first of February. I think of down-pourings of rain and puddles at Coronado; at the same time, of wash-outs and delayed trains, &c., but I also think that when the clouds did roll by, and the sun did come out, which was about the middle of the month, it came out to stay, and I cannot recall having to use my umbrella in Southern California after that.

This leads me to speak of the rainy season, for which California is famous, and which, to quote from a writer on Southern California, "Usually begins in November, though slight showers may have occurred in October, and it lasts until about the middle of April."*

From the same writer, a former member of this Association,

---

* In February of this year the rainfall was 4·77 inches as against an average of 2·05 inches, while the four or five seasons preceding were so dry as almost to dry up the orange crops, and in March there were only two cloudy days.

6

William A. Edwards, M.D., in "Two Health Seekers in Southern California," we learn that an average of twenty-four years, puts the total annual rainfall at 10·23 inches, of which 8·75 inches fell in the four months of December, January, February, and March. But then there are the fogs, which come rolling in from the sea in great banks, and may totally obscure the morning sun until late in the day. Sometimes they obscure it all day long. I have frequently seen the trees drip, drip, drip, as though from a shower, and all from a fog or a heavy dew. In the morning the asphalt on the streets is often black as though from a rain, but really due to fog or dew ; and the moon may shine clearly, and the pillars of the veranda be wet from the same cause. One needs wraps at night, and sitting out of doors is almost out of the question. I am speaking now of the sea-shore, and the winter and spring months.

A comparison shows that this climate, which is a dry sea-shore climate, has a high relative humidity, as compared with that of Colorado, and that its absolute humidity is, in the winter and spring months, about two and one half times as great. This is worthy of consideration, especially in relation to pulmonary disease, and personally I should expect better results in persons in the early stage of this trouble, and of recuperative power, in the drier mountainous region, than at the sea level of Southern California, even if the climate is less rigorous than that of most places along the Atlantic sea-board, or vastly drier than Florida, and around the Gulf.

It has been well said, with reference, to quote another subject: "They reckon ill who leave me out," and so the man who leaves out of the consideration of this climate its fogs, which do exist, which are cold and nasty, and depressing to mind and body alike, does not reckon aright. While this is pre-eminently a region of sunshine, one may lose the feeling of buoyancy and exhilaration experienced in the rocky mountains, especially in the early morning, caused by a clear sun, a blue sky, and warm air, all because of the fog. But equality is the keynote to the climate of Southern California. The writer above quoted, says: "There is little seasonal change in the extreme southern part of the State. . . . . We do have cold days. We also have those that are altogether too warm for pleasure and comfort; but we almost never have sufficient cold to injure or kill the most delicate vegetation; nor, on the other hand, is the heat ever prostrating or dangerous to the individual or his animals."

For my own part, I was wont to walk in a golf suit, and frequently the perspiration would stream off me in drops, as on the Maine coast in summer, and I would see shirt waists and fur boas, straw hats and Derbys, in the same crowd. The Marine band from the U. S. S. Iowa, would give open-air concerts in February, and the crowd of several hundreds would sit or stand around, or even lie on the grass, in perfect comfort, and listen to the music for an hour and a half, from 3 to 4.30 in the afternoon. Yet notwithstanding this, it was advisable to have an overcoat at hand, and to be in the house in the evening. This was at sea-level. I found the mountain region somewhat drier, but there, too, the same rule held, though not so forcibly.

The daily motion of wind is slight, and at the sea-shore did not interfere with plans, though higher up in the mountains I experienced several dust storms that would have done credit to a region severely criticised on their account, and a housekeeper at Redlands complained of the difficulty of keeping the house clean.

To sum up, my strongest impression is of sunshine, a dry soil, and mild temperatures. I found this a land of contrasts, novel and interesting, but of contrasts just the same. Orange blossoms and ripe fruit on the same tree. The place, the country, the atmosphere, was pacific and soothing; some found it enervating. People from Colorado came to California for relaxation, while on the other hand, some went from California to Colorado for invigoration. Equally with the surrounding atmosphere, the social tone would vary, from the crowd on pleasure bent, to one of simplicity and refined retirement. One lived in flannels all day long, and fished, hunted, rode horse-back, or played golf; or he sat listlessly around and gaped at the crowd—composed of statesmen, diplomats, admirals, generals, handsomely dressed women, wealthy men—just as the spirit moved. One man remarked: " I thought we had to go to the Riviera to find this."

There seems to be two distinct seasons in the hotel life of California. In the winter comes the tourist from the East; in the summer the migration of the Californian himself; and I am very generally told that the summer is the choice season.

The distance intervening between the Atlantic and the Pacific Oceans seems appalling to many; but some of our best railroads run into Chicago, and from that place to Los Angeles in less than three days, which may be spent in a sump-tuously appointed train that, in elegance and comfort, will bear a favourable comparison with those farther east.

[The discussion of this paper will be found after the fol-lowing paper.]

THE CLIMATE OF SOUTHERN CALIFORNIA.

BY NORMAN BRIDGE, A.M., M.D.

LOS ANGELES, CALIFORNIA.

CLIMATIC conditions are those of the atmosphere we breathe. The atmosphere far above the surface of the earth is substantially the same everywhere, but at the surface it varies somewhat, the variations being determined by the physical conditions that mostly operate locally, and the variations are few in number. I should say that in the study of climate we ought first to consider temperature; second, moisture, including the manifestations of storms and fogs; third, the weight of the air, the barometric pressure determined by altitude, by moisture in the air, and by movements of storms, and, perhaps, by other influences to a slight degree; fourth, the amount of sunshine, which affects the temperature of the air as well as of the earth's surface; and fifth, dissemination of gases, microbes, and dust. The variations are due to the differing physical conditions of different regions, and as physical conditions vary with the parts of the earth's surface, it may be said that there are no two climates exactly alike; it is practically impossible that there should be. The physical features that are the chief factors in determining these elements of climate are altitude of the surface of the earth, latitude, and large bodies of water—oceans, and lakes and rivers. It is substantially impossible that for any two regions of considerable size and extent, these physical features should be identical.

If we study the climate of Southern California on this basis we shall find conditions that I think are somewhat remarkable;

certainly they are unique in the geography of the earth's surface. There is a coast line running in a general direction from north-west to south-east; and back of it, near by, are high mountains. The Pacific Ocean is an enormous body of cold water, there being no warm currents that touch the coast in this region. Here is a range of mountains averaging 5,000 feet elevation, extending in general direction from near the coast easterly; then southerly, leaving between it and the ocean an irregular plateau, varying in width from 2 to 60 miles, and in altitude from sea level up to 1,500 feet elevation at the foot of the mountains. It is this plateau that is inviting as a place of residence for both the sick and well, and it is this that is usually meant whenever the term Southern California is used as a place to live. In latitude the country is only a little north of that of Cairo in Egypt. We rarely consider the far south latitude of the region in our calculations about Southern California. These physical peculiarities inevitably produce certain qualities of climate, and just what they are could have been almost predicted without actual observation of them. It is so far south, that when the sun strikes the earth it heats it remarkably and the air on the surface is warmed, and rises. Other air rushes in to take its place, usually colder air from the ocean; this finds less impediment in such a movement than desert air from north and east of the mountains would. Hence we have an ocean current of air flowing most of the time north-east by day, a large part of the time.

The atmosphere of Southern California is dryer than that of the east, and drier than that of most sea coast countries; it is very much drier north and east of the mountains. The relative humidity is lower much of the time, and the water in the air is actually less. As a result of this fact, as soon as the sun goes out of sight, the radiation from the surface of the earth is so great, that the air stratum above it cools rapidly, especially so on the higher levels; it becomes heavy in consequence, and flows down towards the sea all night. This gives a very curious situation as to regular air currents; the air flows landward all day, and seaward all night, nearly every day of sunshine throughout the year, and the exceptions are due mostly to storm movements of some kind. If it were not for the physical conditions described, this region, so far from being a land of comfort, would be uncomfortable. But the contiguity of high mountains and cold ocean, with a strip of habitable land between—for this latitude, an unique situation—makes it, along the coast, a very comfortable region at all seasons of the year.

There are some drawbacks to continuous comfort in the shape of occasional stiff winds, most in the fall and early winter; and at those points farthest from the sea the temperaure is sometimes disagreeably warm in the middle of the day in summer. The nights are nearly always cool—cool to human sensation even in summer—especially in houses well ventilated in north and south directions. Looking at the map one can readily see the peculiar and providential adjustment of the sea to the mountains, a physical arrangement calculated for the production of a climate that is favourable to man in a most remarkable degree. The air is relatively clean; it comes from over the ocean, the desert, and the mountains, and is uncontaminated by any disease-producing thing.

The physical discomforts incident to living in this region are about twenty-five per cent. of those experienced in the east and middle west. The pleasureableness of the several seasons differs by the estimates of different people; but within twenty miles of the coast a consensus would probably place spring first, autumn last, and summer and winter about equal. Farther inland summer would be put down as least pleasurable.

East of the mountains is a low region, where the surface of the earth is at some points below the level of the ocean. This is the Colorado desert. The desert region is very dry, and in summer very hot and uncomfortable, that people always shun if they can. North-east of the plateau of comfort is another desert, the Mojave, which is always very hot in summer.

Within twenty or thirty miles of the sea coast the summers average very much less disagreeable than they are in the east. Mid-day is liable to be hot, but the heat is tempered by the ocean breeze, and the nights are substantially all cool by the breeze from the mountains.

The rainfall in Southern California is about one-third what it is in the Mississippi Valley and lake regions, and falls mostly in the winter and early spring. There are fogs occasionally in this region, when the atmosphere is for the time saturated with moisture. Most of the time the percentage of moisture in the air is considerably less in this region than it is in the east. It is greater, however, than it is in Arizona, New Mexico, or Utah.

The barometer moves very little. In Los Angeles the range is only one-fourth as much as in Chicago or Buffalo. Just why this is so, is too large a problem to discuss here. The fact is evident, and is probably beneficial to the sick. The temperature of Southern California is higher than that of the Mississippi Valley by an average of 5 to 10 degrees in summer, and by 20 to 30 degrees in winter; and yet the relative humidity is so low that the sensible temperature is $7\frac{1}{2}$ degrees less than it is in the Mississippi Valley and east of it. With an actual summer temperature of 5 to 10 degrees higher than in Chicago, the sensible temperature is $7\frac{1}{2}$ degrees lower; that is, the sensibility of the human body to the presence of heat shows it to be less by that measure. In the regions east of the Rocky Mountains the temperature averages in summer 55 to 75 degrees F.; west of and including that mountain range, it is 50 to 65 degrees.* The rule is that relatively the temperature is high in the sunshine, and low in shadow, and at night, by reason of the rapid radiation of heat from the earth due to low

---

* These figures are taken from the publications of the Weather Bureau, and represent a method of calculation that has, I learn, been abandoned as being subject to some inaccuracy. But as to the figures here given, I believe they correspond with the experience of people so far as they are able to state their physical experiences in figures.

humidity. Whenever you find low humidity there is a rapid change of temperature when the sun goes out of sight. The amount of water in the air is so small, that the stars at night are seen perceptibly more clearly than in the east, where the humidity is greater. The dryer air has more the quality of diathermancy.*

A subject of endless debate and confusion is the fogs of Southern California. These seem to flow in from the ocean in the night or early morning after a warm day; they can be seen to travel landward, so people naturally guess that the ocean has something to do with them. It does have, but the fog is not from the ocean; rather, the cold air from the sea lowers the temperature of the warmer and moister land air, till saturtion point is reached, and a fog results; but at the instant of precipitation there is less moisture present than there was five minutes before. Before the fog the warm air contains, say, four grains of water to the cubic foot; the cold sea air holds, perhaps, three-and-a-half grains, while at the instant the fog appears there is from the mixture of the two, not more than three and three-quarters grains to the cubic foot, less by one-fourth grain than the clear air held at first. As soon as the sun comes up and warms the earth and air the fog disappears by being dissolved again, to become the invisible moisture of the atmosphere.

The table here presented, shows at a glance the relative temperature, humidity, cloudiness, rainfall, and barometer range for the south-west region in comparison with Denver and Chicago, which cities may, as to climate, be regarded as

---

* Diathermancy of the air at Sierra Madre (16 miles north of Los Angeles) in summer. Average of repeated observations. Observations made early in the afternoon.

Elevation above sea level	Difference between temperature in the shade and in the sun, standard thermometer, average :	Difference as shown by black bulb thermometer incased in long test-tube, corked, average :	Highest point registered by black bulb thermometer, average :
1,250 feet.	33° F.	74·5° F.	162·5° F.

(Paper by the Author, *Transactions Association of American Physicians,* 1891.

typical respectively of the highest altitudes in the dry belt
and of the moister regions east of them.

TABLE.

	Mean Summer Temperature—F.	Mean Winter Temperature—F.	Humidity—relative. Mean percentage of saturation	Humidity — actual. Grains water to cubic foot of air	Cloudiness — percentage of by day	Rainfall — inches per annum	Barometer range, in fractions of an inch—average
Chicago	68	22	72	2.80	51	38	·565
Denver	69	29	53	2.14	38	15	·395
Prescott	70	37	74	2.20	24	14	—
Yuma	90	55	46	4.12	17	2	·264
Los Angeles	69	54	66	4.00	34	15	·142
San Diego	68	54	69	4.19	42	10	·174
Eastern Foothills: (Redlands, Riverside, San Bernardino)	75·3	54·7	64·4	—	28·9	15	—
Western Foothills: (Sierra Madre, Pasadena) ...	71	52·6	65	—	30	16	·300

The influence of the climate of Southern California on the
health of people coming to it, is both potent and peculiar. It
is a paradise of the aged and of children. Old people
pass and piece out happy lives because of the relief from
extremes of weather. . Children are singularly free from mortal
diseases peculiar to them; they have fewer such than in any
place I have ever known; especially is this true of the bowel
troubles incident to the sumer season.

The great majority of invalids that go to Southern California
are of the tuberculous class. They recover in encouraging
numbers, in such proportion indeed, that it is a strong argument
against the theory that high altitudes are of any indispensible
value for this disease. Altitude improves nutrition sometimes
by increasing the number of red blood corpuscles, and perhaps
otherwise also; but experience with the surgical treatment of
lung tuberculosis, and I believe the medical treatment as well,
has shown that the intense expansion of the lungs in these cases
is detrimental rather than otherwise. Altitude can do no sub-
stantial good in this way.

The experience of Southern California in tuberculosis also supports the contention that intense dryness of atmosphere is not so important as it has been thought. Of course, relatively, Southern California is more dry than the eastern regions of the United States, but it is not nearly as dry as Arizona. In Arizona patients who had expectorated much fluid sputum, experience a lessening of this symptom, but I am not sure of any proof that the tuberculosis fails to travel on, much the same as when the expectoration is more fluid. Absence of cough, however, means more stillness of the diseased lung, which is a positive benefit. Another advantage of Arizona climate is the fewness of stormy days that keep patients indoors; but I have known of many recoveries directly on the sea coast where the humidity is not low. The quality of climate that pre-eminently is needed for tuberculosis is such as enables patients to live practically out of doors much of the time day and night. This, I am sure, is a correct theory, and Southern California fulfils the conditions in a large measure.

Many patients come to the south-west with chronic bronchitis, catarrh, and asthma. Those with chronic bronchitis do well; many with catarrhs of the throat improve, and some with beginning deafness improve greatly. Some of the cases of pure nasal catarrh do not improve, but these cases are harmless anyway, and portend no harm; and we ought to be chagrined at ourselves for having allowed the public to make such a bugbear of them for so long, as we ought to be ashamed of ourselves for having tinkered them locally so much. Asthma is always an interesting study in California, because some cases improve markedly in one region, and only a few miles distant do badly. Some of these, if they stay near the mountains, are free from their wheezing. They can go down towards the sea during the day with impunity, but they must get home before darkness, or be seized with a paroxysm of wheezing.

Quite a number of patients have come for relief from chronic rheumatoid troubles, and nearly all have recovered or improved.

There is frequent complaint among newcomers of neuralgic or myalgic pains. ' Such patients must learn to clothe themselves properly nights and during the cloudy part of the day; the pains often result from lack of clothes. This trouble is frequently called rheumatism. It is not rheumatism, and it does no particular harm, but it is disagreeable. The rest of the world seems determined to make the great mistake of supposing that Southern California is a tropical country where one may always go thinly clad.

I have never been able to identify a case of thermic fever, otherwise, sunstroke. I have known of numerous cases of persons somewhat overcome by heat, but they never have elevation of temperature, and the symptoms that go with what we call thermic fever, and they never die. Hydrophobia is almost unknown, though one case did occur last year in Pasadena. Another curious fact is the relative absence of ordinary lobar pneumonia among the resident population. I have lived in Southern California three-fourths of the time for ten years, have seen a great number of patients with all sorts of pulmonary troubles, including catarrhal pneumonia, but these were substantially all tuberculous in origin. Only a possible two cases have been true lobar pneumonia, and they were in people just arrived from the east.

DISCUSSION.

Dr. SHURLEY: I would like to ask Dr. Bridge if those two cases of lobar pneumonia originated at Los Angeles?

Dr. BRIDGE: One was a woman who was attacked by the disease before leaving Chicago, and the other was a man who had come from Massachusetts, stopped for a few days at Colorado Springs, and developed his fever four or five days after arrival at Pasadena.

Dr. PHILLIPS: I am very much interested in the question of sensible temperature. Some years ago I presented a paper before this Association on this subject, in which I endeavoured to consider what we knew of sensible temperature, and I came to the conclusion that we knew nothing at all about it. I know that the wet bulb thermometer has been used extensively in the west, and that, by some accident, this method was adopted by some one as giving a standard of sensible temperature. I think Professor Harrington, perhaps, proposed this standard and for a while the Weather Bureau lent countenance and aid to it, but after a somewhat awkward experience the Bureau decided to abandon the wet bulb thermometer as an index of sensible temperature.

The PRESIDENT : I presume the gentlemen from Colorado are reserving their ammunition for discussion of the home treatment of tuberculosis, and yet Dr. Bridge has shaken the red rag in the face of the bull.

Dr. HART : I want to ask Dr. Bridge whether the patient who stopped in Colorado Springs was supposed to have developed his trouble while there, because recently I had a case of the same kind in a patient who came from Pasadena to Colorado Springs ?

Dr. BRANNAN : As comparing the two climates I remember particularly the members of one family living in Southern California that came regularly every year to visit Colorado Springs, and believed they derived great benefit from the altitudes. I also remember that during my four years' residence there we had cases that were not doing particularly well, perhaps, in Colorado, and decided to try California, but my recollection is that the majority of them came back worse than when they left. The impression I gained was that if you were going to try the two climates it was well to go to California first and then Colorado. That was sixteen or seventeen years ago and my memory may be at fault, but the impression remains with me that the climate of California, after having experienced that of Colorado, is debilitating to patients, and is rather a dangerous thing to try.

Dr. SOLLY : The gentlemen from Colorado seem to be struck with a modesty that I had never noticed about them when they were at home. I do not think there can be any contest between California and Colorado, as one is the complement of the other. The only grievance I have against California is her pretence to dryness in a strict sense of the word. It is dry in the middle of the day, but seldom dry in the morning and evening. As to the value of the climate as compared to Colorado I think they apply to different cases, except that both apply to early cases of tuberculosis. The great advantage of California for such early cases is that they can live out of doors as they do in Colorado, and in both they get a large amount of sunshine and fresh air and can live out of doors both day and night. I saw a photograph of a physician's house in Pasadena, and the doctor lives and sleeps in his room without any windows in the frames. We have the same conditions prevailing in Colorado, but the effect upon serious cases of tuberculosis may be very different in the two places, and this depends very much upon the nervous system ; some cases are benefited by sedative climates while some require stimulating ones. Patients with chronic fibroid conditions, after the disease has been arrested, often do better in Southern California than they do with us, and for persons in good health who are overworked, tired out, I do not know anything better than to go to Southern California.

Dr. REED : It seems to me there is more contest between the advocates of the different climates for tuberculosis than there should be, and we overlook too much the fact that the great advantage is to be found in the life out of doors in the sunshine in almost any climate. The amount of oxygen to be taken in is of more importance than the degree of dryness. It is unfortunate that we can not have a completely unbiassed report on the climates of different places. Most of us have been living at health resorts and are naturally more or less biassed by that fact. It seems to me that this Society might well appoint a committee from among members not residents of climatic resorts to investigate and make a report after a year or two on the comparative merits of the principal localities recommended as climates for tubercular cases.

Dr. EDSON : I think the question that has come up without being definitely raised, concerns particularly the relation of climate to altitude. There are many patients who, even with dry air and sunshine, do not thrive at a high altitude because of embarrassed respiration, but do well in lower altitudes. In my own experience I meet with such patients constantly, patients that do not thrive well at Denver, but who improve in the lower altitudes, and Dr. Bridge has received some of these.

Dr. THOMAS W. HARVEY : Perhaps you will allow one who has to act mostly as a guide book in these climatic matters to give the impression he gets from patients that come back from different parts of the country. We find that it is not only a question of climate but also of the patient. If we could read our patients better, and sum up the factors that make up his illness perhaps we could better choose the resort for him, and if we could have before us with more detail the conditions of these varying climates, so that we could put each patient in the right place, we could get along very much better. It would be very nice if these gentlemen at the health resorts, in sending our patients back to us, would tell us why there seems to be a difference between the climate there and that which the patient needs. Another thing that might be considered in this matter is the question of progressive change. To take a patient immediately from an altitude of say 500 feet to one of 5,000 feet may cause a good bit of suffering at first, and I have been in the habit lately of advising a gradual change. I send them to Colorado by way of the lower altitudes of New Mexico and Arizona.

Dr. MINOR : I think there is a great mistake made by many doctors who send their patients away for their health in supposing that the very fact of going to a climatic resort insures their having the conditions the doctor desires for them. Patients going to a resort and living, as so many do, in their own way without any attention to detail of any kind will natur-ally not get the desired results, and will come home disappointed and to disappoint the doctor who sent them. The home doctor has a right to ask of the resort doctor to whom he should refer his patient, unless he expects him to be turned over to his own tender mercies and care for himself, a careful watching of the case and a faithful study of local conditions, so that the home doctor can with some reasonable certainly know what he can expect for his patient. But even with such data, which it is the duty of resort physicians to collect and publish for the benefit of the rest of the profession, the suitability of any special locality to a given case will always be a matter of experiment by the local man who watches the case for the home doctor, and a month and often more are needed to decide whether the special place suits the case. It is only as we get the co-operation of these two men, an unprejudiced study and report of the progress of the case by the resort doctor, and a willingness on the part of the home doctor to trust this man with his patient, and let him do what is best under local conditions that we shall get the best results. Yet a great many good men give their patients the idea that the curative power of climate is so marvellous that the simple going to some resort without any local supervision, and while living just such a life as they live at home will suffice to restore them to health. This can only result in disappointing the patient, and in giving the home doctor a false idea of the possibilities of climatic cure, which, like all other remedies, must be intelligently used to yield results.

Dr. BONNEY : It seems to me the gist of the whole matter is that there is no one type of climate applicable to all cases of tuberculosis. The gentlemen of Colorado wish to acquiesce in the statement that California exercises a very beneficial influence over certain cases of tuberculosis. Now, I have been sending quite a number of cases to California, cases that had a great deal of bronchial disturbance, cases of emphysema, cases with certain forms of heart, kidney, or rheumatic troubles, and I have been very much pleased with the results. There is a prevailing opinion I find among physicians and patients that nervous patients do not do well in Colorado. These patients come with the idea that they will not sleep and that their neurasthenia will be aggravated, and with that idea once in their heads it is a difficult thing to get it out. I do not think it is a question of altitude at all, but one of environment and of personal attention to detail. I fail to find after a considerable experience that nervous cases are at all aggravated in Colorado. One of the gentlemen spoke of the ill results that happen from sending consumptives to high altitudes suddenly. The only cases that I have been able to assure myself are injured by such a trip are those that have had hæmorrhages before starting. They come to Colorado in a hurry, perhaps bleed on the train, and that class of cases does not do well to come so quickly.

Dr. FISK : It may seem singular that a Colorado man should write up Southern California, but having spent three months there this winter, and never having been there before I was curious to see what the effects would be, and to study my results. I was sent to Colorado many years ago by Dr. F. I. Knight, and he has often met me on the street since and remarked, " Who would ever think, Fisk, that I sent you to Colorado to die ? " I believe I am loyal to Colorado, and I think that incipient consumption does better in that State than anywhere else. I think the climate there is stimulating, while that of Southern California is soothing ; some find it enervating. The relative humidity, as compared with Colorado, is about twice as great

and there is a fog, there is no use denying it, and a fog is a fog, no matter
where you meet it. I have been on the coast of Massachusetts, in the
Berkshire hills, have lived for years in Colorado, and have spent some
months in Southern California, and I find a fog is a fog in all of these
places. We had some of it here last night, and the dampness affected me
so that I wondered whether I could continue at this meeting. I find that
consumptives are affected by dampness in all of these places. You can
theorise upon it as much as you please ; Colorado has its inhabitants by the
tens of thousands that have gone there, like myself, and are living and doing
the work of life there. Most of us Colorado men here are men that went
to that State because we were obliged to go on account of some trouble
inside our chests. At the same time there is no reason why we should not
favour the climate of Southern California. " There is one glory of the sun,
and another glory of the moon, and another glory of the stars, for one star
differeth from another star in glory."

Dr. BRIDGE : I wish to thank Dr. Phillips for having corrected me as to
the value to be placed upon the former records of his own department of
the Government. I used them because I thought everything that came from
that department was correct. I suspect I should have had some misgivings
about it had it not come from that office, but I was rather of the belief that
I could confirm its correctness by my own feelings and those of many people
I had known. I fear some of the gentlemen have included me with the
health resort doctors. As far as I am myself concerned I wish to be considered as a plain, common doctor, and I am interested in any good climate
that helps the sick. I believe in the climate of California or I should not
have joined with some gentlemen in putting money into the establishment
of a sanatorium for the treatment of tuberculosis. I cannot agree that the
climate of Southern California back from the coast has the qualities that
usually produce enervation. I have never experienced it, and most of the
people I have known as patients have not. I do not think that it is harmful
to send patients with incipient tuberculosis from one climate or altitude to
another. I have repeatedly seen them go from one to the other without
harm that I could say was due to the change. My own advice has been to
many patients from the east to stop in Colorado and see if that agrees with
them, and if it does not to come on to New Mexico, Arizona or Southern
California. Some of the patients have not done well in Colorado and have
gone to Phœnix or to Southern California, and some have reversed the
order, and have obtained more benefit in the later place than the other. I
have endeavoured to state the exact facts about Southern California in this
paper, and had not the least idea of enticing sick people to go there. I
would not do that by the slightest colouring of the facts.

THE INFLUENCE OF THE COLORADO CLIMATE UPON PULMONARY HÆMORRHAGES.

S. G. BONNEY, A.M., M.D.

DENVER, COLORADO.

A COMPLETE discussion of this subject should include the preliminary introduction of certain physiological considerations, followed by the collaboration *en masse* of clinical facts.

The physiological interest centres chiefly in the respiratory and circulatory changes produced by the diminished barometric pressure. Relative to this in health, much valuable information has already been advanced. It seems sufficient for present purposes, to call attention briefly to the increase in the depth and frequency of the respirations, and in the rate and vigour of the heart contractions. From this there results a considerable degree of vesicle dilation, increased chest expansion, greater lung capacity, together with an acceleration of the blood flow, and an equalising of the circulation throughout the body. The tendency to local stasis or capillary congestion in the lungs is thus avoided. The peculiar changes in the blood itself incident to the altitude, consist in an increase of the hæmoglobin, and in the number of red blood cells.

It is reasonable to suppose by virtue of these influences, that the tendency to pulmonary hæmorrhage in high altitudes should be distinctly lessened in cases judiciously selected with reference to other considerations. It remains for the correctness of this to be demonstrated ultimately by the established facts of clinical experience, and such shall be the scope of this paper.

In presenting the results of my personal observations, it

is my desire to refute any prevailing opinion that elevated regions are unsuited for hæmorrhages in general. It is my conviction, however, that hæmorrhages *per se*, constitute neither an indication nor a contraindication for moderate altitudes. The hæmorrhage, let it be remembered, is but one of many outward manifestations of the disease, occurring at any stage of the infectious process, due to a variety of causes, with widely differing pathological conditions, associated with all manner of concomitant symptoms, and representing but a single component and perhaps unimportant part of the clinical picture as a whole.

While it will be seen that hæmorrhage cases with certain modifications have done exceedingly well in Colorado, it is insisted, nevertheless, that the choice of climate must be made with reference to *all* the several phases and conditions, without especial attention to hæmorrhage itself, save under the specific circumstances to be hereinafter described.

My observations are derived from my private work in Colorado during a residence of nine years. I have selected from my list of recorded patients a series of 900 cases seriatim, who may be said to fairly represent the character of cases sent to Colorado taken as they come, and who have remained sufficiently long under observation to permit at least approximate conclusions.

I make no effort at this time to classify the cases with reference to physical conditions and prognosis at time of arrival, as such distinctions do not appear pertinent to this inquiry. It should be said, however, that the very incipient cases were but seldom observed, and that the great majority belonged to the category of advanced infection. The patients required no admission blanks to gain entrance to Colorado, and many are thus included with a prognosis utterly hopeless from the beginning. I have thought it best to embrace even these in the list, in order to secure an authentic and established basis upon which to compute further statistics. As briefly illustrative of the general character of the cases, I will refer to one of my previous papers,* in which it is stated that "out of 546 cases 71 per cent. of the patients arrived in the State with distinct evidence of tubercular infection in each lung, and with a total average period of delay following the definite onset of the disease before arrival of over eighteen months, affording abundant opportunity for advanced pulmonary and constitutional impairment."

With many of the cases it has been possible to maintain for prolonged periods, a strict supervision of daily life and habits, fully equal to that observed in any well-regulated sanatorium. A suitable *regime* has been quite as closely adhered to here as is possible in the latter institutions, but a tremendous handicap has been experienced from the advanced nature of the cases as a class. A very large number of the list, however, despite extensive infection and doubtful or grave prognosis, I have not been permitted to observe under the best conditions of life or management, on account of peculiarity of temperament, habits of dissipation, domestic relations, and financial distress. Many have been compelled to practise the strictest economy, others to work daily. Some have been burdened with family responsibilities, and still others have indulged in the most reckless dissipation. It is apparent that this series as a whole comprises an exceedingly heterogeneous class, and differs widely from the selected cases representative of sanatorium results. The cases have been conscientiously recorded, and the computation of the following statistics has been conducted personally, and with as much care and pain as possible. With reference to results obtained, I have made two broad classifications, *i.e.*, those who have shown improvement in Colorado, and those who have grown worse or died. By improvement, I refer to a material lessening of the activity of the tubercular process as disclosed by physical

* "Observations upon Pulmonary Tuberculosis in Colorado," *Boston Med. and Surg. Journal*, Sept. 16, 1897.

signs, diminution of cough and expectoration, also of pulse and temperature, increase of appetite, digestion and weight. It is hardly necessary here to further classify the various stages of arrest. I am frank to admit that I am reporting as improved several who are now dead, but had exhibited a progressive and material gain until suddenly overcome by intercurrent disease, accident, or other extraneous and direct causes. On the other hand, several are reported as not improved, whose loss following an initial gain, is easily attributed to a return east, resumption of work, disobedience of instructions, or other indiscretions. In a work of this kind it is recognised that everything depends upon the integrity and authenticity of reports, and I have thus endeavoured as far as possible to eliminate sources of error.

Number of cases improved 618
Number grown worse or dead 284
Percentage of cases improved ... ... 68·5

Generally speaking, over two-thirds of the cases coming to Colorado, independent of the question of hæmorrhage, but in all stages of advanced infection, may be expected to gain. This is certainly a very large proportion in view of the indiscriminate character of the cases, but furnishes a basis from which to draw further conclusions relative to hæmorrhage. Four hundred and fifty-seven cases are found to have had a hæmorrhage at some time during the course of the disease; of these 308, or 67·8 per cent., are reported as improved. It then appears that about one half of the entire number are hæmorrhagic cases, and approximately the same proportion have improved in Colorado as the non-hæmorrhagic, each class having about the same per cent. of improvement as the entire list. This comparison in itself fails to indicate any specific influence of the climate upon hæmorrhage cases in general. Much of interest and value attaches to the time of hæmorrhage relative to residence in Colorado. One hundred and seventy-five cases present the history of hæmorrhage as the first symptom distinctly referable to the disease, or as supervening immediately upon appearance of cough and beginning loss of weight. Thus about 20 per cent. of all the cases of consumption are found to experience a hæmorrhagic onset of the affection. In these the bleeding almost necessarily took place before the development of any very extensive destructive change in the lung. These cases have usually sought climatic relief early, and it is in precisely such conditions that an equalising of the circulation by high altitude should be attended by the best results. It is not surprising therefore to find that 127, or over 72 per cent., have done well. Three hundred and eighty-six, or over 82 per cent. of the hæmorrhage cases occurred before arrival in the State, including those with hæmorrhagic onset. Of these 253 are reported as improved, establishing a per cent. of 65½, which is quite up to previous standards.

Of the 386 with hæmorrhage before arrival, only 97, or 1 in 4, have suffered subsequent recurrence in Colorado. Among those who did experience a recurrence, but 59 are found to have done well, effecting a percentage of 60. On the other hand, out of 289 with previous hæmorrhage and no recurrence, 201, or 70 per cent., have shown improvement. The logical deduction is, that among the comparatively small number who do have a recurrence in Colorado of their previous hæmorrhage, the chances for recovery are somewhat below the average, while those who do not experience such a return are correspondingly favoured with better than average prospects. It must be remembered that among these with previous hæmorrhage and subsequent recurrence, many are included who had a distinct hæmorrhagic onset, and although without extensive destruction of lung tissue, had experienced, nevertheless, a considerable circulatory disturbance from slight causes, and who might well be expected early upon arrival, with the usual nervous temperament and erethetic habit usually common to such cases, to suffer a temporary return.

It is further of interest to note, that of the 97 recurrences,

34 were in individuals who had experienced a hæmorrhage within two or three weeks before arrival, and in whom it is reasonable to suppose the direct results had not been fully overcome. In fact, nearly half of those had their hæmorrhage on the train or at the time of starting ; 22 of the recurrent hæmorrhages in Colorado were in these people in whom the bleeding took place immediately before arrival, and the recurrence within a very few days thereafter. It is obvious that such cases should not be embraced among hæmorrhages in Colorado as the specific cause was put in operation before arrival. Should these be excluded, and rightly so, the percentage of recurrences in Colorado would be materially diminished. On the other hand, 47 cases are found to have bled more or less profusely, and often repeatedly so, within one or two weeks before arrival, yet have not suffered a return since residing in the higher altitudes ; 71 experienced their last hæmorrhage in Colorado. Of these, 33, or 46·4, have done well. An explanation of the small percentage of improvement is found in the fact that 40 of these were associated with very extensive and advanced infection, such conditions being present as would be likely to occasion hæmorrhage anywhere. Thirty-one took place in the midst of a general gain, but in these, without exception, a distinct external cause could be assigned, and usually improvement was later continued.

Taken altogether, including the initial and the recurrent hæmorrhages ; 168 have bled in Colorado ; 68 very shortly after arrival, usually preceded by others immediately before coming. Of the remaining 100 cases, 48 are found to have occurred as a result of accident or great indiscretion. The great majority of the balance—52—took place in the midst of a general decline, associated with more or less extensive cavity formation, syphilis, or kidney disease, entailing a poor prognosis in any locality.

Of the 168 cases, there were 58 easily recognised cavities, nearly one-third of the whole number arriving as advanced cases, and usually with a history of a previous attack.

The character of the hæmorrhage has been severe and copious in 65 instances; moderate in 103. As a general rule, they are stated to have been considerably more severe and harder to control than any previous attack at or near sea-level. Four have been instantly fatal. In 13 death has resulted in a very few days; 21 have survived but one or two weeks. The remainder rallied sufficiently to continue the struggle, only finally in some instances to succumb as a remote result of the loss entailed by the hæmorrhage. Many have suffered no permanent ill effects, often rallying from the very alarming attacks, and some have exhibited most remarkable improvement following it. Of the latter class 14 are conspicuous examples. My conclusions are:

(1) That hæmorrhage by itself, save with few exceptions, furnishes no criterion upon which to base a choice of climate, the indications for high altitude in complicated, and in not too far advanced cases being highly imperative, independent of this single manifestation.

(2) That an exceedingly small proportion of recurrences may be expected in Colorado, although not necessarily reflecting accurately the degree of ultimate improvement secured.

(3) That recurrences are more likely to result, and that quickly, in those cases with hæmorrhage immediately preceding arrival, and hence the wisdom of a short delay following the hæmorrhage before leaving home, and unusual precautions as regards rest upon arrival.

(4) That primary hæmorrhages are comparatively rare in Colorado, and usually take place incident to a rapid progressive destructive change in cases already with hopeless prognosis, or as a natural result of some external assignable cause, which under proper *regime* could be avoided.

(5) That hæmorrhage while less likely to occur in Colorado than at sea-level, is, nevertheless, as a general rule, more severe, and associated with greater shock.

(6) That the avoidance of hæmorrhage, particularly in the

early months of Colorado life, demands a most rigid compliance
with detailed instructions.

DISCUSSION.

Dr. SOLLY: I agree with Dr. Bonney's results generally that hæmorrhage is not a counter-indication to high altitudes, and that such cases do
not do worse there than elsewhere ; but I think that after hæmorrhage
pneumonia results more frequently in Colorado than elsewhere. I have
thought of analysing some cases with a view of ascertaining that, although
it would be difficult to compare them with cases in the east. Our cavity
cases that ultimately die live longer than they do in the east, and during
that time it is probable that there comes an aneurismal condition of the
arteries in the cavities, and we get sudden and unexpected hæmorrhages in
the cavity cases in Colorado; I think in the advanced cavity cases hæmorrhage is more frequently the termination than it is elsewhere. I was
called once down to La Honda to see a man apparently dying from profuse
hæmorrhage. He was returning from a visit to Boston back to New
Mexico, where he had lived for a while and had been taken from the train
the night before. In three days I moved him up to Colorado, where he got
entirely over his hæmorrhages and is living to-day in Silver City, New
Mexico. He had a large cavity, but his general condition was good. In
another case I was called to Kansas City, Missouri, to see an old patient,
a man who had returned to Boston for a brief visit. He was taken with
a violent hæmorrhage on the 'train as he approached Kansas City and I
found him very weak. In three or four days I took him back to Colorado.
He had a large cavity with fibrosis, but he got well and is now living in
New Mexico. So it is not always the advanced cases that come to
Colorado with hæmorrhage that will die from them.

. Dr. BALDWIN: I would like to ask Dr. Bonney if he has made any
notes in regard to the hæmorrhages as to whether they occured more frequently at one season of the year than another? One recent writer on
that subject discovered more hæmorrhages in the spring and in August,
and at Saranac we have noticed it more frequently about the month of
March. I was very glad to hear this paper, which illustrates how fallacies
may be destroyed little by little. I have always felt that it was a mistake
to suppose that a medium high elevation was a counter-indication for
hæmorrhagic cases, and Dr. Bonney has proved that bleeding is no more
frequent in Denver, with its high altitude, than it is in Saranac with an
altitude of only 1,600 feet.

Dr. MINOR: I, also, want to thank Dr. Bonney for putting out knowledge of this subject on a firm basis. I believe the mistake originated in
England, and was simply a result of theorising on known effect upon the

heart-rate of going to high elevations. Speaking for my elevation of 2,200 feet, I have observed very similar results.

Dr. FISK : Dr. Bonney's experience coincides with my own. Years ago, back in the early eighties, Dr. Jacob Reed, of Colorado Springs, a keen observer and a man of large experience, reported to the State Medical Society of Colorado, a collation of his cases, from which he drew the same conclusions which Dr. Bonney has reached, that altitude was not a contra-indication for hæmorrhagic cases. In 1898 I collated some cases from which I arrived at the same conclusion, and I think Dr. Solly has confirmed it. I have not regarded the presence of hæmorrhage as necessarily an element of unfavourable prognosis. Cases where hæmorrhages have not occurred at all, have, in my experience, done quite as badly as those with hæmorrhage. In reference to the question Dr. Baldwin asked, my experience has been decidedly in favour of what is known as the "spring thaw," at which time hæmorrhage is more apt to occur in Colorado.

Dr. SOLLY : The opening of spring seems to have the same effect in Switzerland.

Dr. CURTIN : In 1889 I read a paper on hæmoptysis in chronic lung diseases, in which I expressed the belief that with care, altitude was no contraindication in hæmorrhagic cases. The subject was discussed at the time pretty thoroughly by the Society and the general impression was in accordance with the view I have expressed. Since that time I have sent a number of hæmorrhagic cases to elevated resorts in the United States. All have been benefited, and some have come back apparently cured; none of them died.

Dr. MCGAHAN : I beg to state that about fourteen years ago I noticed that more hæmorrhages occurred in the spring of the year than at any other time. I tried to determine whether atmospheric pressure had any effect upon producing them, and I consequently observed the barometer very carefully, and found I was unable to lay any connection between them. When I was at Cœrbersdorf I saw the observatory which Brehmer had erected to test this question, but he was unable to decide that they had any bearing upon each other.

Dr. EDSON : I would add a brief clinical note in regard to the pulmonary hæmorrhagic cases at Colorado. I think the amount of blood lost is not usually accurately measured. I had this spring a young man, aged 20, with very marked lung conditions, who had come to Colorado five months previously after having had several hæmorrhages. He had some spitting of blood for a few days afterwards, but gained weight though he was running a temperature. He began to have hæmorrhages again, and at the end of the third day had reached such a condition that he had to be placed in the charge of a trained nurse who measured the amount of blood lost. During the first few days the hæmorrhage measured from 3 to 4 ozs. each time, and the total on the three last days was 20, 21 and nearly 23 ozs. He was absolutely blanched at this time, unable to talk or make signs, but after the last hæmorrhage referred to had no more spitting of blood. He recovered sufficiently to sit up in bed, but died five weeks later of acute disseminated tuberculosis. It is my only experience of having actually measured the amount of blood lost.

Dr. NEWTON : I spat blood myself in Colorado and never had anything at all the matter with my lungs. I should think that if a healthy man may spit blood after going up into the mountains, it is a matter for consumptives to carefully guard against.

Dr. HARVEY : I have had the experience three times in three years of spitting blood on going down to Kansas City, but I do not know that it was the result of going into a low latitude.

Dr. BONNEY : As I intimated in my paper I think it is the cases that bleed immediately before arrival that occasion the rather alarming frequency of hæmorrhages in Colorado. I have been impressed by the comparatively large number that bled on the train just before arrival. I have noticed that there are more hæmorrhages occurring in the spring than at any other time, but these hæmorrhages have been usually slight ones, more of an oozing than an aneurismal hæmorrhage, and I have attributed this to the winds and dust. During the summer in Colorado, patients in the mountains do very much better than all the rest of the time put together. When they return to Denver and get the wind and dust they have more or less bronchial irritation, and hæmorrhages may occur. I have been so impressed with this fact that I have been sending sixty to seventy-five patients during this period to an altitude of 7,500 feet, and I have not had a hæmorrhage occur at that place. They are twenty-five miles from a railroad or telegraph station, and I recognise the responsibility of sending a patient to that sort of place.

THE BLOOD COUNTS IN HIGH ALTITUDES.

BY W. A. CAMPBELL, M.D.; ASSISTED BY H. W. HOAGLAND, M.D.

COLORADO SPRINGS, COLORADO.

THE study of the blood and its changes are extremely interesting. You will pardon the writer for again calling your attention to its consideration. We were made familiar with the number, size, colour, shape, and physiological functions of the red blood corpuscles twenty-five or more years ago, in the beginning of our medical reading. Renewed interest has been taken in the study of the blood in recent years. Now the hæmatologist would have us look to him for the diagnosis of many diseases; and as general practitioners we are glad to seek his aid where formerly we were content to rely upon physical examinations.

We wish to present but one phase of the subject of the blood to-day, viz., that of the red corpuscle count in high altitudes. A number of years ago Paul Bert called the attention of the profession to the discovery he made, that the number of red corpuscles was increased in high altitudes. Since he announced his discovery many physiologists and scientists have confirmed it. The object of our paper to-day is not to add another confirmation to those of other observers, but to give a few investigations that we have made as to the permanency and transitory phases of this increase. For convenience of consideration we will divide the subject into two divisions, viz., those who have lived for some time at a high altitude, and those who go for only a few hours.

The question of an increased blood count in residents of

high altitudes may be considered as conceded. Prominent among those who have made this subject a study, we find the names of Viault, Egger, Wolf, Herrera, Lope, Solly, and others. The following table compiled by Herrera and Lope from data of many observers, will show the gradual increase in the blood count as we ascend in altitude.

At Christiana ...	...	... sea level ...	... (Iaoche) ...	... 4,970,000
,, Paris ...	...	... 78 metres	... (Hayem) ...	... 5,000,000
,, Gottingen ...	...	... 148 ,,	... (Schaper) ...	... 5,225,000
,, Tubeingen ...	...	... 314 ,,	... (Reinert) ...	... 5,322,000
,, Zurich ...	...	... 412 ,,	... (Stierlin) ...	... 5,752,000
,, Anerback ...	...	400 to 450 ,,	... (Wolf & Koppe)	... 5,748,000
,, Reiboldogrun	...	... 700 ,,	... ,, ,,	... 5,970,000
,, Arosa ...	...	... 1,800 ,,	... (Egger) ...	... 7,000,000
,, Mexico City	...	... 2,280 ,,	... (Herera & Lope)	... 6,500,000
,, Morococha ...	...	... 4,392 ,,	... (Viault) ...	... 8,000,000

We note that they found the average at the City of Mexico 6,410 feet, to be 6,500,000 per cm.. Solly, in counting the blood of twenty-five students of variable length of residence in Colorado Springs, altitude 6,000 feet, found the count to be 5,927,000. In four natives, and three who came to Colorado under seven years of age, the average number was 5,724,550. Our own observations on twenty subjects gives us an average of 5,700,300. Thus we note there is a decided increase in the count of 6,000 feet over that at sea level. At Morococha, 14,274 feet, Viault found the count to be 8,000,000. There are no records of blood counts of people who have been some time on the summit of Pike's Peak, except that made by Dr. Holmes, of Denver. He examined the blood of a man who had remained on the Peak almost continuously for six months, and found the count to be 6,788,000. We note the marked difference between the blood count taken at Colorado Springs and those taken at the City of Mexico at practically the same altitude. This may be due in part to the instruments used, but we believe it to be due in a greater degree to the warmer climate of the City of Mexico. Heat is one of the important factors in producing a permanent rise in the blood count.

To demonstrate the permanent increase, we took three Belgian hares to 10,000 feet altitude, and two to the top of the Peak. The following tables will show the result of the experiment :—

No.		6,000 ft.		On arrival. 10,000 ft.		After 3 wks. 10,000 ft.		Mesentery
1	...	6,070,000	...	6,880,000	...	7,462,000	...	7,715,000
2	...	6,480,000	...	6,500,000	...	7,382,000	...	7,920,000
3	...	6,470,000	...	6,620,000	...	6,500,000	...	6,667,000
Av.	...	6,340,000	...	6,467,000	...	7,148,000	...	7,434,000

In Nos. 1 and 2 we note quite an increase in the number of corpuscles from a three weeks' sojourn at an increased altitude of 4,000 feet. No. 3 did not show the increase, but remained at about the same number. The rabbits taken to the Peak did not do well. The keeper of the Summit House tells us that they became very sick after ten or twelve hours, crying pitifully, and panting for breath. Before morning one of them died, demonstrating that Belgian hares can sicken and die at high altitudes. The following is the report on the remaining rabbit after three weeks' stay on the Peak: Count, 6,000 feet, 6,280,000. On arrival at summit, 7,200,000. After three weeks on the summit, 7,280,000.

We note the rapid rise on going to the Peak. This rise was only slightly increased by three weeks' stay on the Peak. We observed quite a number of microcytes in the count after the three weeks at a higher altitude. The size of the corpuscles varied. No measurements of the corpuscles were made, but the variation was quite noticeable to the eye.

To what shall we attribute this permanent increase in the count? There is one chief cause, viz., diminished barometric pressure. There are many auxillary causes. Among these we might mention the greater number of clear days, hence the increased amount of sunlight; the purer atmosphere, hence less obstruction to the sun's rays; the lessened humidity, both absolute and relative; the outdoor life of the people permitted by the foregoing conditions. *Apropos* to this subject, we note the conclusions of Herrera and Lope on the modification of the human body from a residence in elevated regions : —

" Increase in number of respirations.
      "   "   "   " pulsations.
      "   " capacity of respiratory organs.
      "   " mobility of the walls of the thorax.
      "   " number of red blood corpuscles and all principles fixed in the blood in general.
      "   " density of the blood.
      "   " density of the urine and all economic liquids in general (secretion of milk, &c.).
" Diminution of the intravascular tension of the blood."

We note these changes throughout the system, and our observations during a residence of eleven years confirm their accuracy. As a result of the diminished barometric pressure, we have a diminution in the amount of oxygen or a " reduction of oxygen pressure." The animal economy requires a definite amount of oxygen to maintain its equilibrium, hence changes must take place in the body to meet these requirements. The red blood corpuscles are the hæmoglobin carriers, hence they would be the first to multiply to meet the necessities of the body. Therefore the blood corpuscles remain permanently higher to compensate for the less amount of oxygen in the atmosphere.

The length of time required to establish an equilibrium in the circulation is short. As noted in our experiments on rabbits taken to the Peak, referred to later in our paper, we see the increased count is at first at the expense of the abdominal circulation. In our rabbits after three weeks the count is increased in general, and is as high in the mesentery as in the peripheral capillaries.

We will now call your attention to the rapid increase of blood corpuscles as we ascend to a higher altitude. The facilities for making these observations are as good, if not better, in Colorado, than anywhere in the civilised world. Our city of Colorado Springs, located at the base of Pike's Peak, has an altitude of 6,000 feet. We are connected by rail with the summit of the Peak, having an altitude of 14,147 feet. Without any exertion we can be elevated to the summit of the Peak in one and a-half hours. This gives us an opportunity to observe the blood changes and effects of altitude without having to eliminate the element of exercise. The cog-road running to the summit of the Peak is well built, and there is comparatively no excitement to cause changes in the circulation. We are indebted to Mr. C. W. Sells, manager of the road, for courtesies shown us, and much valuable information given. He informs us there has never been a death on the Peak since the road was open, and comparatively few persons complain of the effects of altitude.

As preliminary work, we took to the Peak during October, 1900, seven young and vigorous men, to see whether we would find the blood count increased by an increase in altitude without exertion. We found a material one in five out of the seven, and thought we made mistakes in the technique of the other two subjects. These observations inspired us to go further into the investigation of the subject, and try to account for this sudden increase. The great amount of labour involved in these observations is only appreciated by those who try to carry them on, and at the same time attend to the regular routine of a general practitioner. Owing to this latter fact, I have limited this paper to the consideration of the blood count alone, and have drawn on outside sources for my authority as to blood pressure and other facts. Our observations were not limited to the blood counts alone, but we have not had the time to investigate other features of the subject, and we do not give our paper as a complete thesis on blood changes at high altitudes.

I have interested in this work Dr. H. W. Hoagland, to whom I am indebted for a great portion of the practical work and many valuable suggestions.

A few words concerning the technique of our blood counting will suffice. Our examinations were all made with the Thoma-Zeiss apparatus. We were very exacting in all details. Two counts were made from two separate drops of each specimen, and the average taken. The blood was mainly obtained from the tip of the finger. In the experiments done during massage, the blood was taken from the skin of the forearm. The blood was not encouraged to flow by squeezing or stretching the skin, as we found early in our work that these methods changed the count, and would furnish unreliable data. The counting was done in Colorado Springs, the pipette being filled at the desired altitude, and carefully carried to our office. Being aware of the criticism of the Thoma-Zeiss apparatus (Gottstein) at high altitudes, or under diminished barometric pressure, we thought best to make all counts at one altitude. Gower's solution (sod. sul., acet. acid and aq.) was used as the diluting medium.

We found the rabbit to be rather an unreliable animal for experimental purposes in blood counting. It is difficult to draw blood on the surface of the body unless an extensive laceration is made, except in the ears. They are timid and impressionable, and the circulation in the capillaries of the ears vary greatly under different degrees of excitement, hence they are to be carefully handled.

In our preliminary work we found that the blood count was 250,000, to 500,000 more per cubit millimetre in Colorado Springs than at the sea level. We found an increase of from 300,000 to 500,000 corpuscles per cubit millimetre by ascending Pike's Peak on the cog-road without exertion. Was this a fictitious increase, or was there a true multiplication of red corpuscles? This is a mooted question, and it was for the purpose of trying to solve it that the following experiments were made during the past few months. We do not claim originality in all the experiments, but we will say that they were all original with us as far as the conception in our minds was concerned. We knew not that others had investigated along the same line until the most of our experiments had been made (*Journ. Amer. Med. Assoc.*, April 20, 1901).

Being convinced that the rapid multiplication of blood corpuscles in our preliminary examinations was not a permanent one, we made the following experiments to see if the' count could not be varied by many influences not accredited to altitude. The following table will show the effect of running one-half mile : —

No.	Name	Age	Wt.	Pulse Rest	Pulse Ex.	Time after meal	Dist. run	Time in run	Tem. of room	Blood-count Rest	Blood-count Exercise
1	C	44	190	82	132	3 hrs.	½ mile	8 min.	65°	5,510,000	5,610,000
2	H	27	150	82	148	3 ,,	,, ,,	7 ,,	,,	6,460,000	6,360,000
3	W	24	147	88	134	1 ,,	,, ,,	5 ,,	67°	5,380,000	5,820,000
4	H	31	145	78	114	2 ,,	,, ,,	8 ,,	,,	5,950,000	6,400,000
5	M	22	164	66	132	2 ,,	,, ,,	5 ,,	62°	5,330,000	6,570,000
6	C	18	134	82	150	2 ,,	,, ,,	5 ,,	,,	5,780,000	5,690,000
7	C	18	135	84	148	2 ,,	,, ·,,	5 ,,	,,	5,260,000	5,690,000
8	B	18	136	60	132	2 ,,	,, ,,	4 ,,	68°	6,570,000	6,660,000
9	B	14	87	78	142	2 ,,	,, ,,	5 ,,	,,	5,410,000	6,270,0co
10	W	15	154	90	148	2 ,,	,, ,,	6 ,,	,,	5,830,000	6,000,000
Av. ...		23	144	79	138	—	—	5 min.	—	5,748,000	6,132,000

The exercise, with one exception, No. 2, increased the blood count. The average count was increased about the same as an ascent to the Peak without exertion. The heart's action was increased, and the peripheral capillaries dilated, as shown by the ruddy color of the skin, and the moisture from perspiration. We cannot here account for the increase of count by the multiplication of corpuscles, although some investigators might do so by the abstraction of water by sweating.

Finding that general exercise of the body increased the count, it occurred to us to investigate whether the count could be increased in one member of the body over that found in a corresponding member of the same body. We made seven tests of this character. One arm was kept at perfect rest while the other arm was massaged and rubbed vigorously for ten minutes. At the same time the subject opened and closed the hand

8

continuously. By these methods we sought to increase the circulation to as great a degree as possible. The counts were made simultaneously in both arms. The following table will show the results of our experiments :—

No.	Age	Wt.	Pulse	Time after meals	Arm at rest	Arm exercised
1 ...	18 ...	136 ...	60 ...	2 hrs. ...	5,980,000 ...	6,320,000
2 ..	15 ...	154 ...	82 ...	,, ...	5,830,000 ...	5,940,000
3 ...	18 ...	160 ...	78 ...	,, ...	6,000,000 ...	6,490,000
4 ...	18 ...	136 ...	60 ...	,, ...	5,810,000 ...	6,010,000
5 ...	17 ...	145 ...	84 ...	,, ...	5,770,000 ...	6,000,000
6 ...	44 ...	190 ...	75 ...	,, ...	6,260,000 ...	6,510,000
7 ...	44 ...	188 ...	78 ...	,, ...	5,480,000 ...	5,550,000
Av. ...	25 ...	158 ...	74 ...	— ...	5,875,714 ...	6,117,143

We note quite a material increase, 241,429, in the blood count. This can only be accounted for by the increased flow of blood in the arm, due to massage; although a possible difference might be produced by an accumulation of carbonic acid in the blood, the result of the violent exercise of the muscles. Cabot tells us that poisoning from carbonic acid gas will increase the blood count. Nevertheless, we believe the increased count was due to vaso-motor conditions. There is considerable fatigue to the subject during this experiment. The circulation is slightly quickened, and we note a higher count in the quiet arm than in the same subjects on other occasions when the blood was counted when the whole body was at rest. Dr. J. K. Mitchell, of Philadelphia, in an interesting paper on "Massage and the Blood" (*Amer. Jour. Med. Sc.*, vol. 107), has shown that the count is invariably increased in massage unless the subject had been physically fatigued immediately before receiving the treatment. Here again we have a changed condition of the cutaneous blood vessels due to manipulation, provided that they had not been previously dilated by exercise.

Having satisfied ourselves in our own experiments, and by the experience of others, that the blood count could be increased by causing a dilatation of the peripheral capillaries by exercise or manipulation, it occurred to us that we might be able to diminish the count by causing a contraction of the capillaries. We made three counts with the results as shown in the table following, after packing the arm to the elbow in snow.

No.	Age	Wt.	Time after meals	Normal	Arm in snow 10 min.	20 min. late
1 ...	44 ...	190 ...	2 hrs. ...	5,510,000 ...	5,140,000 ...	5,430,000
2 ...	18 ...	135 ...	,, ...	6,570,000 ...	4,545,000 ...	5,000,000
3 ...	15 ...	154 ...	,, ...	5,830,000 ...	4,915,000 ...	5,280,000
Av. ...	25 ...	159 ...	— ...	5,970,000 ...	4,870,000 ...	5,257,000

We made three counts of each individual, one in hand not experimented with, one simultaneously in the hand in the snow, and one after reaction had partially taken place. As noted in the table, we were able to materially decrease the count, and it gradually came back towards its normal count as reaction took place. It also occurred to us to try what effect intense heat would have on the count, knowing that it would produce contraction of the blood vessels similar to the intense cold. We accepted the proffered courtesies of Dr. B. B. Grover, of this city, and tested five subjects in the Betz hot air apparatus. The table will show the degree of heat applied, and the results on the count.

No.	Age	Wt.	Pulse Before	After	Degree of heat	Length of time	Blood-count Baked arm	Outside arm
1 ...	44 ...	190 ...	78 ...	88 ...	325° ...	15 min. ...	4,690,000 ...	5,710,000
2 ...	18 ...	136 ...	60 ...	88 ...	350° ...	10 ,, ...	5,460,000 ...	6,050,000
3 ...	15 ...	154 ...	90 ...	100 ...	,, ...	,, ,, ...	5,570,000 ...	6,070,000
4 ...	16 ...	152 ...	88 ..	100 ...	,, ...	,, ,, ...	5,500,000 ...	5,800,000
5 ...	15 ...	148 ...	96 ...	88 ...	,, ...	,, ,, ...	5,800,000 ...	6,480,000
Av....	22 ...	156 ...	82 ...	93 ...	— ...	— ...	5,404,000 ...	6,022,000

The count will be seen to have been materially lessened in the arm subjected to the intense heat. As noted in the experiments where one arm was massaged the general count was increased, owing to the subject becoming quite warm. The arm baked perspired quite profusely, and the skin was shrivelled by the sweat when removed from the apparatus. The blood count being lowered under such an amount of abstraction of watery elements, would indicate that the increase of blood counts can not be due to the abstraction of water from the surface of the body.

· The late spring snows delayed us from making as many experiments as we would like to have done on the top of Pike's Peak before submitting the report of our observations to the society, but we feel that they have been sufficiently numerous to demonstrate certain features in regard to blood counts. We would call your attention to the following table :—

| No. | Age | Wt. | 6,000 ft. | | 10,000 ft. | | 14,147 ft. | | 6,000 ft. | |
			P.	Count	P.	Count	P.	Count	P.	Count
I	44	189	78	5,760,000	84	6,070,000	84	6,100,000	78	5,790,000
2	27	150	80	6,420,000	104	6,440,000	96	6,510,000	82	5,840,000
3	17	135	80	5,740,000	80	5,700,000	84	5,730,000	78	5,670,000
4	16	150	82	6,150,000	88	6,280,000	80	6,390,000	80	5,970,000
5	19	160	90	6,040,000	84	6,150,000	88	6,240,000	85	6,420,000
6	18	145	60	5,890,000	62	6,750,000	78	6,960,000	60	5,500,000
7	19	120	80	5,680,000	86	6,340,000	92	6,380,000	78	5,575,000
8	40	123	78	6,120,000	80	6,105,000	88	6,485,000	76	5,700,000
9	51	112	84	5,480,000	88	6,670,000	90	6,170,000	80	5,090,000
10	20	140	84	5,170,000	88	5,790,000	96	5,955,000	82	5,790,000
Av.	27	142	80	5,845,000	84	6,229,500	88	6,292,000	78	5,734,500

The last four subjects were ladies.

As stated in the beginning of our paper, we want to confine our consideration of the study of the blood to the blood count alone, and its probable cause. We made·other observations, but will leave them for future consideration. We note from the table that the average blood count at 6,000 feet is 5,845,000; that it increases to 6,229,500 at 10,000 feet; and that there is still further increase on top of the Peak, 14,147 feet, to 6,292,000. When we returned to 6,000 feet the count again dropped to the normal for this elevation, or even below it. We want to say for the subjects of these experiments, that they were all healthy, and had been in Colorado for variable lengths of time. The first count was made in the morning before breakfasting, as it is claimed that the count is modified during digestion. The second and third counts, taken at 10,000 feet and 14,147 feet respectively, were made while seated in the railroad carriage, thus doing away with any element of exercise. The only other influence that could have made any impression was the mental excitement incident to the ride up the steep ascent. The subjects were accustomed to mountain life and travel, and were as little excited as it is possible for one to be, hence this element was reduced to a minimum. The fourth count was made on return to Colorado Springs after a light lunch. We have tried to eliminate all sources of change of the blood count except those due to altitude. From these observations, we are convinced that the count is increased in the peripheral blood vessels as we ascend, and again falls to its normal condition when the original altitude from whence we started is reached.

To further demonstrate this we took three rabbits to the Peak. We examined their blood before starting and immediately on arrival on the Peak. We note the increase in the peripheral count. We also made a count from the mesenteric circulation, which shows a marked diminution as compared with the external capillaries, as it also does to what it was on starting from Colorado Springs. The blood for the mesenteric count was taken as follows : The rabbit was fastened to a board. With one stroke of the knife the abdomen was laid open. After drying the surface, from which the blood was taken to avoid the possible error of diluting the blood with peritoneal secretion, a small vessel was punctured, and blood taken therefrom. The length of time consumed in getting the blood into the pipette was ten to fifteen seconds. The following table will show the results of the experiment : —

No.			6,000 ft. Count from ear			14,147 ft. Count from ear			14,147 ft. Count from mesentery
1	...	...	6,210,000	...	...	6,636,000	...	...	5,760,000
2	...	...	6,530,000	...	...	7,040,000	...	...	6,230,000
3.	...	...	5,520,000	...	...	6,230,000	...	...	5,700,000
Av.	...	...	6,087,000	...	...	6,635,000	...	...	5,897,000

This shows a marked increase in the blood count on rapid ascent, 548,000. It also shows that this rapid increase is at the expense of the internal circulation, as the external capillary count shows a plurality over the internal of 738,000. We further note the marked decrease of the internal count, 190,000, compared with the count at Colorado Springs before starting. We are convinced that this rapid increase in the blood count is not a true multiplication of blood corpuscles, but a fictitious one, due to the calling of the blood to the surface of the body, incident to diminished barometric pressure and increased heart's action.

Herrera and Lope have shown by extensive experiments that the arterial tension is diminished as the barometric pressure is lessened. They have given us the following law : " When certain conditions are equal, the vascular tension is in direct ratio with barometric pressure." It is not necessary here to outline their experiments, but they have been extensive, and their deductions seem conclusive.

A. Mosso, who has experimented extensively in the Alps (" Life of Man on the High Alps," p. 187), recognises the dilated condition of the external blood vessels and the results thereof. He says: " The rapid changes in the pulse observed during ascents, and more especially during mountain sickness, are due to the state of the blood vessels. When these dilate the resistance opposed to the circulation of the blood is diminished, and the heart beats more rapidly."

Our experiments lead us to the following conclusions as to the rapid increase in blood count as we ascend :—

(1) The blood count increases as we ascend (without exertion at the rate of 50,000 corpuscles, per cubic millimetre of blood, per thousand feet.

(2) The pulse rate increases in the same ratio as the blood count, the count rising as the pulse rises, and in like proportion falling when pulse rate falls, showing that the heart seeks to overcome the changes brought about by the lessened barometric pressure.

(3) The increase is not a true multiplication of the blood corpuscles, but is due to a changed vaso-motor condition in the peripheral vessels incident to diminished barometric pressure. This condition of vaso-motor control of circulation and blood count was demonstrated in the various experiments made, where it is shown that the count can be increased or diminished by any means that will dilate or contract the peripheral capillaries.

(4) This is further demonstrated by the experiments on the rabbits, which showed the same increase as man, and by the mesenteric count demonstrated that the external capillary count was increased at the expense of the internal abdominal circulation.

(5) The increase in blood count disappears and the heart's action returns to the normal when we return to the altitude from whence we started. This is another confirmation of the fact that the increase is a fictitious one, and is due to a diversion of the blood current incident to diminished barometric pressure.

(6) The dilatation of the external capillaries (skin and lungs) would not alone account for all the increase, but with this dilatation we have another effect of diminished barometric pressure, viz., diminished arterial tension. With vessels of an increased calibre and a heart with diminished force, we can plainly see that we will have more or less of a temporary stasis in the dilated capillaries. In course of time nature seeks to adjust an equilibrium in the economy of those who live at high altitudes. The heart becomes more forcible by the strengthening of its muscles, and the circulation becomes more equitable, hence the gradual decline in the blood count (Solly) of those who have remained for some time at a high altitude.

(7) The want of increase of hæmoglobin in proportion to the increase of blood count in ascents, is accounted for by the fact that blood corpuscles, the carriers of the hæmoglobin, are not increased at once in high altitudes. After remaining some

time at a high altitude, the true increase in blood corpuscles takes place, and with it the increase of the hæmoglobin.

DISCUSSION.

Dr. F. SAVARY PEARCE: This paper has been very interesting to me in confirmation of the experiments that have already been done, and also in support of the ideas I hold as to the way in which high altitudes help certain patients. The sensible perspiration undoubtedly carries off much of the waste products from the body, and in this way, it seems to me, great benefit is obtained in nervous individuals when auto-intoxication exists. Thus toxines are thrown off in excess, even though the blood does not circulate more rapidly. If a greater amount of blood is permitted to reach the surface, as at high altitudes, an increased sensible and insensible perspiration occurs, according to the moisture or dryness of the air. The average case of simple general nervousness or essential neurasthenia will do better at low levels however.

Dr. BALDWIN : I just want to express my appreciation of Dr. Campbell's careful work which I feel we must all consider a valuable scientific contribution. Last year Dr. Solly called attention to the dearth of researches in that line in the Rockies, but I think he can no longer have any qualms of conscience on that score.

Dr. MINOR : I would like to add a word to what Dr. Baldwin has said, and would like to suggest that the doctor might hereafter in addition to the blood counts, test the specific gravity. One question that arises to my mind is whether it is possible in opening the abdominal cavity to avoid producing practically peripheral conditions and whether it would be necessary to make deep punctures instead ?

Dr. CAMPBELL : We tried to limit the influence of air on the internal circulation as far as possible. I hardly think it is possible to make a deep puncture with any degree of accuracy as to where the blood is coming from. By having everything ready, however, and two men working, as we did in this instance, the exposure was so brief that there was no material change in the circulation, although theoretically, those twelve to fifteen seconds form a considerable portion of the time it would take to cause a complete change in the peripheral circulatory conditions of the rabbit. I believe, from my experiments of the past three months, that the diminished barometric pressure is the most important factor in altitude so far as the blood count is concerned. Increase in the peripheral vessels brings to the surface, as Dr. Pearce has said, an increased amount of blood to be exposed to the sun, light, and air, and in this way we get increased oxidation and better nutrition, especially in pulmonary cases.

Adjourned.

FURTHER NOTES UPON THE DIAGNOSTIC TEST OF TUBERCULIN.

BY EDWARD O. OTIS, M.D.

BOSTON.

––––––

AT the meeting of this Association in 1899, I presented a series of tuberculin tests, published in the *Transactions* of that year. I have now to present sixty-two more tests, undertaken with two objects in view, first to determine how many cases of known syphilis react to tuberculin, and second to determine how reliable the test is in suspected or incipient tuberculosis, both of the lungs, and of other organs or portions of the body. The tuberculin used was Koch's original, imported, and diluted as used to a one per cent. solution, one-tenth of a cubic centimetre of which solution being one milligramme of the original product. The injections were all given in the back, under aseptic conditions. The patients were those of an ambulatory clinic, but from former experience I have learned that results so obtained are reliable, and such also was the experience of Dr. R. C. Cabot, who pursued a similar course in his series of tests, referred to in my previous paper. Fränkel also agrees that the test can be satisfactorily made in an ambulatory clinic.[*]

In none of the cases herewith reported were there any

[*] "Polikliniken für Lungenkranke," *Zeitschrift für Tuberkulose und Heilstättenwesen*, April, 1901.

serious or alarming symptoms as a result of the injection, so that
I am still further confirmed in my opinion previously expressed,
that no injurious results follow the diagnostic test of tuberculin
in doses up to 10 milligrammes. There was invariably a little
soreness complained of at the point of injection for one or two
days following. In most cases the general reaction was depended upon only, but I am inclined to think that there are
some few cases of tuberculosis which, for some reason or other,
do not give any general reaction, but do give a marked and
definite local one, as in case No. 4. The dose was 2, 5, 7, or
10 milligrammes, never over 10. All the cases were practically
afebrile at the time of the injection.

If from six to twenty-four hours after the injection there
was a rise of temperature, and the patient complained of
marked weakness, sensations of heat and cold, nausea or
anorexia, pain in the back and limbs, headache, sweating, either
sleeplessness or somnolence, a general " miserable " feeling, a
reaction was considered to have taken place. I do not think
that any special temperature can in itself be relied upon without
some or all of these other symptoms. Sometimes a slight rise
of temperature was accompanied by marked constitutional disturbance. Each patient was given a thermometer to take home,
and requested to hold it under the tongue for five minutes at
6 o'clock at night, upon going to bed, and in the morning on
getting up, and then to report the following forenoon. In this
way the maximum temperature was obtained, at whichever of
these three periods it occurred. As the class of patients were
more or less ignorant, no attempt was made to teach them how
to read the thermometer, the plan just stated was considered
a surer, as it was a simpler, one.

The diagnosis of syphilis was carefully made by Dr. C. M.
Smith, of the Skin and Syphilis Department of the Boston
Dispensary, and I desire here to express my thanks to him for
so kindly furnishing me with the material for these tests.

I present first thirty-six cases of the tuberculin test in

syphilis, or, throwing out No. 11, the only doubtful case, thirty-five. The smallest amount of tuberculin used was 2 milligrammes, the largest 10 milligrammes. There were six undoubted reactions, and five what I have called abortive reactions, where there were temporary symptoms of a reactive nature, but which I do not think could be called genuine reactions. Considering only the six undoubted reactions, we have 17 per cent. of reactions; including the abortive cases, we have 31 per cent.

In the discussion upon Dr. J. M. Anders' paper upon " The Value of the Tuberculin Test in the Diagnosis of Pulmonary Tuberculosis," presented to this Association last year, Dr. Baldwin quoted Beck as showing in his experiments that about one-half the cases of syphilis in which he used the injections reacted in tuberculin. My cases give a much smaller number, only about a sixth, or at most less than a third. From my experience I cannot think that however large the number of cases experimented upon, as large a proportion as a-half would react, or anything near that number. Still, in using the tuberculin test we must always bear in mind the fact that syphilis, at whatever stage, does give a reaction. Further, there does not seem to be any guide in the activity or quiescence of the syphilic infection, as to whether or not a reaction is likely to occur. In the most violent reaction I had, where the temperature went up to 104 degrees, the case was one of many years' duration, and with no active manifestations.

Second, I have twenty-six cases of suspected or proved tuberculosis which give some interesting and perplexing results. Taking the eight cases in which the physical examination showed sufficient evidence of tuberculosis, or where tubercle bacilli were found in the sputum, we have four reactions and four failures to react. In the three cases in which tubercle bacilli were found in the sputum two did not react; in one 7 milligrammes were used, and in the other 5 and 10 milligrammes. In the third case, in which 2, 5, and 8 milligrammes of tuberculin were successively used, only a local reaction was obtained. I have no explanation to offer for these unexpected and disappointing results. Of the remaining eighteen cases of suspected tuberculosis, there were six reactions and twelve failures to react. In no one of those cases which failed to react could tuberculosis be more than suspected with greater or less probability by the physical examination. The case of lupus of the face, besides giving a general reaction showed a very pretty local one. In a case of chronic laryngitis, where either syphilis or tuberculosis might have been the cause, a reaction was obtained, thus leaving the origin doubtful as before. In using the tuberculin test for suspected tuberculosis, experience would teach us to carefully look for syphilis.

"One swallow does not make a summer," nor should one be discouraged by a few failures, yet I must confess that when a case of tuberculosis not far beyond the incipient stage, with tubercle bacilli in the sputum, fails to react, one's confidence in the test is, temporarily, at least, a little shaken, but it is well to bear in mind that in all such investigations as the above there is always a chance of error, and as yet we do not know what the minimum efficient dose is, and not unlikely it may vary for each individual. One thing I feel sure of, that up to 10 milligrammes there is no injurious result to be feared.

[The discussion of this paper is included in the discussion of the succeeding paper.]

TUBERCULIN TEST IN SYPHILIS.

No.	Condition—Stage	Sex	Age	Temp.	Pulse	Dose in mg's.	Result	Temp. at reactive epoch
1	Syphilis; early stage ...	M.	23	98·6	100	5	No reaction ...	97·2
2	„ pustular syphilide on shins	F.	20	99·3	88	2	„ „ ...	—
3	Late syphilis: tubercular syphilide	F.	37	99·1	76	2	„ „ ...	98·4
4	Syphilis; no active manifestations	M.	28	98·5	72	8	„ „ ...	99·5
5	Syphilis; few small papules in brows	M.	34	98·9	100	8	„ „ ...	98·4
6	Syphilis; early secondary	M.	29	99·7	80	5	„ „ ...	99·2
7	Early syphilis	M.	30	99·4	88	5	„ „ ...	91·4
8	Early syphilis; abundant eruption	F.	19	99	120	5	Reaction ...	102·5
9	Syphilis; late manifestations	F.	29	99·8	96	2	No reaction ...	99
10	Syphilis (old); no acute manifestations for several months	F.	29	98·9	96	2	Abortive reaction...	99
11	Probable syphilitic lesion on cheek	M.	9	99	86	2	No reaction ...	99·8
12	Early syphilis; abundant eruption on body	M.	28	98·2	88	5	„ „ ...	99
13	Syphilis of year's duration	F.	23	98·4	96	3	Reaction ...	104
14	Early syphilis	F.	40	99·6	96	5	No reaction ...	98·4
15	„ „	F.	22	98·9	100	5	„ „ ...	99·2
16	„ „	F.	21	98·3	92	5	„ „ ...	96·3
17	„ „ mucous patches	M.	18	97·8	80	5	„ „ ...	98·9
18	„ „	M.	...	99·4	92	5	Abortive reaction...	99·7
19	Late syphilis; gummatous lesion	M.	...	99	80	5	No reaction ...	99
20	Early syphilis; mucous patches	M.	...	97·4	76	5	Abortive reaction...	99·5
21	Early syphilis; initial sore on chin	M.	...	98	78	5	Moderate reaction	100·6
22	Late syphilis	M.	27	98·1	64	5	No reaction ...	99·5
23	„ „	F.	20	99·2	92	5	„ „ ...	99·2
24	„ „	F.	43	98·6	76	5	„ „ ...	99·3
25	Early „	F.	31	99·6	104	5	Reaction ...	100·2
26	Late „	M.	37	98·4	88	10	„ ...	101·3
27	Early „	M.	28	99	72	10	„ ...	100·8
28	„ „	M.	28	98·2	76	10	Abortive reaction...	99
29	Late „	M.	46	98	96	10	No reaction ...	98·4
30	Early „	M.	38	98·4	80	10	„ „ ...	99·8
31	„ „	M.	29	99	108	10	„ „ ...	99·4
32	„ „	M.	39	98·4	72	10	„ „ ...	99
33	„ „	F.	25	99·4	96	5	„ „ ...	99·2
34	„ „	F.	20	98·4	88	5	„ „ ...	98·5
35	„ „	F.	37	99·1	78	5	Abortive reaction..	100
36	„ „	F.	43	99·4	108	7	No reaction ...	90·5

SUSPECTED OR PROVED TUBERCULOSIS.

No.	Condition	Sex	Age	Temp.	Pulse	Dose in mg's.	Result	Temp. at reactive epoch
1	Suspected tuberculosis of urinary passages	M.	40	99	74	5	No reaction ...	98·4
2	Enlarged suppurating glands of neck, both sides; dulness over left apex	F.	20	99·5	112	2	Reaction ...	103
3	Cough; slight dulness in right back	F.	23	99·8	100	2	No reaction ...	97
4	Dulness above and below clavicle on left sides; moist râles; T. B. in sputum	M.	52	99·4	100	2, 5, 8	No general reaction Marked local reaction with 8 mg.	99·8
5	Dulness over right apex; bronchial resp.; few moist râles on cough	M.	39	99·2	68	5, 8	No reaction ...	99
6	Suspected renal tuberculosis	M.	19	98·4	64	5	,, ,, ...	98·4
7	Fine moist râles below left clavicle; diminished resonance, prolonged exp.; T. B. in sputum	F.	38	98·6	81	7	,, ,, ...	99·6
8	Dulness left axilla, and few moist râles on deep inspiration	M.	28	97·8	62	10	,, ,, ...	99·6
9	Suspected renal tuberculosis	M.	36	98·8	80	5	,, ,, ...	99·5
10	Moist râles at both apices	M.	30	98·8	70	8	General and local reaction	101·3
11	Suspected tuberculosis of wrist	F.	40	98·6	74	5	No reaction ...	98·4 .
12	Suspected tubercular laryngitis	F.	23	100	99	5	,, ,, ...	99·8
13	Lupus of face	F.	29	99	114	5	General and local reaction	101·2
14	Suspected tuberculosis of anus	M.	50	98·8	80	5	No reaction ...	98·4
15	Dulness of right apex ...	M.	42	98·4	80	10	,, ,, ...	98·4
16	Suspected tubercular epididymitis	M.	30	99·5	90	10	,, ,, ...	—
17	General tubercular condition; above spine of scapular in left lung a few fine moist râles	M.	41	100·2	100	5	Reaction ...	102·1
18	General evidence of tuberculosis; a few dry râles on left side below clavicle; harsh respiration ...	M.	39	99·6	105	7	,, ...	104·2
19	Suspected tuberculosis of finger and hand	M.	3	99·8	110	1	No reaction ...	98

SUSPECTED OR PROVED TUBERCULOSIS.—*Continued.*

No.	Condition	Sex	Age	Temp.	Pulse	Dose in mg's.	Result	Temp. at reactive epoch
20	Dulness above and below left clavicle; fine râles after cough; harsh respiration	M.	...	98·3	72	7	No reacti ...	97·1
21	Syphilis or tubercular laryngitis	F.	16	99·1	104	2	Reaction ...	100·2
22	Suspected tubercular laryngitis	M.	56	97·5	72	5, 10	Abortive general reaction; local reaction	98
23	Suspected tuberculsosis of septum of nose	F.	40	97·7	88	5	General and local reaction	101·7
24	Few fine moist râles at left apex	M.	52	98·7	90	10	Reaction ...	103
25	Dulness over both apices; moist râles; consolidation on right side; T. B. in sputum; fistula in ano	F.	22	99·2	112	5, 10	No reaction ...	98·6
26	Possible tubercular infection at the right apex	M.	39	98·2	72	10	,, ,, ...	98

CASES IN WHICH THE TUBERCULIN TEST SEEMED JUSTIFIED AND DECISIVE.

BY W. E. CASSELBERRY, M.D.

CHICAGO.

———

IN an experience, the trend of which is largely toward the upper as well as the lower respiratory tract, it should be one's constant effort to establish the real diagnosis in the earliest demonstrable stage of pulmonary tuberculosis. This infection, when present in a latent form, during a slow and insidious onset and during periods of partial arrest, by impairing the general vitality, predisposes to other and more conspicuous complaints, prominent among which are catarrhal conditions of the upper respiratory tract. With an irritable throat, a hacking cough, a tendency to hoarseness, and an inclination to rhinitis, the patient of this class is often ready to believe, and sometimes even to insist that he has only "throat trouble" or "catarrh." To demonstrate in such a case an unmistakable underlying tuberculosis in the earliest, perchance remedial, stage, is to render an immeasurable service. Others, again, who may be suffering affections actually limited to the throat or from non-tuberculous broncho-pulmonary conditions, are not infrequently in constant dread of tuberculosis, and demand of their consultant a positive and speedy opinion which shall either confirm their fears or ease their troubled minds. To announce tuberculosis even tentatively to such a patient, when in reality it does not exist, is perhaps to work an irreparable injury.

One meets with no inconsiderable number of patients in whom it seems of paramount importance to positively exclude tuberculosis. It is conceded that to this end, in the majority of cases, a consideration of the symptoms and of the physical condition is entirely adequate, yet in an appreciable minority this evidence, because of its scantiness and of possible variations in its interpretation, is not conclusive, and conversely, the typical steadily progressive case of pulmonary tuberculosis may be gauged by a tyro, while the atypical cause, by reason of minuteness of foci of infection, diminished virulence, increased resistance, favourable environment, latency, fibroid, inclusion, arrest, or confusion with other pathogenic infections, may leave an uncertainty in the mind of the expert.

There is a prebacillary stage in the sense that the sputum examination may be negative without disproving the existence of tuberculous infiltration. Confusion arises between the normal relative dulness and the harsher respiratory murmur of the right infraclavicular region and the slightest signs of initial tuberculosis at that apex. The temperature when other symptoms are obscure is not always decisive, and would best be observed over a period of weeks, even months, if one would attach to it a positively diagnostic import. Subacute inflammatory attacks in the upper respiratory tract, influenza and its after effects, empyema of the nasal accessory sinuses, prolonged convalescence from acute pleuritis or pneumonia, and the primary and secondary stages of syphilis, are the conditions which I have in mind as simulating for a time the unpronounced tuberculous febrile reaction. This is especially true when these affections occur in individuals of relatively light weight, deficient nutrition, sedentary life, poor thoracic development, and adverse hereditary tendencies. And then there are prefebrile, interfebrile, and postfebrile periods in which the tuberculosis, supposedly, for the moment, in a state of inactivity, fails to register above 99 or 99·5 degrees F., which does not exceed an occasional maximum normal. There are persons in varied states of simply impaired health, or in the midst of an exhaus-

9

tion incidental to a strenuous life, whose afternoon temperatures commonly reach that point.

So also with the rapidity of the pulse, when there is progressive activity of the infective process the resulting toxæmia quickens the heart, but in intermediate periods and in latent tuberculosis the pulse rate may not rise above 80.* Stress has been laid upon the inalterability of the rapid pulse rate by position and the characteristic sphygmographic tracings,† but one would expect these also to vary in accordance with the degree of activity as does the rate itself. Attention is also called to the fact that the arterial pressure in tuberculosis is low, as it is in other forms of anæmia, but that blood examinations, with special reference to the low specific gravity of chlorosis, while not an unerring guide, may aid in differentiating the anæmias.

Therefore, while it is not contended that the fallacies herewith enumerated are of very frequent interposition, and while it is admitted, even urged, that the conclusiveness of the customary methods of examination can be broadened by superior skilfulness and a keen appreciation of certain of the finer phases, such as skodaic tympanitic apical resonance, a heightened pitch of the prolonged expiratory murmur, the relation of height to thoracic perimeter,‡ Röntgen ray photography, &c., nevertheless it happens from time to time that cases present themselves in which it is impossible to assert the presence or absence of pulmonary tuberculosis despite a conscientious resort to all of these means, and in these cases it would seem that the careful injection of tuberculin as a test is both justifiable and decisive. I say justifiable because, notwithstanding the commendations of all who have recorded a practical use of the test, including B. Frankel,§ Trudeau,‖ Beck,¶ A. C. Klebs,** Otis,†† G. W. Webster,‡‡ Whittaker,§§ Anders,‖‖ and numerous others, there is still an aversion to the deliberate injection of the organic toxines of a pathogenic organism such as the tubercle bacillus, an aversion which by laymen is based upon the mere uncanniness of the idea and by physicians upon the double apprehension that tuberculin may carry virulent tubercle bacilli, and that its injection may generalise or re-excite a previously circumscribed, quiescent tuberculous deposit.

These apprehensions have been definitely answered anew by B. Frankel,§ who affirms that the tuberculin of Koch is heated in a water bath to a consistency of one-fifth its volume and then filtered, that therefore it can contain no living thing. The fear of generalisation and re-excitation he ascribes solely to the observation that during the early use of tuberculin as a cure, dissolution was apparently hastened in certain advanced fever-stricken cases, but now, by reason of the many thousands of test doses which have been given without detriment, he holds it for proven that the careful application of the tuberculin test can result in no harm.

In the midst of an undue conservatism the decisive value of this test was first forcibly impressed upon the writer by the following case :—

Mrs. J. A., aged 35 when first examined in 1890; weight 90 lbs.; height 5 feet 4 inches; anæmic; persistent cough; expectoration negative regarding tubercle bacilli; afternoon temperature 99 degrees F., never above 99⅔ degrees unless having acute rhino-bronchitis; pulse 90 to 110, weak and compressible. Pronounced hypertrophic rhinitis, follicular pharyngitis, and laryngeal irritation. Chest emaciated, slightly pigeon-breasted, narrow at the apices, periphery 26½ inches. Respiratory murmur at left apex approaches broncho-vesicular, percussion resonance impaired, but these signs were then so slight as to be noted with a question mark. They had become more pronounced in 1892, when also the murmur over the right infra-clavicular and mammary regions lacked breeziness and strength. Certain features were absent, but a provisional diagnosis of partly latent tuberculosis seemed reasonable. The following winters were passed at Colorado Springs, Asheville, and Las Cruces, New Mexico, where skilled physicians concurred in the diagnosis. The physical signs did not progress, and later the disease was supposed to be "arrested." About 1895 certain neurotic symptoms appeared, hysterical aphonia, high-pitched voice, twitching of the facial muscles, leucoderma, and œdematous ethmoiditis. A few nasal polypi were removed in 1896, with the comment that these were unusual in tuberculosis. Soon, during an attack of acute rhino-bronchitis with digestive derangement, irregular asthmatic symptoms developed,. which further clouded the original diagnosis. About this time, during my temporary absence, Dr. Boomer injected tuberculin, and later I repeated the test, both times without reaction. The final diagnosis is bronchial asthma and pulmonary fibrosis, both of mild degree. At present all symptoms are in abeyance, except cough and malnutrition. Weight reduced to 81 lbs.

CASE 2.—Rev. H. R. O., aged 30. Well-nourished, thick-set, and of good colour. Loss of energy, persistent morning cough and mucopurulent expectoration for nine months. Afternoon temperature 98⅖ to 99⅓ degrees F., pulse 80. Three negative sputum tests by Winnipeg Government Laboratory and several indecisive physical examinations. Resonance and vesicular murmur at right apex impaired, but scarcely more than the relative difference. Also dulness over a limited area at the left base. No râles. Skiagraph inconclusive. Wants a positive opinion on which to base action regarding choice of climate and pastorate. Tuberculin ·003 caused little reaction, but ·006 at 4 p.m. sent the temperature to 100⅘ degrees F. by 11 p.m., together with malaise and chilliness.

The next two cases are of special interest, aside from the negative tuberculin tests.

CASE 3.—Mr. F., aged 32 ; weight 137 lbs. ; height 5 feet 11 inches ; temperature 98⅔ degrees F. ; pulse 65 ; always anæmic. Felt well till two weeks ago ; then confined to bed two days with cough and pain in right side. At business since, but conscious that right lung fails to inflate. Inspection shows right diminished, and left exaggerated expansion, but no interspace retraction or bulging, or adhesive collapse of side. Respiratory murmur over whole right lung deficient, distantly tubercular, but with a light vascular character when forced, as if adequate air failed ordinarily to enter the lung. Vocal fremitus intensified towards the base. Resonance impaired, but nowhere flat or decidedly dull. No râles or creaking. Aspiration negative. No tumour or cause of occlusion of main bronchus. Probable diagnosis, restriction of expansion from thickened and adherent pleura following pleuritis. He applied chiefly for an opinion concerning tuberculosis, and willingly submitted to the tuberculin test, which was negative.

CASE 4.—J. E. T., aged 41 ; height 5 feet 9 inches ; weight 128 lbs. ; former weight 150 lbs. ; temperature 99⅔ degrees F. ; pulse 96. Syphilis twenty years ago. Cough and right pleuritic pains for two years. Murmur over right lower lobe elicited only by forced inspiration, weak, distant, not bronchial, and with subcrepitation like the creaking of thickened pleura. Resonance impaired, but not flat. No fluid. Fremitus increased. Sputum negative. Repeated tuberculin tests negative. Rapid amelioration of cough. Pain and dyspnœa under potassium iodide. One year later, weight 144 lbs. ; pulse 80.

Other instances in which the test proved of value, include positive reactions in two cases of early laryngeal tuberculosis (Cases 5 and 6), in which the pulmonary involvement was so slight as to be doubtful. In one the disease progressed but slowly ; the test induced submission to suitable treatment, and the patient still survives, well nourished, of good colour, fair strength, pulse and temperature normal, but with cough, hoarseness, and an infiltrated larynx. A few tubercle bacilli have since been found in the sputum.

CASE 7.—H. E. O., aged 23, but youthful in development ; height 5 feet 11 inches ; weight 125 lbs. ; pulse 99 ; temperature 100 degrees F. Two sisters affected by tuberculosis. He applied for an opinion while suffering from an acute laryngo-bronchitis. Chest flat and small, shoulders sloping. Murmur at apices deficient, puerile and jerky. After a few days his temperature and pulse had regained the normal. Sputum examination and tuberculin tests both negative. He remains well now two years after.

CASE 8 concerned a physician's wife (Mrs. W.), in whom hypertrophic rhinitis and laryngo-tracheitis had long been permitted to masque an apical tuberculosis. Temperature 99⅖ degrees; pulse 79. The positive reaction of the tuberculin test proved sufficiently convincing to induce a correct mode of treatment. Tubercle bacilli subsequently found.

CASE 9.—Dr. W. A young woman hospital interne, who by study and confinement had lost flesh, strength, and colour, and in whom incipient tuberculosis was suspected by her colleagues because of cough and deficient respiratory murmur. Was given assurance by a negative tuberculin test, by which relinquishment of position was avoided. Recovery ensued through better care.

I have used the test satisfactorily in still other cases, but those described represent conditions in which it proved an essential aid to prompt and precise diagnosis, therefore seeming especially justified. Other circumstances under which it was proposed as suitable, but was rejected by the patients, mostly through interference by other physicians, include a case of hæmorrhage, possibly pulmonary, but lacking in positive physical signs; one of early circumscribed dry pleuritis, in the person of a young physician, whose life might have been saved by a timely demonstration of tuberculosis; another of circumscribed dry pleuritis of one month's duration, with pain and friction sounds, all of which disappeared in a week under counter-irritation and sodium salicylate, leaving the fundamental cause in doubt; and one of tuberculous family history, with rapid pulse and normal temperature, with ratio of chest perimeter to height and corpulence reduced, but without other rational or physical signs, except slight cog-wheel respiration, and perhaps a trifle more than relative dulness at the right apex.

The test quantity of tuberculin is usually stated at ·005, although the first dose should be less, in order to provide against a supersensitiveness or extreme debility of the patient.   In this precaution lies the element of safety.   The fact that hypodermic syringes are not usually graduated in the metric system has deterred some from using the test.   A simple method is to prepare afresh at each injection, a 2½ per cent. aqueous solution of Koch's old tuberculin, of which one minim, representing approximately ·0015, may be the initial dose for a debilitated person, or two minims, representing ·003 for one of good size and strength.   Failing to obtain a positive reaction, the test is repeated after three days, being trebled in the first instance, that is, 3 minims injected, representing ·0045, or doubled in the second instance, that is 4 minims injected, representing ·006.   Thus a conclusion is reached by two injections.   The reaction consists of a rise of temperature of about 2 degrees in from five to twenty-four hours, supplemented usually by malaise, slight chilliness, and increased cough, which all subside within twenty-four to thirty-six hours.

Is the tuberculin test always decisive?   If one were compelled to answer by an unqualified yes or no, it must be admitted that there are variable factors, such as special susceptibility, exceptional resistance, habituation to toxines, and even a close similarity of other pathologic processes to tuberculosis, which are capable of precluding absolute accuracy of results. Since Koch's description*** of a typical reaction in himself by an injection of ·25, it is known to be merely a matter of sufficiently large dose to cause any person, either normal, indifferently ill, or tuberculous, to exhibit a characteristic general reaction.   In the non-tuberculous, as a rule, the dose must considerably exceed ·01, while the special affinity of tuberculin for tuberculous tissue, causes a reaction to be elicited by a dose under ·01, usually ·005, or less.   It is conceivable that in exceptional instances a natural supersensitiveness towards tuberculin might be found, just as certain persons are extraordinarily impressionable by cocaine, turpentine, quinine, &c.; but while such a heightened susceptibility might underlie a very small percentage of errors, it cannot be made to account for 8††† or 9 per cent. of reactions, said to have been produced in healthy persons. The most reasonable explanation of this large discrepancy lies in the recollection that autopsies disclose previously unsuspected foci of tuberculosis in even a larger proportion, and that the bulk of the 8 or 9 per cent. therefore were tuberculous.

Practically, heightened susceptibility is less apt to vitiate the results, for the reason that the test with reference to pulmonary and laryngeal conditions is needed only when it is a question of incipient, latent, or unpronounced tuberculosis, in which the patient, not being habituated to large quantities of the toxine already generated in the body, reacts to quite small test doses. For the same reason it is readily appreciated, that in advanced tuberculous toxæmia, reactions are excited only by large doses, with corresponding lessened safety and dubious results. In such cases the test is not commended, and should be but rarely required.

The course of events in the limited series of cases herewith described, tends to support the decisive character of the test, but a demonstration from any human statistics is obviously impossible. Verification by autopsy is the only universal proof, hence the value of bovine records. The Illinois State Board of Live Stock Commissioners§§§ in a synopsis for the year 1899, shows the smallest percentage of errors yet attained. Of 3,655 cattle officially tested, 560 were condemned, of which all but eight were found tuberculous at a careful, but ordinary macroscopic autopsy, and of these, three had given only partial reactions, thus reducing the actual failures to five, or less than 1 per cent. Eight other cows which had failed to react to tuberculin were killed, on account of actinomycosis, mammitis, &c., and found free from tuberculosis. The latter is a small number, but as far as it goes, it tends to substantiate the negative value of the test. But it is argued, man suffers from other diseases not present in cattle, which are said to react to tuberculin, notably syphilis and lepra. Additional evidence that this allegation concerning syphilis is correct, has just been presented by E. O. Otis.‖‖‖ It is true that tuberculosis exists not rarely in conjunction with syphilis, yet the proportion of reactions in syphilis is too large for this explanation to be complete. One must therefore otherwise exclude syphilis, in case of positive reaction, from tuberculin. An imperfect reaction is said to occur in certain cases of sarcoma and carcinoma, but the same liability to the coexistence of tuberculosis should be remembered. Lepra is closely related to tuberculosis, and a reaction in it, which is said to occur, would seem not unreasonable.

REFERENCES.

* R. H. Babcock.
† E. F. Wells, *Medical News*, September 21, 1895.
‡ H. P. Loomis, *Medical Record*, December 10, 1898.
§ B. Frankel, *Berliner Klin. Woch.*, March 19, 1900.
‖ Trudeau, *Medical News*, May 29, 1897.
¶ Beck, *Deutsche Med. Wochenschrift*, February 23, 1899.
** Klebs, *Boston Med. and Surg. Journ.*, August 5, 1897 ; reprint.
†† *Journ. Am. Med. Assoc.*, October 28, 1898.
‡‡ *Chicago Med. Journ. and Examiner.*
§§ *Cincinnati Lancet Clinic*, 1897 ; cited by Anders, *New York Med. Journ.*, June 23, 1900.
‖‖ J. M. Anders, *New York Med. Journ.*, June 23, 1900.
*** R. Koch, *Deutsche Medicinische Wochenschrift*, 1890, No. 46a ; 1891, No. 3 and 43 ; cited by Frankel, *loc. cit.*
††† Guttstadt (quoted by Trudeau), cited by Anders, *New York Med. Journ.*, June 23, 1900.
§§§ Bulletin No. 1, Series of 1900, Tuberculosis and the Tuberculin Test by the State Board of Live Stock Commissioners of Illinois, Springfield, March 29, 1900.
‖‖‖ See page 121.

DISCUSSION.

Dr. REED : Eight years ago, when I was practising in Thomasville, Georgia, and later in Atlantic City, I had much experience with this agent, but I was led to abandon it because of the wide-spread and unreasoning prejudice against it by the profession. I am very glad to see that with the lapse of time this feeling has become much less, and that now there is a largely increasing opinion in favour of the use of tuberculin diagnostically. I would like to ask whether these gentlemen have seen any reaction to tuberculin in the fever which is occasionally found in hysteria? I have an indistinct recollection of having read that such has been observed.

Dr. BALDWIN : I have very little to say because I think the tuberculin question is still in the experimental stage, and I do not feel quite ready to say very much about the work we are doing in that line. I am very much interested in the limitations of tuberculin, and until we get something better as a diagnostic agent, there are certainly some cases that would seem worth testing with tuberculin, although we do not see very many in the Adirondacks in which we need tuberculin to make the diagnosis. In regard to the reactions in hysteria, I might answer that question in one way. On several occasions there were patients who had symptoms of tuberculosis but no physical signs, and they were thought by some physicians to have hysteria· In one or two instances, instead of using the tuberculin Dr. Kinghorn gave them first a dose of salt solution, and in one case simply a dose of the carbolic acid solution used to dilute the tuberculin. In one instance he found a temperature of 99½ degrees in a patient who had previously a normal temperature. It showed enough of the influence of expectancy on the part of the patient to give a slight reaction ; but still I do not think the real tuberculin reaction, which is very pronounced, could be obtained in a hysterical patient unless a very large dose was given. In the work we are doing at Saranac I have endeavoured this winter to determine two or three things by experiments on animals. The first was : What is the earliest day on which the reaction can be obtained after the infection of the patient? That is a difficult point to determine in the human being, but experimentally we can determine it, and at present it seems probable that the reaction may occur within a few days after infection, but is more likely to occur uniformly about the twelfth to the fifteenth day. We know that that is about the time necessary for the infection to become an actual tubercle. Another point to determine was how long after the removal of a tuberculous focus by surgical or other methods would the susceptibility to tuberculin remain ? In several experiments in this connection rabbits were inoculated in the eye, and after the disease had become pretty well advanced they were tested with tuberculin. They all showed the reactive power, and then, while a number of these rabbits were taken as controls, a certain number had the eye enucleated so as to remove every particle of tuberculous tissue so far as possible. At the end of two weeks, upon testing these rabbits, it was found that they failed to give any reaction. I do not consider this as conclusive, but it points to the possibility that removal of the infected tissues soon removes the susceptibility to tuberculin. This has an important bearing upon surgical tuberculosis, as where joints or bones are to be operated. There are several other questions that might interest us, and I wish I were in the position to answer them positively: for instance, whether the tuberculin reaction indicates whether the bacillus is alive or dead? whether the bacillus is encapsulated or not? Those are questions that may be determined with some degree of accuracy by experiments on animals. A great deal of our clinical work is useless until we can get more sound pathological knowledge in regard to the reaction of tuberculin.

Dr. BOWDITCH: Two or three years ago Dr. Klebs gave us a very interesting paper at Boston on this question, and at that time I had to take a position which I thought myself was ultraconservative. I announced that I had never used it for diagnostic purposes in tuberculosis because I had such a repugnance to it. Although I still have that feeling of repugnance, I have changed my position somewhat, feeling that possibly I was carrying my prejudice too far, and to the detriment of the patient. I have used it in forty cases at the Rutland Sanatorium, where I felt that the circumstances of apparent doubt in diagnosis justified it. In three of these cases, however, I believe that I made a great blunder in discharging them because of a lack of reaction to 10 milligrammes of Dr. Trudeau's tuberculin. There was a lack of definite physical signs in these cases, and yet their general symptoms were such as to make them probably tubercular not long after discharge. One of these patients spat up bloody sputum and had symptoms of incipient disease, and the others I feel should have remained longer because their general symptoms were suspicious. I mention these cases now simply because I think it is well to emphasise the fact that even when we do not get a reaction with 10 milligramme doses we cannot safely conclude that that patient is without tuberculosis. I should like to mention an interesting fact with reference to the use of another substance in the same cases. My assistant at Rutland, Dr. H. B. Dunham, used theobromine with salicylate of sodium, and secured exactly similar results to tuberculin in several cases. Some were negative, but those that were positive to tuberculin were also positive to theobromine.

Dr. KLEBS: I was very much interested in these two papers, and think they are most valuable, because any additional help we can get in diagnosing tuberculosis we should be grateful for. I agree fully with Dr. Baldwin in regard to the rarity of the cases in which we need to use it, but in those few cases it is of the utmost value to the patient and to the physician. It is also of great value to us to know in what other diseases we can get a tuberculin reaction, and I think the contribution Dr. Otis gives us in regard to reaction in syphilis is most important. There is still a great difference of opinion as to what constitutes a reaction, and I can repeat the same opinion I expressed three years ago; that it depends very much on the preparation used. Dr. Bowditch spoke of using the preparation of Dr.

Trudeau. He did not tell us what sort of reaction occurred in the theobromine tests. It is important to know exactly what constitutes the reaction because, as Dr. Baldwin points out, 2 degrees of temperatuie may follow the use of salt solution. We must have a more decided reaction, at least 2 degrees I should say to constitute the reaction.

Dr. BOWDITCH : When our results were under 1 degree it was not considered positive, but in most of the instances it did not exceed 2½ degrees.

Dr. KLEBS: That is very interesting indeed, and should lead to further investigation.

Dr. BALDWIN : I would like to say in connection with Dr. Bowditch's remarks about theobromine, that I have been trying to find out what other substances would produce this reaction. I have not experimented upon human subjects, and animals do not seem to be so susceptible to these other substances. It has been found that many animal and vegetable albuminous substances have been known to produce quite a marked and similar reaction to that of tuberculin. Pilocarpine is one of the substances that seems to produce such a reaction. It has been noticed both clinically and experimentally that the reactions are similar in kind but not in degree. Intestinal intoxication, produced in the course of an indigestion, may produce in a tuberculous patient the typical symptoms of a tuberculin reaction, and to my mind it is not improbable that the reactions spoken of may be due to the absorption of some of these poisonous substances from the intestine.

Dr. SOLLY : I would like to ask if the doctor has made any experiments in the line of tuberculin causing reactions in other affections, such as influenza?

Dr. BALDWIN : I can only answer that by saying that I have tried experiments with some diseases in animals, but I cannot yet state very accurately what the results are.

Dr. QUIMBY : Koch's original statement regarding tuberculin was that it caused death of living tubercle tissue, and from this I formulated for myself the theory that the fever of this reaction is analogous to that which we get whenever there is death of tissue in the body, that is, that it is the fever of a necrosis. Dr. Otis' report that the same thing occurs in syphilis seems to bear out this theory. A peculiar clinical fact that I have noticed bearing on the point is that the reaction has seemed to be more acute and produced with smaller doses in that class of patients in whom the process was acute or progressing rapidly, showing that the tissue was ready to be killed by a small amount of tuberculin. It seems to me that we can tell by the amount of reaction the rapidity with which the process is likely to go on. I would like to ask if Dr. Otis noticed any relation of the kind?

Dr. NEWTON : I would like to ask if theobromine does not produce the same reaction in healthy subjects.

Dr. BOWDITCH : In several cases in which we used it there was no reaction whatever?

Dr. BALDWIN : It is well known in experimental therapeutics that this is largely a question of doses, and that most of these alkaloids will produce the reaction in healthy subjects if you give enough of it.

Dr. OTIS : I am very glad to hear it said that the profession is showing a greater willingness to use tuberculin with less apprehension of untoward results. My investigations, however, would seem to show that it has its limitations. As Dr. Bowditch says, in certain cases which he was convinced were tuberculous, it did not show the reaction ; but as time goes on it is to be hoped that we shall have more definite knowledge of the proper doses to give, and then I trust the results will be more exact and certain, and we shall use it more frequently. In regard to Dr. Reed's question concerning hysteria, I have not seen such a reaction ; I have never happened to have a case that would enable me to answer that question. In regard to the cases of syphilis which I reported, of course it is possible that they may have had latent tuberculosis, but there was no evidence of it, and I feel convinced that a certain number of cases of syphilis will react, but what the number is and what conditions of syphilis react we do not yet know.

Dr. CASSELBERRY : I wish to say, and I think Dr. Otis will agree with me, that we are pleased, as the writers of these papers, to have brought forth such an interesting discussion and such valuable information from Drs. Bowditch and Baldwin.

THE ASSOCIATION OF TUBERCULOSIS AND SYPHILIS.

BY FREDERICK I. KNIGHT, M.D.

BOSTON.

" SYPHILIS is not infrequently a predisposing cause to pulmonary tuberculosis. To regulate prostitution, and thus diminish the danger of venereal infection, by humane, but strict laws, must of necessity become a portion of the public prophylaxis of consumption."*

" I believe that in the future an inoculation will be made of a vaccine of syphilis, which is amenable to treatment, in order to save the human race from the terrible malady phthisis, which is decimating it."†

Ever since the two diseases have been known, the belief has been well-nigh universal, as stated by Landouzy, that among the infectious associations there is none worse, none more formidable than the combination of syphilis and tuberculosis. The second of the above quotations shows that at present there is at least some doubt about the truth of this belief.

Before the discovery of the tubercle bacillus, the diagnosis between pure syphilis and tuberculosis of the lung was difficult, and syphilitic patients who developed an affection of the lung were usually considered to have consumption, to which they

---

* Knopf, " Pulmonary Tuberculosis," Philadelphia, 1899.

† Pourtalis, *Bericht über den Kongress zur Bekämpfung der Tuberculose als Volkskrankheit*, Berlin, 1899.

had been predisposed by syphilis. Hiller,‡ however, has shown by analysis of eighty-seven such cases, with autopsies, that fifty-eight of them were cases of pure syphilis, and twenty-nine cases were doubtful (either pure tuberculosis or a combination of syphilis with tubercle or cancer). Even now with the presence of the tubercle bacillus in the sputum, it does not necessarily follow that the pulmonary lesions are due to tubercle rather than syphilis, and I have no doubt that in many syphilitic cases which have developed pulmonary signs, anti-specific treatment has been abandoned for simple supporting treatment, to the everlasting detriment of the patient, who has succumbed, oftentimes unnecessarily, to so-called consumption. Neisser, of Breslau, at a meeting of the section of Dermatology and Syphilography, of the last International Medical Congress, in August, 1900,§ said that he believed that if syphilis very often complicated tuberculosis, it is because it is not properly treated. He said that he had never seen anti-syphilitic treatment aggravate tuberculosis. There is no doubt that the local lesions of syphilis in the respiratory tract offer an easy entrance to tubercular infection, as in the case of Renzi,‖ who reports a primary tuberculosis of the larynx in a syphilitic subject, or that the lesions of the two diseases may go on in the same body, as shown by the autopsies reported by Hiller, and by the clinical reports of many observers. Cases in which the two diseases have been observed in the larynx at the same time have been reported by J. D. Arnold,¶ Helmes,* Irsai,† and others, and are of special interest.

‡ *Charité Annalen*, ix., s. 184.

§ *La Presse Medicale*, September 15, 1900.

‖ " Revista clinica e terapeutica," Fasc, 10, 1886, *Centralblatt für Laryngologie, &c.*, Band iii., s. 344.

¶ *Pacific Medical and Surgical Journal and Western Lancet*, vol. xxxi., p. 70, February, 1888.

* Inaugural Diss., Leipzig, 1890, *Monatsschrift für Pract. Dermatologie*, Band xiii., s. 77.

† *Pest. Med. Chir. Pr.*, 1891, No. 46.

Whether the one pathological process may under any circumstances, or in any stage of either disease, exert an inhibitory influence upon the other, is a question worthy of consideration. The inhibitory influence of one of the infectious diseases of childhood upon another, is a matter of common belief. Guidone[‡] says that tubercular infection of the lungs after syphilis runs a rapid course, and that it seems as if the syphilis which preceded the tuberculosis, loses in virulence, and becomes latent. Jacquinet[§] studies the evolution of pulmonary tuberculosis in syphilitics, and concludes that if syphilis supervenes in individuals already afflicted with pulmonary tuberculosis, it aggravates the latter, and hastens its progress. If, on the contrary, tuberculosis supervenes in a case of syphilis, it behaves in two different ways. It develops very rapidly if the syphilis is in the secondary stage, while on the other hand, it pursues a slow, sluggish course, if the syphilis is in the tertiary stage. Bernheim,[||] from a study of clinical reports of forty-three cases, among other conclusions, says that the progress of this morbid association varies when a consumptive contracts syphilis, as contrasted with a case in which a syphilitic contracts consumption. The influence of the syphilitic infection of a patient who has tuberculosis depends upon the stage of the tuberculosis. This influence is almost unnoticeable in the " pre-tubercular " stage, and in patients in the first stage, whose general condition is excellent. The effect is, on the contrary, deplorable in tuberculous patients weakened by excess or the ravages of the disease (tuberculosis).

If syphilis supervenes in a case of outspoken tuberculosis, the latter may or may not be aggravated. Stieffel relates the

‡ Rif. Med., 1893. No. 230, *Monatsschrift für Pract. Dermatologie,* Band xviii., s. 294.

§ *Thèse de Doctorat,* Paris, 1895 ; *L'Union Med.,* 1895, p. 263.

|| Thirteenth International Congress, *Journal of Tuberculosis,* October, 1900 ; *Journal des Maladies Cutanées et Syphilitiques,* October, 1900 ; and *Journal of Tuberculosis,* April, 1901.

case of a woman who had coughed for four years. She contracted syphilis, and immediately became worse; she could not
tolerate anti-syphilitic regimen, and soon succumbed to phthisis.
Bernheim thinks it a rule, with but few exceptions, that in confirmed phthisis the supervention of syphilis has an aggravating
influence. When tuberculosis attacks a syphilitic subject in the
primary or second period, the prognosis is very grave. Jacquinet, Stieffel, Pidoux, Galliard, Fabry, and others, have
reported observations which bear out this claim. Thus, Fabry
saw a case of hybrid ulceration of the penis, which could have
been nothing else than a tuberculous syphilitic chancre. The
inguinal bubo which accompanied this lesion suppurated, and
Koch's bacillus was found in the pus. Secondary syphilis
developed with great violence, and at the same time both lungs
were attacked by subacute tuberculosis, and the patient lived
but a few weeks. The course is milder in the tertiary period.
This mildness is due more to the sclerotic tendency of that
period than to the exhaustion of the syphilitic virus. Specific
medication is badly tolerated by the tuberculous syphilitic in the
first two stages of syphilis, but it is necessary to surround the
patient with excellent hygienic conditions, and to administer to
him hypodermically a salt of mercury in small doses, repeated
at distant intervals. It will be noticed that this author agrees
with Jacquinet in the slower progress of tuberculosis engrafted
on a syphilitic subject in the third stage of the disease. The
editor of the *Journal of Tuberculosis*, points out that Bernheim
goes too far in denying the existence of antagonism between
infectious diseases, as Mauriac and others have reported numerous instances of the radical cure of tertiary syphilitic lesions by
erysipelas, a streptococcus infection akin to that which com-
plicates advanced phthisis.

In recent years some reports of cases have been published,
both in this country and in Europe, with the purpose of showing
that syphilis has a beneficent action on the course of tuber-

culosis: R. Abrahams¶ reports the case of a Pole, aged 35, who had come to this country about five years before Dr. Abrahams' report, in excellent health. After working in a coal mine for a year he contracted a cough, which was followed by profuse hæmorrhage. He showed marked signs and symptoms of pulmonary tuberculosis, with tubercle bacilli in the sputum. He improved somewhat under creasote, though the lesion in the lung remained unaltered. He contracted syphilis. Well-marked secondary symptoms followed. He received fifty mercurial inunctions. Very often iodide of sodium was added, and was continued occasionally afterwards. He also took some cod liver oil. The syphilitic symptoms vanished under this treatment ; but what was more wonderful was that from the very start of the evolution of the secondary period, and all along through this energetic specific treatment, all the symptoms of consumption disappeared, the physical signs also disappeared, and the sputa failed to show bacilli. The patient returned to Poland, and has occasionally reported that he was enjoying the best of health.

F. W. Ross* reports the case of a young man who came to him in 1886, with incipient pulmonary tuberculosis, attended with hæmorrhages. A year in the pine woods of Michigan arrested the disease. He returned apparently well. About a year later there were more hæmorrhages, cough, sputa, night-sweats, and all the physical signs of pulmonary tuberculosis. In December, 1888, he acquired syphilis, had secondary symptoms, and was put upon mercurial inunctions and iodides. Dr. Ross was in despair, but to his surprise, the pulmonary symptoms began to improve ; all symptoms ceased gradually. He had constant anti-syphilitic treatment for about one and a-half years. When this report was made, seven years and a-half after the initial lesion of syphilis, the patient was well and healthy.

¶ *New York Med. Record*, December 28, 1895.
* *Ibid.*, February 15, 1896.

Pourtalis[†] reports upon twelve cases, which he had seen in fifteen years, of the grafting of syphilis upon phthisical patients. All of these patients had symptoms of the second stage of phthisis more or less marked. They all improved, and the disease was finally arrested, as if completely cured. The same author reports[‡] the case of a student, whose studies were constantly interrupted by symptoms of phthisis, cough, night-sweats, hectic, hæmorrhages, &c. No physical signs are given, and it was before the discovery of the tubercle bacillus. After a serious hæmoptysis, this young man gave up his studies and went into the country. There he acquired syphilis, and immediately began to improve. As the syphilis developed his general condition improved; he felt stronger, more tranquil, gayer; and, as if by magic, the characteristic cough, the night-sweats, and the evening fever, all improved, and finally disappeared. He resumed his studies, and has been in active practice for nineteen years. Pourtalis also reports details of four other cases. Whether these are included in the twelve mentioned above I do not know, as the details of the latter were not given in the report of the Congress at Berlin. I will make an abstract of the first two cases, in both of which the improvement was striking.

CASE I.—A man, aged 36, with advanced phthisis, bacilli in sputum; he had severe attacks of dyspnœa several times daily. He came to Pourtalis with a history of syphilis of eight months' duraton, with which he was quite contented, as he said that since he had had the chancre he was relieved of all his symptoms except hoarseness. Examination of sputum showed no bacilli, though three previous reports which he brought did show them. Under specific treatment he regained his voice, and appeared strong and well.

† *Bericht über Kongress zur Bekämfung der Tuberculose als Volskrank-heit*, Berlin, 1899.

‡ *Zeitschrift fur Tuberculose und Heilstättenwesen*, vol. i., pp. 112, 199.

CASE 2.—A man, aged 47, whose three brothers and one sister died of consumption; had cough at the age of 23, expectoration, and fever, diarrhœa, &c. Was said to be phthisical, and sent abroad. He spent the winter in Egypt without improvement. On his return he acquired syphilis in Geneva. All the symptoms of phthisis began to improve, and the cough, fever, and sputa disappeared, and he grew strong. He was treated for syphilis nine months, returned to Constantinople, and married. His wife had two miscarriages, one still-born child, and one living child, with marks of hereditary syphilis. The father is stout and well, except for general arterio-sclerosis. Pourtalis' conclusions are as follows:—

(1) Syphilis engrafted on a phthisical patient arrests the progress of the phthisis.

(2) Syphilis engrafted on a phthisical patient becomes of a mild type.

(3) The antagonism of the bacteria of syphilis and phthisis should cause their toxines to neutralise each other.

(4) When the bacterium of syphilis is discovered and cultivated, and its toxines obtained, a serum may be obtained by inoculation with which consumptives may be rendered immune and cured.

(5) We believe that the inoculation of the blood serum of patients in the third stage of syphilis may be of much benefit to the phthisical.

M. I. Monteverdi§ observed a case in which syphilis infection, far from aggravatng the pre-existing pulmonary tuberculosis, appeared to have determined its rapid and complete cure. It concerned a young man in whom the existence of bacillary lesions at the summit of one lung could not be doubted. He had dulness under one clavicle, cough, nummular sputa, containing Koch's bacilli, hæmoptysis and night-sweats. He acquired syphilis, and from the moment its manifestations

§ *Gazz. degli. Osped.*, July 30, 1899 ; *La Semaine Med.*, 1899, p. 281.

appeared, the symptoms of pulmonary tuberculosis began to retrocede. The fever diminished, and finally disappeared; night-sweats ceased, as did the cough. The sputum lost its purulent character, became simply mucous, and bacilli could no longer be detected in it. The general condition and physical signs of the lesion at the apex improved simultaneously, and soon the patient could be considered cured. Six years have passed, and the cure persists.

These cases, with one exception, could apparently be roughly classified in the second stage of the tuberculosis. One case was advanced. All are said to have improved at once and rapidly on the manifestation of the secondary symptoms of syphilis.

Of course it is not to be expected that these few cases, though supported by very strong opinions on the part of their reporters, will do more than to cause a more careful observation of cases of combined tuberculosis and syphilis, and it is for this purpose that I bring the subject before the Association. To be of the greatest value, such cases should be studied and recorded with this special object in view. In my own personal experience I can recall comparatively few cases of the combined diseases, and the notes I have—not being taken with the object of studying this association in view—are not of much value for the elucidation of this question; but those that I do recall have pursued a decidedly chronic course, attended with signs of fibrosis of the lungs, which is regarded as one of the conservative agencies in arresting pulmonary tuberculosis, and in producing which, it is possible in these cases that syphilis was a factor. I have under my care at the present time a young gentleman, who, in the early summer of 1896, contracted syphilis, and during the next year acquired tuberculosis. According to Bernheim, the prognosis in this case was very grave, but its history has been a quiet one, seldom attended with fever or other serious symptoms. He came to me in the early autumn of 1897, with the history of many colds, with cough, in the previous winter, and one attack of " grippe " in the spring, which confined him to the house for two weeks. He had had cough off and on ever since. He had lost flesh. He had no signs of consolidation of lung, but had moist râles under both clavicles, extending in the left front as low as the fourth rib. The sputum showed fairly numerous tubercle bacilli in every field, and some elastic fibres. On inspecting the throat I noticed an ulceration of one tonsil and pillar of the palate, when I was informed that the patient had contracted syphilis fifteen months before, and had given up treatment for about two months as cured. He was put upon mixed treatment, and immediately began to gain. He kept up specific treatment for a year longer without any inconvenience. He spent a year and a half away from business, one year of it in Colorado. When I saw him in June, 1899, he reported that there had not been much cough or expectoration for three months. Pulse 88; temperature 98·4 degrees a.m.; weight 151½ lbs., ten pounds more than at the time of leaving for the West. There was now dulness at top of left lung to third rib, with some moist râles to nipple. Moist râles here and under right clavicle. There certainly has been ard kept at it until last December (1900), when being tired out, and the cough increasing, he went West for another winter. He remained away till May of this year. Examination on his return showed pulse 92; temperature 98·6 degrees. Fibrosis of left upper lobe as shown by flatness on percussion, with feeble bronchial respiration and bronchophony. Some moist râles here and under right clavicle. There certainly has been no virulence in the development of this case.

There is at least some reason to believe that other diseases, which tend to produce fibrosis, as, for example, acute rheumatism, are more or less antagonistic to the development of pulmonary tuberculosis. May the same possibly be true of syphilis.

DISCUSSION.

Dr. ELSNER : Unfortunately I did not hear the first part of Dr. Knight's paper. We must agree with his conclusions. A thorough study of the cases seen in private and hospital practice shows a surprisingly small percentage in which tuberculosis and syphilis have been associated. It is true that in some of our cases the syphilitic infection may have remained unrecognised. It is equally surprising and interesting to note how few cases of judicially treated syphilis finally develop tuberculosis where there is no preceding diathesis. Tuberculous patients who contract syphilis do badly as a rule ; this is particularly true of alcoholics. The combination of tuberculosis, syphilis and alcoholism is unfavourable because of the rapid disorganisation and degeneration of the invaded tissues. Mixed infection does not long postpone the end. The disease runs a rapid course in tuberculous subjects past fifty years of age who contract syphilis. In these cases the lung tissue seems to melt away.

A case of tuberculosis which was sent to Saranac, in which syphilis was suspected, did well on climatic and anti-syphilitic treatment. Tubercle bacilli originally found have disappeared. After between five and six years, the disease at the apex can only be recognised by an abnormally high pitched note.

The study of the literature of this subject is remunerative. In Nothnagel's recent work, two cases are quoted in which the reporters believed that the syphilitic infection exerted a favourable influence when grafted upon the tuberculous. This has not been my experience.

The subject introduced by Dr. Knight opens a field for future study and investigation.

Dr. CURTIN : I have been very much interested in this paper as the subject is an important one, and I have seen a great number of cases of tuberculosis associated with syphilis in the Philadelphia Hospital. I have observed, in the twenty-one years that I have been on duty there, that tuberculosis when engrafted on a case of syphilis and specifically treated has generally a slow progress, but when the syphilis is secondary to the tuberculosis during the active period, the progress is apt to be extremely rapid. I have also noticed that the secondary symptoms are very apt to be mild when tuberculosis is engrafted upon syphilis, and the nervous symptoms are very apt to be more marked than in simple tuberculosis.

In 1884 I read a paper before this Association on the influence of sea air upon syphilitic phthisis, and reported a number of cases that were benefited by going to sea. Now we know that tuberculous cases as a rule are not benefited by an ocean climate, but these cases were immediately benefited, and both diseases were held in abeyance while they were at sea, but as soon as they began to live inland the diseases again progressed with their former rapidity.

Dr. SOLLY : I would like to speak of my impressions concerning syphilis and tuberculosis. They agree with what Dr. Curtin has said, that if the syphilis

comes before the tuberculosis it appears to make the latter slower in its progress, but if the syphilis comes after tuberculosis it makes the latter more
severe and rapid. We see some interesting cases occasionally in Colorado of
throat affections in the tuberculous who are also syphilitic. The appearances
are sometimes misleading, and it is only by the use of iodides that you can
tell what you have to deal with. I have had one case of what resembled a
syphilitic tuberculosis at the top of one lung, with very high fever, and he
became perfectly well under anti-syphilitic treatment, except for a dulness
at the top of the lung. There was another case where a man had evidently
a gumma in his lung which would occasionally break down, with high fever
and expectoration of pus, in which there were no bacilli ; that is, the pus
brought up at the time contained no bacilli, although he had bacilli in his
sputum at ordinary times. He was a tuberculous patient with syphilis, his
father had syphilis and he had two sisters who were tuberculous and presented signs of syphilis. They were all benefited by anti-syphilitic treatment
as well as tuberculous treatment, but one developed exophthalmic goitre
and did not live long.

Dr. BALDWIN : I would like to mention an incident that occurred in my
experience. A physician told me that he had advised two young men, who
were sons of a tuberculous father, to acquire syphilis as a precaution against
tuberculosis, and he asked whether I had had any experience with such
cases. Neither of these men developed tuberculosis, but they acquired
syphilis. The physician was a much older man than myself, and I could
not say all I thought, but I told him that statistics were all against the
position he had taken, and I advised him to treat his patients with anti-
syphilitic treatment.

Dr. NEWTON : I would like to give my personal impression that syphilis,
which is so frequently characterised by extreme anæmia, is likely to pre-
dispose to almost any disease. Having served my time in the New York
City Hospital, where practically everybody, except a few favoured members
of the house staff, was syphilitic, I concluded that the tendency of syphilis
is to render the character of other diseases worse.

Dr. ROBINSON : I would cite the history of a family of three children
with inherited syphilis, which did not develop until after twelve years of age.
The treatment was continuous, but one of the sons, aged 18, developed
tuberculosis and died ; a daughter, now aged 23, has been under anti-syphilitic
treatment for ten years, but developed tuberculosis a few months ago, and
is now dying ; and the older daughter now has symptoms of consolidation
at the apex of the left lung.

Dr. FISK : In Denver, whether because we have a large number of young
men under observation, or from whatever cause, it seems to me we meet
the association of tuberculosis and syphilis frequently. I have seen many
cases myself, and a physician here tells me that he has seen four cases in
the last nine months. Personally I always feel relief in my tuberculous cases
suffering with syphilis when I find that the tuberculosis was engrafted on
the syphilis. I have in mind cases of rapid tubercular affections, where

the patient was pulled down by syphilis beforehand, that have yielded well to specific treatment, and I now recall a case of hæmorrhage with consolidation of the left apex where, as soon as I found that the patient was syphilitic I put him on treatment and the case healed rapidly. I remember a case, with an affection of the knee-joint, which I supposed was rheumatic, others thought it tuberculous, but a diagnosis of syphilis having been made, and being treated accordingly, he got well at once. I have in mind cases in which the syphilis was engrafted on the tuberculosis, and in those, where the patient was very much pulled down by the first disease, he did not react well, but if he was in pretty good condition he got along first-rate. In other words, where tuberculosis is engrafted on syphilis, I look for good results, but where syphilis is engrafted on tuberculosis it has à bad effect, unless the patient had not been much pulled down by his lung trouble.

Dr. J. C. WILSON : I have not looked up this subject from the records, but I desire to state my impressions, in support of which I can recall a number of cases at this moment, that the development of pulmonary tuberculosis is not at all rare in young individuals during the secondary period of syphilis, and that in most all the cases I have seen in which this has occurred the course of the disease has been rapidly progressive to a fatal issue. I think we can all, perhaps, recall cases of young prostitutes who have developed tuberculosis in the early stages or secondary period of syphilis, in whom the tuberculous process has run a very rapid course.

With reference to the therapeutic test in the matter, it seems to me we cannot attach too much importance to the iodides, since a certain proportion of cases of pulmonary tuberculosis, especially those in which the administration of iodides is followed by improvement of nutrition, do well under this treatment in the absence of any syphilitic infection.

Dr. EDSON : I can remember a number of cases, two coming on the same day, in one of which the syphilis had antedated the development of tuberculosis some nine months, and in the other case the syphilis appeared at least six months after unmistakable evidence of active tubercular trouble. Unexpectedly the man whose syphilis antedated his tuberculosis has done very well. The other three cases have run, so far as I can see, a course which, with one exception, has been unaffected by the combination of diseases. One had involvement of the entire right lung and upper part of the left, but he has, to my surprise, run along better than I expected. One of the cases that has nasal and pharyngeal ulcerations from a very active syphilis, that came on six months after the tuberculous disease, improves so far as his nose is concerned, when put on mercurial treatment, though his cough and tubercular symptoms increase, but if I take him off this drug his general condition improves, but his nose and pharynx begin to break down at once. This man is in a very bad way.

A FOREIGN BODY IN THE AIR PASSAGES SIMULATING RAPID PHTHISIS.

BY JAMES B. WALKER, M.D.

PHILADELPHIA.

FOREIGN bodies in the air passages are neither rare nor unique. Medical literature, remote and recent, is full of accounts of such truants. Something further must exist to justify me in asking your attention to a single case. The cause of offence in my case was a water-melon seed. In this I cannot claim originality, for I find two other cases recorded of the same material, while the seeds of almost all fruits have figured in the various cases reported. Orange, plum, date, cherry, have contributed with their pips to harass the unwary swallower; while grains of corn, the bean and pea, head of grass, peanut shell, pieces of meat; while from the organic kingdom, and from the inorganic a list almost interminable can be given, including carpet tack, nail, dime, gold coin, half sovereign, half franc piece, flexible and silver tracheotomy tubes, &c.

The *time* elapsing between the ingress and egress of the offender in my case was two months. This is quite length enough to retain a foreign substance in one's bronchus, but it is short in comparison with many, whose records are open to investigation.

Jackson reports* a screw expelled after three years. An umbrella ferrule is reported impacted in left bronchus for two months. A silver tracheotomy tube, loosened from its holder,

---

* *Boston Med. and Surg. Journ.*, 1855.

lodged in left bronchus for seven weeks before its removal. A head of rye was found at an autopsy twelve years after its introduction. Bridge reports[†] the removal of a button three years after its introduction. Eldridge[‡] reports removal of a foreign body twenty-three years after. Henry H. Smith, of Philadelphia, successfully removed by tracheotomy a grain of corn which had remained seven weeks, and had commenced to germinate. Bartlett reports[§] a case of lodgment and retention of a foreign body in a bronchus for sixty years, with final spontaneous expulsion.

Curtin reported a case—which appears in our own *Transactions*—of a mutton bone, which gave rise to subsequent abscess in the lungs; and Hooker reports two cases with similar results.

The almost complete occlusion of the left primary bronchus, and the similarity of the resultant condition to acute phthisis, makes my case somewhat unique, though no doubt a more thorough search than I have been able to make would have unveiled cases resembling it.

A girl, aged $2\frac{1}{2}$ years, was brought to my attention early in October, 1900. She was suffering from a cough, which had existed for over a month, and was growing worse rapidly. The child was pale and emaciated, with a constant harassing cough, and occasional severe paroxysms, terminating in vomiting. She was feeding badly, and had rapidly changed from an exceedingly rosy and robust infant to her present emaciation. Her temperature on examination was 101·3 degrees F.; pulse feeble and quick, and respirations somewhat laboured. Physical examination of the chest revealed on palpation, râle fremitus over the entire left chest, and with inspection, greatly diminished expansion. Percussion revealed no areas of consolidation, nor appreciable reduction of resonance, nor elevation of note. Auscultation showed submucous râles and greatly diminished

† *New York Med. Record*, 1878.
‡ *Rhode Island Med. Soc. Proc.*, 1860.
§ *New York Med. Journ.*, 1846.

breath sounds : that which existed being simply feeble, without bronchial element. There was no sibilant nor musical note, as of air passing a constriction. The right side was normal, with exaggeration of mobility, &c.

The child was listless and apathetic, and at no time complained of pain, though happiest when lying in the crib or the mother's lap. The appetite was capricious, and the bowels usually constipated, alternating with looseness, with evidences of indigestion in the discharges from the bowels.

The mother had lost her mother, two brothers, and one sister, with pulmonary consumption, all running a rapid course.

The case resembled an attack of *la grippe*, which so often shows a unilateral bronchitis ; or an attack of acute phthisis, arising from disseminated tuberculosis, though its confinement to one side absolutely, with the other entirely free from signs of invasion, rendered this idea unlikely.

Inquiry as to the onset of the attack, revealed the following history : About the 1st of September, while the child was eating a piece of water-melon, it was seized with a choking and coughing spell, the child exclaiming that she had " swallowed " a seed. Inversion and slapping the back were at once resorted to, but the distress was not relieved. The mother hastened with the child to a near-by hospital, at which a mid-day dispensary was in progress, and related her story, when an effort, by the physician in attendance, was again made to dislodge the seed by gravity and succussion, without avail. She was dismissed with some medicine for the cough. A few days later another physician, calling in the neighbourhood, was asked to see the child, when he prescribed for the cough and dismissed it. Since then it has continued to grow worse, until I was shown it as I called on a sick relative living near.

I repeated the process of inversion and succussion without avail, and placing it on appropriate food and supporting measures, watched it. In the next two weeks it had gained some in strength, and ate better, but the physical condition of its lungs remained as before, and I about decided that the melon seed was but an incident, or perhaps an exciting cause, of what was now a tuberculous affection, and directed the mother to send me a sample of the sputum for examination. She was somewhat dilatory in doing this, and in a few days brought the child to my office, with the report that the previous day after a severe paroxysm of coughing, terminating in emesis, the child seemed to experience great relief, and was now breathing easily. On examination I found air entering the left lung freely, though the cough still existed, and some râles were present. The vomited matters had been searched for the missing seed, but none was found. The child now gained each day, and the trouble seemed at an end, though the cough remained. On November 3, another severe coughing occurred; emesis followed, and the seed was brought to light. The cough immediately ceased, and in a very short time the child became, and continues to be, a rollicking, round, rosy infant.

The first relief evidently displaced the seed without removing it; the last attack of emesis (Nov. 3) expelled it.

PIECE OF MEAT IN BRONCHUS; DISAPPEARANCE BY ABSORPTION; RECOVERY.

BY THOMAS W. HARVEY, M.D.

ORANGE, NEW JERSEY.

JOHN C., an American, aged 50; lawyer. Seen first on October 16, 1900. While eating his dinner, and attempting to swallow a piece of meat, he was suddenly seized with a fit of coughing and choking. This was so severe, that he felt certain that he was going to choke to death. After a few moments this sensation passed off, and except an almost continual cough, he had no further difficulty until the next day. He went to town in the morning of the next day, but his cough continuing and increasing in severity, he returned, and sent for me on the succeeding afternoon. He then had a constant cough, and so much dyspnœa that he could not lie down, even when asleep. His pulse was 100; temperature 100 degrees F.; and his respirations 40. Physical examination showed left side normal. Right side down to the level of the nipple gave normal pulmonary resonance and vesicular murmur. Below the level percussion gave a modified resonance, not marked enough to be called dulness, but less resonant than the upper part of the lung. One-inch internal to the nipple, and a little below, by auscultation could be heard a high pitched note, like a whistle; this was heard on inspiration. All over the lung, below the level of the nipple, could be heard sibilant and crepitant râles. For one week these symptoms continued. There was always moderate dyspnœa, but when the patient moved it became greatly exaggerated, but never spasmodic. The pulse varied from 90 to 100; the temperature 98·5 to 100·5 degrees; the respirations gradually sank to 20. The high-pitched musical ronchus at the border of the fifth rib disappeared about the tenth day, and normal vesicular resonance and murmur were restored over the entire lung by the sixteenth day.

Mr. C. was not able to lie down until about the tenth day, and during this time he had a harassing cough and a muco-purulent expectoration, nummular sputa usually floating on the water. This expectoration was examined carefully macroscopically for fragments of the meat, but none were found. The diagnosis of foreign body in the bronchus was based, however, upon the presence of the high-pitched rhonchus, a symptom which I had already observed in a previous case, where a part of a nut shell had lodged in the right bronchus, in the second division, heard over the third rib. In that case the nut shell was coughed up three weeks later through the larynx, after an unsuccessful attempt had been made to remove it by tracheotomy, and the tracheotomy wound had healed.

The question as to the fate of the piece of meat is an interesting one. In my previous case an abscess had formed around the foreign body, and when it was expectorated it was accompanied by about two ounces of pus. There had also been well-marked systemic infection until the abscess was evacuated, and a regular pneumonic process accompanied and followed these symptoms. Complete recovery, however, took place.

I had expected in the last case at least a local infection, with perhaps phthisis as a sequel, but the man has made a complete recovery. Poulet, in his classical work on the subject of foreign bodies, makes no mention of cases that recover, and my acquaintance with the literature of the subject does not help me to theorise on the subject. I suppose that the piece of meat, rendered sterile by cooking, was softened, digested, and absorbed, by the bronchial juices, or perhaps was expectorated in liquified state. I was prepared for several days to open the trachea on the first indication that the foreign body had become loose, and was free in the trachea, but I was not at the time willing to endeavour to extract such soft tissue from so deep a part of the lung as was indicated by the location of the ronchus.

A PLEA FOR AN ACCEPTED NOMENCLATURE WITH REFERENCE TO THE CLASSIFICATION OF PULMONARY TUBERCULOSIS.

PROPER DEFINITIONS OF THE TERMS FOLLOWING AS APPLIED TO PULMONARY TUBERCULOSIS.

(1) PRETUBERCULAR OR PREBACILLARY STAGE; (2) INCIPIENT STAGE; (3) MODERATELY ADVANCED STAGE; (4) FAR ADVANCED STAGE; (5) IMPROVED CONDITION; (6) ARRESTED CONDITION; (7) CURED OR APPARENTLY CURED CONDITION. .

BY DR. J. EDWARD STUBBERT.

LIBERTY, N.Y.

———

IT is not my intention to inflict upon you at this meeting a long paper, to explain theories or statistics; rather to lay before you a few statements showing the inaccuracy of statistics as compiled to-day by various observers in tuberculosis, with the hope that my few words will provoke a discussion which will lead to the adoption by this Society of certain fixed definitions, that may be accepted as the basis upon which all statistics must be built in order to enjoy the confidence of the profession at large, and especially to merit consideration by scientific observers. No one present, I believe, will doubt either the necessity for some positive and common· basis upon which to build statistics and compute results, or the fact that there is no society in this country or abroad, the scope of whose work, or the standing of its members, renders it capable of deciding the question before us.

While statistics are to an extent unreliable, we cannot dispense with them. All conclusions must be derived from them, and yet great confusion exists, not only in conclusions so drawn

II

by widely-separated observers, but among those intimately associated in work. In Massachusetts we find Bowditch and Otis widely divergent upon the definitions " cured," " apparently cured," or " arrested cases "; while in New York we find as wide a difference of opinion between Trudeau, Baldwin, and the writer, in defining the difference between " apparently cured " and " arrested cases." At the meeting of the Medical Board of the Loomis Sanitarium, held in New York, about three years ago, there were present: Doctors Polk, Loomis, A. A. Smith, Walker, Quimby, F. Miller, Chappell, Markoe, Beverley, Robinson, and the writer, and yet no two men held exactly the same opinion as to where the dividing lines should be drawn between the incipient and moderately advanced, or between the latter and the far-advanced stages of pulmonary tuberculosis.

There are, then, two conditions to be classified: (1) The condition of the patient when he comes under observation and treatment; (2) the condition that exists when he is discharged from the physician's care. Under the first heading we have to deal with three, and possibly four conditions: (b) Incipient; (c) moderately advanced; (d) far advanced; and as a possible fourth, but naturally preceding the others, (a) variously designated as the pretubercular or prebacillary stage.

By a large number of physicians, including such names as Baldwin, Trudeau, Knight, Babcock, Bowditch, and others, a pretubercular stage is not recognised, but accepted as a general dyscrasia, such as might precede the development of any infectious disease; or in other words, that would make infection possible. I find, however, that a few, namely, Baldwin, Babcock, Bowditch, Brown, and Janeway, will allow the term " prebacillary," while objecting to the term " pretubercular," although the majority do not think the term necessary. Another physician (Brown) considers the term "prebacillary" as synonymous with the incipient stage of tuberculosis; two others (Loomis and Ingals) see no difference in the meaning of the two terms.

The definition gathered from the different ideas is as follows: One in which tuberculosis is suspected, but where the symptoms are slight, and bacilli cannot be found in the expectoration. None, however, have suggested what name shall be given to moderately or far-advanced cases in which tubercle bacilli are present. Others again, notably Ingals and Hance, affirm their belief in a so-called pretubercular stage, which they define as follows: A condition in which the physical signs are indefinite, and in which there is loss of weight and strength, a rapid heart action, slight fluctuation in temperature, and sometimes a slight hacking cough.

In comparing notes on the definition of an *incipient case*, I find that Loomis, Trudeau, Knight, Babcock, Bowditch, Hance, and Ingals, agree in all essential points, the following being the general idea gained by such comparison: Slight physical signs of limited extent in one or both lungs, with or without bacilli in the sputum; with or without constitutional debility or complications.

Another authority (Hance) recognises such a stage only when bacilli are present together with the usual symptoms; and still another (Baldwin) claims that slight physical signs may be present or absent, provided the rational symptoms point to such a condition.

As to the definition of the term " moderately advanced," I find an agreement in the most important points in the opinions of Loomis, Baldwin, Trudeau, Hance, Knight, Babcock, and Brown. The definition is as follows: More or less well-marked constitutional symptoms with extensive signs in one or both lungs, or where there is only a slight amount of pulmonary involvement, but very severe rational signs.

Another noted physician (Bowditch) is more reserved, and does not allow the term if there is evidence of decided consolidation or cavity formation; while another (Ingals) relies solely on the extent of the physical signs.

There seems to be a general harmony in the definition of

the term "far-advanced," the composite idea being this: A far advanced case is one in which there are extensive physical signs, with or without cavity formation, and in which there is severe constitutional disturbance with or without complicatons.

Once we are finished with a patient, it becomes a question of even greater importance how to properly classify or index him. Shall we declare him "cured," "apparently cured," "arrested," or "improved"? Again we find a wide divergence of opinion among competent observers. Very few are willing to declare a patient cured until a considerable length of time has elapsed without the manifestations of any symptoms of the former disease. Ingals and Baldwin say they require a patient to pass at least two years free from all signs of disease, rational or physical. Another physician (Loomis) has the same require-ment except that no time limit is given. Brown, Hance, Trudeau, and Knight do not use the term; .Ingals and Bab-cock consider the term synonymous with that of "apparently cured." Bowditch classifies all such cases as "arrested." The term seems to be in disfavour with the majority of those whose opinions were received, while that of "apparently cured" seems to be the choice.

Probably the greatest difference exists in the definition of the term "apparently cured." Some observers, such as Brown, Trudeau, and Baldwin, place the time limit at three months— the writer at six months—while two others (Loomis and Hance) give no time limit; another one year; some others two or three years; and one (Babcock) considers the term as synony-mous with "arrested."

A composite definition, leaving out the question of time, would be absence of all rational symptoms of disease, and dis-appearance of nearly all physical signs, or only those that would be indicative of scar tissue. *Apropos* of this subject, I would like to submit the following statistics: Out of a number of cases at the Loomis Sanitarium, there was a reappearance of bacilli in seven cases after having been absent for three months; in three cases after having been absent for four months;

in three cases after an absence of five, six, and seven months respectively; and in one case after disappearing for three and a-half years. However, in this last case, it should in justice be stated. that the patient has never been free from a condition of chronic bronchitis since she was seven years of age.

Now we come to the term "an arrested case." Again, there is great confusion as to the exact meaning of the word. As to the time limit, Knight and Trudeau agree that a quiescent condition should exist for several months, while Babcock and Bowditch say months or years. Baldwin places the time limit at two or three months, while Ingals, Hance, and Loomis make no arbitrary rule.

As to the question of the presence of bacilli in the sputum, Brown, Babcock, Bowditch, Knight, and Ingals, claim that bacilli must be absent; while Loomis, Baldwin, Hance, and Trudeau, declare a case "arrested" while bacilli are still present, provided, of course, the general condition and physical signs justify such a term. A fair definition, compiled from the opinions of the majority, leaving out the question of time, would be absence of all constitutional symptoms, including cough and expectoration, and, therefore, bacilli; and physical signs show no further activity, although the limits of diseased areas may remain the same.

In regard to the last term to which I call your attention, namely, "improved," I am glad to say there is a very general agreement in this respect, a good idea being given by the following: Lessened symptoms, or signs improved (local or general), or both. The only point of difference noticed is that the majority require both local and general improvement; while a few require only an improvement in general condition. Special work among the tubercular has grown so rapidly during the past few years; sanitariums and hospitals for the care of these patients are multiplying so rapidly, it would seem not only wise but imperative, from a scientific standpoint, that now, before the machine becomes too unwieldy, and greater confusion has been created by lack of harmonious work, a more or less fixed definition of these various stages of pulmonary tuberculosis shall be determined upon. Then statistics from all recognised sources can be worked together harmoniously, and deductions of scientific value may be realised.

SUPPLEMENT.

Prebacillary or Pretubercular Stage.

The condition of an individual whose family history, personal appearance, physique, and age, experience has proven, in the majority of cases, antedate the active development of tuberculosis. This stage is generally marked by persistent chlor-anæmia, uncontrollable digestive disturbance, inexplainable rapid heart action, and progressive loss of weight.—Dr. Loomis.

Prebacillary, meaning " closed " or non-ulcerated tuberculosis, could include all cases described by certain writers as pretubercular, which, according to their own description, are nearly always already infected, and the symptoms clearly secondary to such infection. Prebacillary likely to confuse, as some very acute bad cases reveal bacilli; should prefer to use in a very narrow, restricted sense, or dispense with it altogether. Definition : No symptoms and no bacilli. " Pretubercular " stage not necessary.—E. R. Baldwin.

Not recognised.—E. L. Trudeau.

Terms synonymous. Definition : Slight hacking cough, with some langour and emaciation, but no expectoration, and no distinct physical signs.—E. Fletcher Ingals.

Pretubercular Stage.—Designates the time antecedent to that in which physical signs and microscopical examination indicate disease ; evidences of impaired health, loss of weight, strength, rapid heart action, slight fluctuation in temperature, general malaise, anæmia, &c.—I. W. Hance.

Does not think term should be used; not properly applicable to any infectious disease.—F. I. Knight.

No pretubercular stage. There may be a prebacillary stage, if by this term is meant a stage in which no bacilli are contained in the sputum, but if there is tuberculosis, there are certainly tubercles. Always supposed that by a pretubercular stage was meant a latent tuberculosis.—R. H. Babcock.

Great objection to term "pretubercular." "Prebacillary" stage permissible. because of cases in which tuberculosis is suspected, but no bacilli can be found, or only after a length of time. Does not like to use the term "prebacillary."—V. Y. Bowditch.

Prebacillary (excluding tuberculous pneumonia and miliary tuberculosis). Definition: Incipient stage before ulceration. Pretubercular not necessary; often erroneously applied to the early part of incipient stage.—Laurason Brown.

A prebacillary stage is one in which tubercle bacilli are absent, and very often expectoration also. In the majority of cases there will be found by blood examination, a certain amount of anæmia, with which there may be loss of weight, possibly digestive disturbances, and in which physical signs are totally, or almost totally, absent. By X-ray examination there must be shown a very slight haze, generally at one apex. Very often in these cases suspicious sounds may be elicited at the apex, which would not be detected without attention having been first called to them by the aid of the X-ray, and would not be positive enough to base a diagnosis upon alone; unless a shadow were discovered by the X-ray we would not be justified in diagnosing them as cases of tuberculosis. I have never seen a case where suspicious physical signs were accompanied by a slight haze, shown by the X-ray, in which the subsequent history of the patient did not prove the correctness of the original diagnosis. Does not recognise the term "pretubercular."—J. Edward Stubbert.

Incipient.

Slight localised lesion, with or without bacilli, and but little constitutional disturbance (fever, loss of weight, &c.)—H. P. Loomis.

Symptoms with or without early physical signs of limited extent in one or both lungs; with or without bacilli in the sputum; with or without slight constitutional debility or complications.—E. R. Baldwin.

Cases in which both the physical and rational signs point to but slight local and constitutional involvement.—E. L. Trudeau.

Involvement of apex low as the first interspace; a few râles, feeble respiratory murmur, and moderately harsh expiratory sounds.—E. Fletcher Ingals.

Physical signs and rational symptoms are both slight; tubercle bacilli are present, and evidence of toxic infection small.—I. H. Hance.

Same as Trudeau.—F. I. Knight.

A stage in which symptomatology and physical signs point to tuberculosis without mixed infection.—R. H. Babcock.

Very slight signs in one or both apices; exceptionally in one spot elsewhere; little or no fever, and general symptoms are not those showing that the disease has taken any general hold upon the patient.—V. Y. Bowditch.

Slight local, with little or no constitutional involvement.—Laurason Brown.

Slight localised involvement of the lung, with or without constitutional disturbances.—J. E. Stubbert.

Moderately Advanced.

Lesion involving one lobe of one or both lungs, and in which there may be excavation; constitutional disturbances, anorexia, and loss of weight present.—H. P. Loomis.

Symptoms are more or less marked, with extensive signs in one or both lungs, beginning or actual cavitation with or without constitutional debility or complications.—E. R. Baldwin.

Cases in which the localised disease process is either extensive or in an advanced stage, or where, with a comparatively slight amount of pulmonary involvement, the rational signs point to grave constitutional impairment, or to some complication.—E. L. Trudeau.

Involvement as low as third rib, or a corresponding amount in another portion of the lung.—E. Fletcher Ingals.

All rational symptoms present in severe form; evidences of a very active disease present over varying areas; may have small areas of disease with very severe rational symptoms, or the lesions and rational symptoms may both be great.—I. H. Hance.

Same as Trudeau.—F. I. Knight.

Stage in which there is mixed infection with signs of softening, but not any considerable destruction of lung tissue.—R. H. Babcock.

Well-marked symptoms of a catarrhal condition in the lungs, with evidences of decided consolidation, or still less of cavity formation.—V. Y. Bowditch.

Localised disease process extensive or in an advanced stage, or slight local pulmonic invasion, with rather marked constitutional involvement, or with complications.—Laurason Brown.

More general consolidation of the lung with more marked constitutional disturbances and beginning of softening, or a single cavity without very marked constitutional disturbances, and with a small area of lung involvement.—J. Edward Stubbert.

Far Advanced.

Extensive involvement of the pulmonary tissue, generally more than one lobe in each lung. Marked constitutional debility, and often complications are present.—H. P. Loomis.

Symptoms of long standing with extensive signs, with or without large cavities; marked constitutional debility and complications.—E. R. Baldwin.

Cases in which both the rational and physical signs warrant the term.—E. L. Trudeau.

Involvement as low as the fifth rib, or lower, with cavities. —E. Fletcher Ingals.

All rational symptoms of severest type present; destructive process and progressively increasing areas of disease present in lung; complicating tubercular diseases in other organs.— I. H. Hance.

Same as E. L. Trudeau.—F. I. Knight.

Well-marked cachexia, with or without extensive caseation and excavation.—R. H. Babcock.

No definition..—L. Brown.

Consolidation, cavity formation, and symptoms of general infection are present.—V. Y. Bowditch.

Extensive area of involvement, with softening and excavation, and with marked constitutional disturbances.—J. Edward Stubbert.

Improved.

Local lesion becoming quiescent, and constitutional symptoms decreasing.—H. P. Loomis.

Lessened symptoms or signs; improvement local or general, or both.—E. R. Baldwin.

No definition.—E. L. Trudeau.

Diminution of cough and expectoration, increased flesh, greatly diminished râles, and nearly normal temperature.—E. Fletcher Ingals.

Some bettering of rational symptoms, with little or no progress of pulmonary lesions.—I. H. Hance.

No definition.—F. I. Knight.

Vague and relative term. Would involve a lessening of all symptoms, and a gain in weight, without signs of extension of disease.—R. H. Babcock.

General symptoms, cough and expectoration have diminished, with increase of strength, and possibly weight, there being, of course, different grades of improvement, as slight or marked.—V. Y. Bowditch.

Physical signs showing process less active, or general health improved, with symptoms relieved or abated.—L. Brown.

An improved case is one in which the constitutional disturbances are removed, and signs of activity in the lung are reduced; the temperature is normal, or nearly so, and the patient able to return home and do a fair amount of work without exacerbation of existing symptoms.—J. Edward Stubbert.

Arrested.

Lesion fibroid, with the physical signs of this conditon; constitutional symptoms absent; bacilli present.—H. P. Loomis.

Three months without fever or other symptoms of disease progression; partial or complete recovery of general health, without loss of expectoration and bacilli.—E. R, Baldwin.

Cough, expectoration and bacilli still present, but in which all constitutional disturbances have disappeared for several months, the physical signs being interpreted as indicative of a retrogressive or arrested process.—E. L. Trudeau.

Absence of cough and expectoration; general good health; absence of all râles and marked diminution of dulness, with cessation of much of the broncho-vesicular breathing formerly present.—E. Fletcher Ingals.

Rational symptoms have almost wholly disappeared, and physical signs show no further activity in pulmonary lesions; bacilli still present.—I. H. Hance.

Absence of all constitutional symptoms, pulmonary condition being stationary, and therefore no longer active. Such an improvement must have existed for many months, or even years.—R. H. Babcock.

All cases in which cough and expectoration have ceased,

and where the general condition would indicate outwardly a return to health, regardless of the fact as to the exact condition of the chest itself, even though in many cases, so far as the physical signs themselves were concerned, the term "cured" might possibly be justified. On account of the treacherous nature of the disease, am unwilling to use the term "cured" until after the lapse of two or three years possibly, when no return of the symptoms had been manifest.—V. Y. Bowditch.

No activity in process in lungs, with absence of fever and other constitutional symptoms for at least two months.— L. Brown.

Cases which have previously shown marked constitutional disturbance, but in which all constitutional disturbance has disappeared for several months. Physical signs interpreted as indicative of arrested process.—F. I. Knight.

An arrested case is one in which all signs of activity and all constitutional disturbances have been absent for at least two months. Bacilli may or may not be absent.—J. Edward Stubbert.

Apparently cured.

Absence of bacilli. The local changes recognised only those of complete fibrosis; no constitutional symptoms.— H. P. Loomis.

Three months without any symptoms of disease progression; complete recovery of general health, and absence of bacilli or expectoration during whole period.—E. R. Baldwin.

Cases in which rational signs and bacilli have been absent for at least three months, or who have no expectoration; any abnormal physical signs remaining being interpreted as indicative of a healed lesion.—E. L. Trudeau.

Absence of all symptoms of disease, and disappearance of nearly all signs for a period of two years.—E. Fletcher Ingals.

All rational symptoms have disappeared, and physical signs

show no evidence, or but slight evidence, of scar tissue remaining. No bacilli.—I. H. Hance.

Same as Trudeau, except time limit should be one year instead of three months.—F. I. Knight.

After lapse of two or three years, during which time no symptoms had been manifest.—V. Y. Bowditch.

Practically synonymous with arrested. If lung were fibrose, and tubercles calcareous, condition would certainly be cured. It is possible for old cheesy areas to be incapsulated and thus produce no local or general symptoms, yet the patient could not be said to be cured; it would constitute a relative cure.—R. H. Babcock.

Abnormal physical signs absent or only slight, indicative of healed lesions; absence for at least three months of constitutional symptoms, and of bacilli in sputum.—L. Brown.

One in which the above conditions have existed for six months.—J. Edward Stubbert.

Cured.

Absence of bacilli; no evidence of any localised pulmonary process (even fibroid) changes. Lungs normal.—H. P. Loomis.

Two years without relapse. Not in favour of word.—E. R. Baldwin.

Same as apparently cured.—E. F. Ingals.

No definition.—I. H. Hance.

No definition.—L. Brown.

No definition.—E. L. Trudeau.

No definition.—F. I. Knight.

Synonymous with apparently cured.—R. H. Babcock.

Only after lapse of two or three years. Does not use term; includes all such cases under head of " arrested."—V. Y. Bowditch.

Those in which all constitutional signs of disease have been absent for two years and in which, for some length of time, bacilli have not been found; and in which the physical signs are such as can be justly attributed to scar tissue, or are totally absent. Expectoration may or may not be absent.—J. Edward Stubbert.

DISCUSSION.

Dr. BOWDITCH: As to the use of the term "pretubercular stage," I must confess that I dislike it almost as much as that much-abused term "heart failure." It seems to me that a case must either be tuberculosis or it is not. I acknowledge that the gentlemen who recognise that condition are men whose opinions are entitled to great weight, but I cannot agree with them. As to the term "arrested," I think I stand alone perhaps in not using the terms "cured" or "apparently cured" when the patients are discharged from my care, even when the general condition and physical signs would seem to warrant the latter terms. There will be differences of opinion always on this question, but I have seen so many cases discharged as "cured" or "apparently cured," and yet the day afterwards possibly a hæmorrhage or even death occur, that I have adhered to the more conservative term thus far in my nomenclature. I was somewhat vague in my own reply to Dr. Stubbert as to the length of time after which I was willing to consider the case cured. I am willing, however, to accept the time stated by Ingals and Baldwin, say, perhaps, two years.

Dr. EDSON: Not being Germans we are deprived of the advantages of long words to explain our meaning. It seems to me the term pretubercular or prebacillary stage is a good one. So much depends on the secondary infections *et al.* that the stage in which the tubercular process is slight, one without any breaking down in the covering, as it were, of the inflammatory area, as compared with that in which the breaking down has occurred, and until which period we do not get the sputum, is one that may be substituted for the less wieldy one of "no bacilli in the sputum." Those cases, as a rule, have a longer and a more manageable course as regards comfort and length of life than those in which general ulceration occurs.

Dr. QUIMBY: Ever since I began the study of physical diagnosis I have been impressed with the indefiniteness of the terms used. Some years ago, at a meeting of the Section on General Medicine of the New York Academy of Medicine, to test this question of uniformity in the use of physical diagnosis terms, I brought in several patients with well-marked signs, and, after marking a point on each chest where there was a distinctive sound, I asked the gentlemen present to listen at those points and to write down the name which they would give to each sound, folding the paper each time so that the one following could not see what had been written. Some five or six responded and when the lists were read, incredible as it may seem, no two men gave the same name to any one sound.   At our meeting in Bethlehem, I read a paper on " Definite Records of Physical Signs," believing that such records can be made ; but now we are discussing definitions of things which are undefinable.   Our difficulty, and apparently the cause of our controversy, lies in the fact that, having applied names to confessedly mere probabilities or physical prophecies, we act as though the use of those names affirmed the probabilities to be demonstrated facts.   We are attempting to affirm future conditions from present symptoms, which is, of course, impossible.   Nevertheless, there is a certain something which we wish to talk about, and if we will simply agree among ourselves just what combination of symptoms and physical conditions these several apparently prophetic terms shall be accepted as indicating, we can then discuss these questions intelligently, at least among ourselves, and by sticking to them very likely bring others to accept our definition.   I therefore move, sir, that a committee be appointed to draw up a statement setting forth the combinations of signs and physical conditions which these several terms shall be understood to imply when used by members of this Association.

Dr. WILSON : I want to second Dr. Quimby's motion, and my main object in doing so is that I may say a few words from the standpoint of one who is a general clinician, perhaps in contradistinction to the methods of those more interested in sanitarium work and who feel obliged by the exigencies of their own every-day work to use such terms, in order that a set of definitions may be brought into practice which will pass current among all interested in the subject.   It seems to me the whole set of terms we have been speaking of would indicate a want of recognition of the pathological changes which arise under different circumstances in pulmonary tuberculosis.   In the first place, we do not recognise the fact that pulmonary tuberculosis is, in the beginning, a local infection, and that it often remains so, especially in cases where recovery takes place.   Secondly, that there are cases that live with physical signs that are permanent, and which at no time can be shown to have had the tubercle bacilli in the expectoration.   Then there are other cases of fibroid changes starting perhaps in the pleura and extending to the lung without giving rise to the presence of bacilli in the sputum, but leading to disturbances of the health in a lasting way.   We must think, on the other hand, and I am now speaking of the difficulties we must encounter, of the recovery that often takes place which is permanent, but in which the most marked physical signs remain, such as cavities, deformities of the chest, &c.   When we consider these things, the question of the presence or absence of physical signs must be considered as militating against the use of such terms as " improved," " arrested," " restoration of health," and the like.   I want to say a word in this connection on a subject that has attracted my attention more and more in the last few years, and to which I have learned to attach a great deal of importance, a physical sign that is often the only one of an incipient pulmonary tuberculosis, and that is interrupted respiration.   I have recognised this sound over and over again at a time when there was great question as to the patient's health, and at a time when no other sign could be elicited. I have found it in regions of the chest where other signs have appeared later. In the text-books this sign has been given altogether too little attention. If we entertain the pathologic view that pulmonary tuberculosis is an infection, then it is a mistake to make a subdivision such as "prebacillary stage" and "incipient tuberculosis," for every case that shows the physical signs or rational symptoms due to tuberculous infection is a case of tuberculosis from the beginning.

Dr. MINOR : While willing to second Dr. Quimby's motion, I am rather pessimistic as to its outcome. Words, as the Frenchman said, are a means of concealing thought, and no two men will ever ascribe the same meaning to the chosen words. The reasons these misunderstandings will always remain are that the examinations are made by different men, and while all are able they disagree because of their different mental attitudes. As regards Dr. Stubbert's plan to classify the cases when discharged, that has been tried in Germany and failed, yet, although it seems almost hopeless, it is important to try to form some kind of a classification for those of us who have to report on the condition of our patients on discharge. I consider that two or three years at least ought to elapse before a case is considered cured, whatever the findings, and until then the case can only be called "arrested." I always put my patients before leaving to the test of taking violent exercise to see whether they will show any temperature. I have also laid considerable stress upon the restoration of the normal or nearly normal chest circumference, and a condition of steady weight, a weight which holds although it is not necessarily the weight of previous good health.

Dr. BONNEY : I have been for several years heartily in accord with the suggestion made by Dr. Wilson with reference to the undesirability of the terms that have been used. Four years ago I read a paper before this Association in which I made some allusion to the classification, and I would like to read part of a paragraph of that paper (see volume xiii, page 155). I am sceptical about the practical utility of the terms that have been suggested, and think that each writer in reporting his cases should define his position in order that his readers can have a clear understanding of what he means. I have frequently seen cases that might be reported as incipient where the prognosis I would think was considerably less favourable than other cases that might be reported by the same man as advanced cases, if we depended alone upon the area or degree of pulmonary involvement.

Dr. SHURLY : I am in accord with Dr. Quimby's motion and efforts. There is no use in taking trouble, and "crossing the bridge before we come to it." As long as we have to communicate with one another by language the more nearly we can get it to accord in every particular, the more intelligently we can discuss matters. I think this body is the one to make this effort, and though we may not succeed at first, we shall if we keep at it. Some persons may not want to call a certain muscle the sartorius, while the majority of us would continue to know it by that name sartorius.

Dr. ARNOLD : It seems to me the question before us is whether we should establish a committee to make a report upon each of these terms, and the discussion as to the basis of a classification is not profitable at the present time, even though it is instructive. Can we hope to accomplish anything by having such a committee? I am in favour of making the attempt.

The PRESIDENT called for a vote upon the motion of Dr. Quimby, and it was declared adopted.

Upon motion of Dr. MINOR the Chair was instructed to appoint this committee of five.

Adjournment.

THE SELECTION OF FAVOURABLE CASES OF PULMONARY TUBERCULOSIS FOR SANATORIUM TREATMENT.

BY E. R. BALDWIN, M.D.

SARANAC LAKE, N.Y.

THE continually increasing number of sanatoriums for working people, projected or already in operation, brings this subject to attention more and more; and until reception hospitals are provided for acute and doubtful cases, only the most favourable ones can be treated. It is an economic question of great importance, especially with state and municipal institutions; for doubtless for many years to come the number of applicants will far exceed the accommodations, and necessitate close discrimination in selecting patients for treatment.

In no disease is an accurate prognosis more difficult, and only the broadest distinctions can be made. Many so-called "incipient" ones are decidedly unfavourable, while not a few "advanced" ones are favourable for indefinite arrest, even if not for actual recovery.

It is not infrequently impossible to say whether such cases are favourable or not without a trial; yet so long as no provision is made for acute cases in or near sanatoriums, they will doubtless need to be excluded in the interests of those less ill, who would be depressed by their presence.

Except during hot weather, patients with very acute symptoms, such as chills, high fever, and sweats, are better kept at home if properly nursed, until such time as there may be some reasonable prospect of admission to a sanatorium.

Other considerations than the condition of the patient too often weigh in urging them to apply when too ill for admission, or when too late for recovery ; but some general directions may prevent the extravagant promises occasionally made to them. The stamp of incurability goes with a refusal, and works much cruelty towards those who are induced to apply by their physicians or friends without sufficient thought.

This might frequently be avoided by a more careful consideration of those factors which constitute a favourable prognosis and the opposite.

It is easier to define a favourable case, but manifestly difficult to be concise, and the following attempt should not be understood as aiming to be wholly comprehensive nor free from error in application to certain exceptional cases.

It is prepared in a tabular form to facilitate a grasp of salient points, only those factors being named under " doubtful " or " unfavourable " as are considered such, although it may happen that but one of them is present, and all other indications are " favourable."

It must be admitted that in the light of our present knowledge, most of the early cases cannot be considered incipient when they first consult a physician.

The growing appreciation of this fact should institute measures for the instruction of young persons in the schools of higher grade as to the earliest symptoms, while periodical inspection of employees in the large industries would yield good results in detecting the disease in a curable stage. Especially important is the judicious following of cases of slight blood spitting, and of families in which the disease has already occurred.

Condition	Age	Occupation	Parental History
Favourable ...	Between 15 and 50 (except at menopause)	Open air, or not too arduous indoor	Fairly vigorous, though not necessarily free from tuberculosis.
Doubtful ...	Under 15 and over 50	Confined and dusty. Lead workers, miners, quarrymen, grinders, polishers, tailors, actors, bartenders, seamstresses, &c.	Delicate parentage. Maternal tuberculosis.
Unfavourable..	Under 10 and over 60	... ...	Both parents delicate and tuberculous. Maternal tuberculosis at birth.

Condition	Personal History	Habits and Intelligence
Favourable ...	Previous good health or only illnesses with complete recovery. Good nutrition and digestive functions.	Good; or free from excesses.
Doubtful ...	Delicate constitution. Neurotic temperament. Frequent illnesses.	Dissipated. Careless or ignorant. Wilful.
Unfavourable	Frail constitution and late maturity. Rachitis or severe illness in childhood. Always below normal weight for height.	Depraved. Alcoholic excess. Reckless and despondent.

Condition	Beginning of Tuberculosis
Favourable ...	Not noticeable, or from a cold; "grippe"; bronchitis; mild "malaria"; debility.
Doubtful ...	"Chronic bronchitis"; "pneumonia"; "typhoid fever." Prolonged dyspepsia or occasional diarrhœa with fever. "Bronchitis" following measles. Anæmia. Prolonged chills and fever.
Unfavourable...	"Typhoid" or "typho-malaria" fever, from which complete recovery did not issue. "Unresolved" lobar or broncho-pneumonia. Chronic dyspepsia. Prolonged diarrhœa or frequent looseness. Disease developed during menopause, pregnancy, or immediately after delivery.

Condition	Symptoms
Favourable ...	Symptoms of short duration, or long intervals without any, extending over longer period. Occasional short periods of irregular fever and sweats ; temp. average not over 100°. Slight hæmoptyses. Moderate debility, anæmia, loss of weight and appetite. Shortness of breath only on much exertion. Menstruation ceased only few months.
Doubtful ..	Prolonged debility and fever several months. Hoarseness ; severe cough or hack six months or more. Repeated hæmoptyses of considerable amount, or with occasional chills, fever and sweats. Persistently high pulse. Marked anæmia. Slight cyanosis and hectic flush ; dyspepsia.
Unfavourable ...	Marked debility and long period of fever with or without chills and sweats; rapid pulse (distinguish purely nervous cases). Well-marked dyspnœa ; abdominal breathing due to lack of chest movement. Swollen feet. Complications.

Condition	Present Condition	Complications
Favourable ...	Fair physique, intellect and morale. Deep chest expansion, one or more inches ; normal or only temporarily rapid pulse ; good peripheral circulation.	None, unless superficial ulceration of vocal cords without infiltration. Mild dyspepsia. Slight enlargement cervical lymph nodes. Arrested bone or joint tuberculosis.
Doubtful ...	Delicate or slender build. Depressed clavicular spaces. Deformed or flat chest. Neurasthenic or excitable.	Ulcerated vocal cords and inter-arytenoid space without infiltration. Peritoneal, bone or joint tuberculosis ; otitis media. Slight albuminuria, irrespective of fever. Old syphilis. Chronic cystitis. Mitral heart disease.
Unfavourable ...	Very frail build or tall and slender. Pigeon-chested or markedly rachitic. Kyphotic spine. Curvature of nails ; marked cachexia or chlorosis. Markedly neurotic, despondent or melancholic. Actual melancholia or insanity.	Intestinal, genito-urinary. Tuberculous bones. Deep-seated laryngeal tuberculosis. Infiltrated arytenoids or epiglottis. Generalised lymphatic tuberculosis. Fistula in ano with rectal ulcer. Diabetes. Nephritis. Recent syphilis. Chronic gastritis or entero-colitis. Valvular heart disease, not compensated. Emphysema. Empyema. Pneumo-thorax or hydro-pneumo-thorax.

LESION.

Condition	One Apex	Both Apices
Favourable ...	Cases with slight dulness; prolonged expiration; few râles distinctly localised; slight cough with or without expectoration. Cases with some excavation but entirely or practically arrested, and slight expectoration and fever. Early signs to fourth rib; fair history; no complications	Cases with early signs, well localised; good history, colour, physique, and nutrition.
Doubtful ...	Cases with early signs; febrile; poor physique, &c. Dulness; coarse or bubbling râles; acute symptoms. Cavity with debility, chills, fever and sweats	Early signs; symptoms more marked. Flat chest or poor physique, &c.
Unfavourable ..	Large cavern. Acute pneumonic progressive. One entire side extensively infiltrated	Cases with dulness, coarse or bubbling râles, or cavities with constitutional impairment, or marked mixed infection, as evinced by chills, fever and sweats.

LESION.

Condition	Lower Lobe or Entire Side
Favourable ...	Dry pleurisy only, or with effusion and short period of fever. Thickened pleura; mild symptoms.
Doubtful ..	Slight dulness; harsh breathing; few râles, indicative of slight infiltration. Pleurisy with effusion and long-continued fever. Entire side; scattered signs; good history and condition; mild symptoms.
Unfavourable ...	Extensive infiltration (distinguish thickened pleura, not necessarily unfavourable). Pneumonic consolidation, or excavated middle or lower lobe. Broncho-pneumonic lesion one or both sides. Chronic fibroid phthisis. Miliary pleurisy both sides, acute symptoms. Miliary generalised disease as indicated by vague, not localised, physical signs; rapid pulse; respiration and cyanosis.

ON THE HOME TREATMENT OF PULMONARY TUBERCULOSIS.

BY LEONARD WEBER, M.D.

NEW YORK.

FROM 1879 to 1885, I took occasion to visit some of the well-known sanatoria for the treatment of pulmonary tuberculosis, both here and abroad. When I saw what could be accomplished by physiotherapy in the first and second stages of tuberculosis, and how many well-marked cases of it rapidly improved and were even cured in such institutions, I determined to imitate this mode of treatment in private and dispensary practice, for such patients as could not or would not be sent away from home. Besides physiotherapy, I employ such medicines as have proved themselves most serviceable in combating the tuberculous infection. Pretty careful records of my cases have been kept since 1886, and the care and management of them is based upon a fairly uniform working plan which has been followed in every case, slight individual modifications excepted, and which I have not yet had reason to change. Painstaking and repeated physical examinations, the frequent use of the thermometer, and the examinations of sputa will not often leave us in doubt for many days about the presence of pulmonary tuberculosis. By these frequent physical examinations I confess to have been greatly helped in arriving at the correct estimate of a case, in detecting the advance of retrogression of the apex-lesion on the side first infected, or the sudden manifestations of slight but suspicious catarrh in the other apex, supposed to be sound. I have found in this way, even in the early stage of pulmonary tuberculosis, bilateral affection—unequal in depth and extent, to be sure—more often than I had suspected at the first or second examination. So far as my observations go, these explorations are not even now so generally and carefully made as they might be, yet without them we could estimate correctly neither the severity of the infection, nor the power of resistance on the part of the patient, so as to be able to give a fair prognosis of the case.

And it is so important to find out as soon as possible whether we have to deal with a relatively slight and manageable form of pulmonary tuberculosis that will admit of home treatment, or with the more malignant, rapidly-spreading form, that will end in phthisis in a short time unless the patient be saved perhaps by removal into a climate of high altitude.

In making the statement that by physical exploration, including bacteriological examinations, we can generally soon arrive at the positive diagnosis of the early stage of pulmonary tuberculosis, I mean just so much and no more. Unfortunately however, the early stage in which this can be done, is not incipient pulmonary tuberculosis, it is already more than that. In the incipiency of tuberculosis infection there may be no sputum (*vide* last case reported), or, if any, bacilli may not be found present in it. And it is just in these very incipient cases that we should like so much to make a certain diagnosis. The tuberculin test we do not feel inclined to use on our patients; perhaps the Arloing-Courmont serum reaction recently brought out may prove of great value in the near future. In their report, December 1, 1900, Arloing and Courmont, of Lyons, have alleged positive proofs of agglutination in a large number out of 400 cases, but their results have not been generally confirmed, have even been contradicted by some competent investigators. So long as we have to go without a sure and readily made serum diagnosis for incipient tuberculosis, let us give a suspicious case the benefit of the doubt, and rather treat the patient as if he were infected with tubercle than give him medicine for latent malaria or chlorosis.

Having determined the presence of acute or subacute tuberculous infection, the nature of the disease is explained to the patient and his relatives, the fact of its communicability stated, and printed rules and regulations are handed them which describe the order of the requisite sanitary measures plainly and with particular accuracy, with regard to the disinfection and destruction of sputa, the ventilation and disinfection of rooms, clothing, &c. At the same time it is impressed upon them to take a hopeful view of the situation, and to understand that, though the patient is suffering from an attack of tuberculosis, or tuberculous lung-catarrh, if you please, he is not, by any means, consumptive or phthisical as yet, that he will most likely be very much better in a few weeks, if the treatment to be applied is carried out with intelligence, patience, and perseverence, and that he may have a fair chance of regaining his health and strength, and be able to resume his occupation in the course of time. Shall we call this procedure in question, say that we assume too much by this suggestive presentation of the case, and, perhaps, make the patient too hopeful and careless in considering his own case? I have not found it so in practice. Provided we have gained the patient's confidence by locating his disease and its extent by examination, for which half-an-hour's time is certainly required, reassurance and promise of early improvement which can be given with perfect honesty, will be the very thing to help him in the beginning and continuation of adequate treatment. It is surprising, to say the least, but nevertheless true, that, even at the present time, in a case of recent pulmonary tuberculosis, coming on with more or less febrile disturbance of the system, &c., the patient is not sent to bed and kept there for some weeks for rest and treatment until the acute stage is passed. It may well be said that it is to be regretted that these patients not infrequently do not feel very ill at the onset of tuberculous invasion, and that the tubercle bacillus may occupy quite a bit of territory in one or another of the lungs before the first visit is made to the doctor's office. For the good of the sick, and for the increased success of home treatment, I wish it were otherwise, and that they all felt at the beginning at least as sick as a patient with quinsy, rheumatic fever, acute gastritis, or the like; then many more cases of pulmonary tuberculosis would be recognised in the early stages. It is a pity, indeed, that the tubercle bacillus does invade in so insidious a manner, that we often find considerable infiltration of the apex or elsewhere in cases that look as if they had just begun.

(1) *The first order given in a case of fresh febrile tuberculous infection is that the patient should go to bed and stay there until the thermometer shows practically normal temperature. Rest cure at the outset, to be repeated at intervals according to the circumstances of the case, and careful nursing, are essential for successful treatment.*

(2) The patient's room must be well above ground, must admit plenty of light and air, and be easy to ventilate. The furniture and equipment ought to conform more or less to those of the average private room in a modern hospital. The heating of the room should be done by an open fireplace or grate-stove; heating by dry hot air furnace is to be deprecated; it brings too much dust into the room, and this we know to be particularly obnoxious to people with coughs and bronchial trouble. For collection of sputa I recommend either enamelled iron spittoons, such as Dr. Knopf uses, or glass spittoons, or paper boxes, also the Japanese paper sheets for use when the patient is about. What is collected in spittoons is disinfected with a 5 per cent. solution of carbolic acid, or 3 per cent. formaldehyde solution, or 1-1000 corrosive sublimate. Papers filled with sputa are burned, of course.

(3) Food, selected according to the condition of the case, is given every two or three hours in small quantities, or in the shape of meals four times a day so soon as the patient is able to

take and digest them. That fat-producing materials should be largely taken is self-evident. In the acute febrile stage the patient is sponged with alcohol and water three times daily, and his linen changed as often as required; when he has improved and become convalescent, he is advised to take a cool sponge bath every morning, standing in a rubber tub before the washstand that has a large basin full of cool water in it ready for use, and a big linen sheet for drying by the side of it. Time allowed for this procedure, from two or five minutes. When the patient has made further progress in gaining strength and resistance, or is vigorous at the outset, and but little infected, so that he does not need the rest-cure any longer, he is advised to take the douche—or rain bath—warm or tepid for the first two minutes, cool or cold the next two, every morning. Short procedures and low temperature of the water used are the essentials for successful hydrotherapy in this class of patients.

(4) In the early stages, and at all times, I have found it of great moment to keep down high temperature, and hereby save the patient's strength and body weight. Quinine I have not found as serviceable here as the compound coal-tar remedies. For ten years at least the following formula has been in use in my practice :—

R	Acetanilide	...	...	...	...	...	1 grain.
	Phenacetine	...	...	...	...	...	3 grains.
	Antipyrine	...	...	...	...	...	3 „

M. ft. pulv.

such powder to be given when the temperature goes above 101 degrees F. It has been gratifying to notice the prompt action of this compound in the quantity stated—and even less in some cases—in reducing temperature without depressing effects.

(5) Not very infrequently, particularly in young persons, the disease is ushered in, so to speak, to the horror and alarm of the patient and his relatives, by hæmoptysis of more or less severity

No alarm need generally be felt at all at the first occurrence of
hæmoptysis, though it is a different and more serious affair in
advanced cases with excavations in the lung tissue. In every
acute case I have noted of hæmoptysis, there is considerable
rise in temperature from the second or third day on. The treatment I have followed for this complication has been: Ice
application to the chest in the form of two small ice-bags, left
and right side below the clàvicles; dry cupping with rubber-
capped cupping glasses of suitable size, from eight to a dozen
of them set on the chest, on both sides, from the clavicles to
the ensiform process, and repeated two or three times in
twenty-four hours. The patient rests in bed with the head
well elevated, takes a teaspoonful of table salt two or three
times the first day, and milk and water only for nourishment;
controls cough with one-quarter-of-a-grain doses of phosphate
of coedine. From the second day on for three or four
days, I give them of the fluid extract of arbor vitæ one drachm
in a wineglassful of water three times in twenty-four hours, continuing the ice-bags, also repeating application of dry cups. At
the end of a week the regular home treatment may be instituted.

The use of fluid extract of arbor vitæ for hæmoptysis I
learned from the late Dr. Loomis; it appears to be of service.
Ergot and acetate of lead in large doses are harmful; they are
not indicated for this form of hæmorrhage anyway. To quiet
the anxiety of the patient and his friends, reassuring them
of the absence of danger, and resorting to the simple measures
just described, will be adequate treatment for most cases.

(6) The diagnosis of fresh and more or less febrile tuberculous infection of the lung having been made, the general
irritability, harassing cough, &c., are often such that I have not
found it to be a good plan to resort at once to creosote or other
drugs which may be believed to be inhibitory to the development and growth of the tubercle bacillus, but rather order for
a week or two such remedies as would be appropriate to a
case of acute bronchitis with fever and severe cough. Nothing
has served the purpose better than the following mixture : —

R Chloroform water   ...   .   6 ounces.
   Bicarbonate of sodium   ...   .   1 drachm.
   Sulphate of morphine...   ...   .   1 grain.
   Cherry-laurel water ...   .   1 drachm.
M. Sig.   From one to two drachms in an ounce of water every three hours.

(7) So soon as the acute symptoms have subsided, or when they are absent, as in cases that have an insidious or subacute beginning, creosote is prescribed.   Since 1888, this remedy has been employed by me, and the fair measure of success I have had in the home treatment of pulmonary tuberculosis has been due to the action of this drug, I believe, fully as much as to physiotherapy.   It undoubtedly has an antiseptic and tonic effect, the former particularly in the secondary streptococcus and staphylococcus infections of tuberculosis.   It has greatly helped in a number of cases under my observation to make the soil unfavourable to the growth of the tubercle bacillus, and it has also been demonstrated that a comparatively weak solution of it will inhibit further growth of the bacillus in a culture medium, and produce agglutination.   It is generally well borne by the patient even in large doses.   But few patients have objected to its use, and no harm has come from it in any of my cases.   Capsules containing creosote mixed with oil I have not found of good service; I employ it in solution, and according to this formula :—

R Beechwood creosote ⎫
   Alcohol   ⎬ ...   .   each, 1 ounce.

M. Sig.   10 drops in half a tumblerful of milk or water three times daily an hour and a half after eating.   Double the dose every week until the patient comes up to sixty drops *pro dosi*, which is about as far as I have gone.

The effects I look for, diminution or cessation of cough and expectoration, improved appetite, and gain in weight, have generally been procured in the course of two or three months by the doses mentioned, and I do not recollect getting better results by forcing larger doses.   It is to be remembered that we meet with cases often enough which will not respond to physiotherapy and creosote at home, because the infection is too virulent, and spreads too quickly, and the patient becomes rapidly phthisical, unless saved in time by sanatorium treatment in high and sunny mountain climates.

Of the derivatives of creosote I have made fair trials, also of ichthyol, but I have not been convinced of the power of these for making an impression upon the disease, and I believe them to be inferior to creosote.

(8) The class of tuberculous patients who show phthisical habitus, have poorly-developed muscles, and also weak hearts, need cardiac tonics, such as strychnine, with or without digitalis and quinine in small doses t. i. d. before meals. For the often troublesome dry cough I have found the phosphate of coedine in one-quarter-grain doses of good service.

(9) Whenever a stage of improvement had been reached, where it appeared to me timely and opportune to send the patient out of the city to continue the plan of treatment, with the main points of which he has now become familiar, I have done so. It goes without saying, as to convalescence and eventual restoration to health, that he will make more rapid advance in the uplands than by staying in the city, even with the best possible surroundings and best care. In the course of time I have advised single patients and entire families to remove from the Greater City of New York, to the Oranges or to Morristown and Dover in New Jersey, if they could go no higher up from the sea-level; always admonished them to keep on the lookout for light, airy houses, and to guard against wind and dust as much as possible. I give the preference, however, to the uplands of Ulster, Sullivan, and Greene counties, of New York, which abound in places suitable for incipient phthisis; often, also, I have had very fair results by sending patients to Milford, in Pike County, Pennsylvania, near Port Jervis. When a patient chooses to go so far as the Adirondacks, but refuses to become an inmate of a sanatorium there, I insist on his reporting, soon after arrival, to a physician, and

choosing a location by his advice. It does not seem to me either prudent or right and proper, to let a patient in delicate health go and locate 300 or more miles away from home, and be his own physician.

(10) By Dr. Knopf and others I have been informed that, in addition to caring for the tuberculous poor in private sanatoria to be built up by special societies, founded in several large cities of our country, some of these societies have also taken up educational work by trying to instruct the people as to the meaning and importance of pulmonary tuberculosis. It is good news indeed, that men and women who thoroughly understand the subject of tuberculosis, and have the ability to bring it before the people in such a way as to convince them of its importance, and instruct them with reference to the requisite sanitary and prophylactic measures to combat the ubiquitous and most deadly enemy of mankind, should go forth and do this good and humane work. What I said some weeks ago at the annual gathering of a large body of physicians in the city of New York, I will say here again. It is the business of medical men to give instruction by popular lectures on this and similar important subjects to the people in regular courses, and I believe the time is fully ripe to do this, and do it well, throughout the country. Besides that, every dispensary ought to have now its own special department for the diagnosis and treatment of pulmonary tuberculosis, and a bacteriologist who is to be paid for his services should be one of the officers of the department.

And now, what results have I had? Have they been encouraging enough to continue on this road, and have I been right in advising others to follow as I have done for a number of years?

Leaving all hospital and dispensary cases out of consideration, for the reason that we are but seldom in a position to have cognisance of their subsequent history, I can count about 110 private cases that have been under my observation and care since 1885. All of them have been treated as above described ; for every one creosote was ordered as the remedy to be taken steadily and for a long while, and at least four-fifths of them took it without objection or disgust, and without harm to the kidneys or the gastro-intestinal tract ; about one-fifth could not, or would not, take it, but had carbonate of creosote in capsule, or carbonate of guaiacol in powder in sixteen-grain doses t. i. d. given to them instead. So far as I can tell now, about fifty of the whole number have been restored to health and regular occupation after a course of one, two, or three years' care and treatment. About twenty have been greatly improved, but have remained pulmonary invalids ; about thirty of the whole number have died of phthisis pulmonalis. A few cases have been of striking interest, and with an abstract of their histories I will bring this paper to a close.

CASE I.—There is, first of all, the Shorb family, German-Americans. Father, piano maker, aged 70, living ; not tuberculous ; mother, aged 60, still living ; tuberculous infection at 35. Many hæmoptyses in the course of years, but still in a fairly good condition ; able to do housework. Seven sons, all of whom work in piano factories, and every one of whom developed pulmonary tuberculosis between 18 and 26. The oldest son contracted also syphilis when already consumptive, and died. His wife, young and healthy at the time of marriage, became the mother of two children, which showed signs of hereditary syphilis, but recovered, and are now fairly well, aged 7 and 8 years respectively. The mother, however, died of rapid consumption a year after her husband's death. The six other brothers weathered the first storms of tuberculosis bravely, carried out the treatment persistently, and all are able to work at their trade. For the two most delicate ones I was able to procure employment out in Colorado and New Mexico ; the news from them is satisfactory.

CASE 2.—Two sisters, Mary Ann and Alice B., Americans. Father and mother healthy at the time these girls showed incipient tuberculosis. No other members of this rather numerous family have signs of it. These two patients never went away for a cure, but recovered by home treatment alone.

CASE 3.—Alice F., American, dressmaker. Tuberculosis from her twentieth year. Had home treatment only, and recovered. She married two years ago, and is now the mother of a healthy child, and in good general condition.

CASE 4.—Marcus, Edward, William, and Ida R. The mother of these four patients died of pulmonary tuberculosis at the time they were growing up. The father died of cerebral apoplexy about eight years ago. All four had well-marked attacks of tuberculosis, but made good recoveries by home and open air treatment, and are now well.

CASE 5.—Joseph R., American, commercial traveller, aged 40 ; single ; tuberculosis infection ten years ago. Home treatment and occasional sojourn in the Catskill Mountains for two years, then a sojourn in Colorado for six months. Is now in good health.

CASE 6.—Joseph S., American, aged 34 ; married ; pawnbroker. Severe attack of acute pulmonary tuberculosis concerning the entire upper right lobe ten years ago. Home treatment and sojourn in suitable place in the vicinity of New York for three years ; good recovery.

CASE 7.—C. P., Swede ; carpenter ; married ; aged 32. Tuberculosis of right apex at 28 ; also tuberculosis of calcaneum bone, and the sheath of the tendo Achilles. Home treatment only, and surgical treatment in hospital ; complete recovery.

CASE 8.—Albert T., American, aged 23 ; single ; clerk. No hereditary taint. Last September and October a second and severe attack of pulmonary tuberculous disease, right upper lobe, with pleurisy of the left side. Home treatment for three months, followed by a sojourn at Lakewood, N.J., during February, March, and April. When last examined, two weeks ago, I found he had entirely recovered from the pleurisy, and was greatly improved with regard to the tuberculous infection, free from fever and cough, but his sputa were not yet entirely free of bacilli.

CASE 9.--Josephine W., American, aged 12. Father died of phthisis five years ago. The upper lobe of her right lung showed extensive tuberculous infiltration three years ago, yet she has made improvement in all respects by persistent and carefully supervised treatment at home, and the girl is in a good condition at the present time.

CASE 10.—Mrs. Mary R., aged 30; married. Father died of pulmonary phthisis fifteen years ago. Her right lung became infected two years ago after *grippe*. Tubercle bacilli demonstrated in sputa, though very small and few. Had home treatment only and recovered.

CASE 11.—Charles D., American; single; merchant; aged 46. Became tuberculous fifteen years ago, and acutely so. Had home treatment exclusively for three years, and is quite well and strong to-day.

CASE 12.—Joseph O., German-American; innkeeper; married. A fine and strong-looking man when he became infected at the age of 30. For eight years I managed to see him through various relapses of his disease, and to get him again and again in good shape by home treatment only, but it was impossible to keep him away from the saloons, and he finally succumbed. His wife has not been infected, and is in good health now, but his eldest son took the disease at the age of 19 years, three years ago, and died of rapid consumption.

CASE 13.—Lizzie F., aged 26; single; Irish; no occupation. No family taint; became infected two years ago. Carried out home treatment in a perfect manner these last twenty months, and is quite well at the present time.

CASE 14.—Esther S., Russian, aged 22; single; seamstress. No history. Became infected two years ago. Recovery by home treatment only.

CASE 15.—Martin C., American, aged 24; single; good family history. Measles at 10; chronic otitis media on one side for at least ten years; never very severe; appendicular abscess eighteen months ago, successfully operated on; slow but full recovery, so that, two months ago he looked quite well, and was fully able to attend to business. From April 15 to May 20 of this year he had frequent dry cough, but no expectoration, no temperature, no loss in weight. By repeated examinations a small focus of abnormal respiratory murmurs was finally made out over the right posterior apex, and the patient was put to bed for ten days, when he felt so well that he was allowed to go out again. On May 22, however, he was taken with severe hæmoptysis. His case again proves the insidiousness of pulmonary tuberculosis, as well as the peculiar state of long-continued latency of tuberculous infection. Though the loss of blood was considerable, fully a quart within forty-eight hours, followed by high fever and drenching perspiration, I insisted that there was no cause for alarm; applied the ice-bags and dry cups, gave small doses of the compound antipyretic powder and a little coedine to control cough, and ordered absolute rest and diet. At the time of writing this paper—ten days after the attack—the patient is convalescent.

THE HOME TREATMENT OF TUBERCULOSIS.

BY IRWIN H. HANCE, M.D.

LAKEWOOD, N.J.

THE home treatment of tuberculosis consists of the care of the tubercular patient in some nearby country place, where his environment is wholly changed but the climatic conditions remain the same. The scientific application of all approved methods used in treating this disease, modified so as to suit the patient and his surroundings, form a basis to work upon. In a few words, it·is a praiseworthy effort to extend to the masses what is now granted to those few who are treated in or out of sanatoria at our various health resorts. For those of us who have treated patients in health resorts, all the rules and regulations are well known, but for the enlightenment of those who, we hope, will carry out the home treatment, let us briefly mention all the points of treatment.

The fundamental needs of the patient are threefold : *fresh air, good food, rest.* The first two are needed first, last, and all the time; the third in the beginning, all the time, and then coupled with exercise under the direction and orders of the physician. Fresh air is required every day and every night, the more the better. For winter the patient's bedroom should face the south and west; windows on both sides, so. that one or more can always be open, except while bathing or dressing; open fireplace in room. For summer an easterly exposure, with windows in the south as well, is to be preferred. If patient is bedridden, the above arrangement permits of the easiest solution of the question of fresh air without draughts both by day and night. For winter select a house with southerly exposure, and which has the piazza so placed that the patient gets the largest amount of sunshine and the greatest protection from the prevailing winds of the district. For summer tent life night and day is the ideal one.

From the very beginning the physician should instruct and order what the temperature should be ; how the windows and blinds should be arranged—for night particularly ; how much time the patient should be out of doors ; and his aim should be to so educate and acclimate his patient little by little, that he can be out of doors every day—rain or shine—for from four to twelve hours a day.

In overcoming the erroneous views of family and friends, and the idiosyncracies of the patient, the attainment of this desired end, as regards fresh air, requires more tact, and is surrounded with more difficulties than any other part of the treatment, and at the same time is more fruitful of good results.

Food.—Often to begin with a patient has no appetite ; food is distasteful and repulsive. When such is the case prescribe absolute rest, concentrated liquid food every two hours until 8 p.m., and once during the night ; evacuate bowels daily. By this means you frequently restore naturally a poor appetite, and you are always doing the patient good. Overfeeding is the principle to act upon in all cases, whether feverish or not ; whether incipent or advanced ; and keep it up until patient is up to or above his usual weight. If patient is capable of eating three good meals a day, give some easily digested food between each two meals and at bedtime. For fuller details, the author refers the patient to Dr. Gardiner's book, " The Care of the Consumptive," in which are to be found many other useful and valuable hints.

Food alone improves nutrition ; this state produces increased powers of resistance. This is nature's sole means of checking the excursions of the disease, diminishing its power for evil, and finally producing a condition of arrest which neither medicines nor serums have as yet been capable of doing.

Rest should be absolute in all febrile cases, and in all cases at the commencement of treatment for a period of one to four weeks. The exercise should be under the control of the physician, and its effect upon the patient be watched carefully in regard to temperature, heart action, chills, slight suspicions of blood in sputum, loss of or stationary weight, and a state of distinct over-fatigue. Most of us know how often hæmorrhage cases have proved fatal by rowing too much and riding horseback too hard. The writer can recall many fatalities in cases of arrested disease where too stiff a walk or climb started the patient on her downward course. Remember the bad effects of over-exercise are cumulative, and the physician needs to be very cautious in allowing any great increase in the exercise to begin with.

These are the essentials in the treatment of tuberculosis everywhere ; medicines play a secondary part, and are directed only to the symptomatic treatment of the disease. There is one thing which has not received the attention it demands, viz., the care of the skin.

(1) As regards clothing. The patient should be warm, and never feel chilly from being out of doors. The mistake is made of wearing too heavy underclothing and chamois protectors. The best principle is to dress warmly enough for indoors, and then have very heavy and warm outside wraps, which can easily be put on and taken off. The clothing should never produce sweating when a patient is quiescent, as the writer has frequently observed.

(2) Bathing. A phthisical patient's heart action is never strong, and his capillary circulation is always bad when first applying for treatment. Both these conditions can be improved by the proper use of water, and the bettering of the capillary circulation is an outward indication of an improvement in the general circulation. The writer is convinced that the pale, dry, sometimes lightly cyanotic skin of the tubercular invalid can be speedily and greatly improved by the use of

water. The improvement is chiefly due to a betterment of the general nervous system, and the patient thereby is benefited in a two-fold manner. When proper hydropathic appliances are not at hand, the two measures about to be described are fruitful of great good. Standing in hot water (104 degrees F.) up to the ankles, the patient, if unaccustomed to bathing, sponges the whole body with water at 85 degrees F., daily lowering the temperature until the cold water as it flows from the faucet is used. Vigorous rubbing with coarse towel completes the bath. To begin with the bath may be taken at night, but afterwards it is better given in the morning. After this form of bath has been used for several weeks the dashing of cold water from a few feet above the head over the spine increases its usefulness. For many of the weaker class of patients the following procedure may be selected: the patient lies naked in a heavy blanket; an attendant—not necessarily a skilled one—rubs the body vigorously with a very strong hot (110 degrees F.) salt solution, using along the spine the pure moistened salt to produce a greater reaction; then the whole body is gone over with cold water, beginning at 80 to 85 degrees F., and daily lowering the temperature until 50 degrees F. is reached. The time consumed will vary from thirty to fifty minutes for the whole bath. The hand must always be used; no mitten or cloth, and only one part of the body be exposed at a time. It is best done at night; patient will rest better after such a rub. The effect upon the capillary circulation and the general condition, will often be shown by the cessation of night sweats, even when these are pretty severe.

What results may we look for? Bowditch has clearly proven that sanatorium treatment fifteen miles from the city of Boston, gives most encouraging resuls. The Montefiore Home has followed his example, and shown that good results can be obtained within twenty miles of New York City. Such being the case, one should get similar results from the individual home treatment of tuberculosis. The class of patients will not probably be such as will give the most roseate statistics, for among them will be numbered those of very small means; those who are past the earlier stages; those who feel that they can only rest a short time, and then must give some attention to business; and those whose family duties prohibit their leaving home.

Among those the writer has had under observation for three years, are three patients; one is apparently cured, and two have the disease entirely arrested. Two other young girls have been under treatment six months, and benefited considerably.

The physician in instituting this form of treatment, will have to meet certain objections on the part of the patient. In this present age all patients expect better results from specialists and their advice. There is wanting the force of example which spurs on the slow and the dilatory. The visible results of this form of treatment which encourage the patient are lacking as incentives. Each one thinks climate is the essential part of the treatment. The family by being over solicitous about draughts, fresh air, &c., and from one cause or another, ofttimes reacts badly upon the patient's mental and nervous condition. To overcome these the doctor must have absolute faith in his own treatment, and be capable of dispersing all the patient's doubts. If the doctor has any doubt about his results, or feels, as so many do, that little or nothing can ever be done for tuberculosis except by specialists in proper climates, he quickly becomes discouraged, as will be shown in lack of detail in treatment, and an indifference to the patient's general welfare.

The advantages are great, in the sense that it brings to the individuals at home what was formerly only to be secured in certain localities long distances away, and in special sanatoria. History has handed down to us first the climate or region where tuberculosis was cured; then came the natural evolution of sanatorium treatment; now is added the State care of the consumptive; finally comes the individual, and it behoves us all now to battle for his interests, so that when he is a victim of tuberculosis he may get the home treatment for tuberculosis, and his physician extend to him the value of our scientific knowledge, instead of relegating him to the class of chronics whose fate it is to have all nostrums and new pharmaceutical compounds poured down his stomach *ad nauseam*. In another sense the advantages are great, as those of us who have witnessed the lot of the poor (financially) tubercular invalid in a health resort know so well. His room is larger; he gets more air at night; his food is much better; he does not suffer from loneliness or home sickness; mentally he is happier, since there are not present constantly before his eyes the very sick who nearly always fill the cheaper class of boarding-houses in health resorts; his money goes much further, and he gets more out of it.

In conclusion, the writer offers a theme for discussion *apropos* of his paper. Has the prevailing idea that climatic changes were essential to the treatment of tuberculosis retarded the progress of treating this disease? The majority of physicians consider this the only way to advise such patients, and for this reason have not kept posted on what could be done for tubercular persons, and consequently little or no effort has been made to scientifically apply the knowledge of how to treat tuberculosis.

After five years' residence under Dr. Trudeau, in the Adirondack Cottage Sanatorium, the writer has spent another five years in the country, fifty miles from New York City, and it is his opinion that a rational pre-arranged system of action, such as outlined above, controlled by common sense in dealing with each individual patient, will influence favourably a large number of all cases treated in this way; occasionally your efforts will be crowned with the success of an "apparently cured case," and many will have their disease arrested.

The wider the spread of the knowledge concerning the home treatment of tuberculosis the greater the enlightenment of the patient, his family, and his friends. In this way the prevention of the spread of the disease will have been strengthened, and the treatment result in the advancement of prophylactic measures, along with the benefit of the individual.

THE IMPORTANCE OF AN EARLY AND RADICAL CLIMATIC CHANGE IN THE CURE OF PULMONARY TUBERCULOSIS.

BY CHARLES FOX GARDINER, M.D.

COLORADO SPRINGS.

THE advantages of climatic change to those invalids suffering from phthisis has, as we all know, been observed for many years, but the actual study of climatology in its relation to tuberculosis has been a comparatively recent matter. Now, however, the effect of a complete and radical climatic change, such as from a damp climate of the lowlands to a dry climate of elevated plateaus, upon the cure or arrest of pulmonary tuberculosis, is a fact recognised by climatologists all over the world.

The effects upon a pulmonary invalid making this climatic change that I have mentioned, have frequently been presented to this Association in the most able and thorough manner, but with your kind permission I will briefly review them again. A patient with beginning phthisis, brought from a damp climate of little or no elevation, or the climate of most of our large cities, to that climate of 6,000 feet altitude and very dry, as we find in parts of Colorado, is subject to the following effects due to the climatic change.

The thin or rarified air will gradually expand the often ill-formed and contracted chest, acting continuously to bring this about day and night, and far more effectively than any exercises taken at low elevations, and only occasionally. The circulation in the capillaries is promoted, congested tissue is relieved. The air being sterile and dry, re-infection is limited, and mixed infection from diseased lung tissue is arrested. The specific gravity of the blood seems to be increased, and the formation of the new cells encouraged; in consequence of this nutrition is stimulated, and isolation of tuberculosis tissue occurs more rapidly, due to increased cellular activity; appetite is increased and power of absorption, with gain in weight. The sun's rays act with much more power upon the skin, also warm the air, so that in cold weather it is possible to obtain the advantages of outdoor air in winter, when the cold air acts as a tonic, and not suffer from the dangers of damp air, or soil and wind. The sunlight being not only powerful, but present so many hours each day, is a powerful germicide.

The dryness of the air and cool nights, prevent exhaustion from heat during the summer, so trying and even dangerous to an invalid. The electrical conditions are stimulating, and the complete change in scenery has a psychological value often overlooked.

These effects of climatic change upon the pulmonary invalid have been reported by men who have devoted the most time and study to the question, and live in the climate themselves. It is, therefore, with some surprise that I have seen lately a spirit of scepticism among certain phthisiologists in regard to any curative effect of climate in phthisis. We hear it intimated that quite good results can be obtained in any climate, provided we properly utilise fresh air and food; that as sanatorium treatment has proved the fallacy of climatic treatment, what is the use of sending our patients hundreds of miles away when we can obtain the same results in their back-yards at home by the skilful use of a steamer chair, and good beef?

The claim is also made, that even granting all the advantages of a dry and elevated climate, these advantages will have to be most marked and decided, to at all compensate for the lack of care, poor food, accommodations, and home sickness.

We have, therefore, apparently a difference of opinion among phthisiologists as to the advantage of climate. It seems to me that climate is of as much benefit as it has always been, but the abuse of climate has given a wrong impression. Especially is this true of the dry climates of the West, as in Colorado. Invalids are often sent to resorts in the West, where proper food and attention are difficult or impossible to obtain, and any sanatorium methods impossible to establish; also patients are sent in the last stages, too ill to recover under any conditions, and often in a financial stress, which is an added burden. The climatic treatment of such cases as these is, of course, unfavourable, and to compare such results with those from a sanatorium in a damp climate is misleading, to say the least. Also any comparison of climatic treatment in the West with sanatorium treatment in the East is unfair to climate, for the reason that, with few exceptions, all invalids treated in closed sanatoriums in the East are subject to a close systematic and skilled examination by trained men, to weed out the unfavourable cases, and only leave the favourable or curable cases, those in the incipient stage of the disease, for treatment in the sanatorium; and from these carefully selected cases so taken and placed under a perfect system, having in most cases better food and more pure air than they ever had before, the percentage of arrested cases is taken and compared with cases treated by climate alone, with no system at all. It is no wonder that unaided climate suffers by this comparison, and the inference is drawn that climatic treatment is worthless.

When, however, any kind of a fair comparison is made, the result is striking. Take cases treated in the first stage in Colorado without the aid of any specially closed sanatorium, but in boarding-houses, in their own homes, or in general sanatoria, and the percentages of arrested or cured cases is from 76 to 90 per cent., the sanatoria in damp climates showing 70 per cent.

The truth of the matter seems to me to be that in the climate such as exists in the dry high plateaus, near the Rocky Mountains, we have undoubtedly a powerful aid in the cure and arrest of pulmonary tuberculosis; that although a closed sanatorium is the best place in which to treat a tubercular invalid, if other things are equal, in parts of the West other things are *not* equal, hence climate comes in as a factor, and such a powerful one, that with ordinary methods at invalids' homes in Colorado, the results in incipient cases will show as good, and better results, by 15 per cent., than cases treated in closed sanatoriums in the East. Besides, many cases will not go to a sanatorium in any case, but prefer to live in a home with their families. Such invalids should have the advantages of the proper climate, which increases their chances for cure by 15 per cent.

As for poor food and accommodations at Colorado health resorts, this objection is simply a question of climatic ignorance. There are resorts in Colorado where the markets are excellent, the houses well built, and where there are good physicians and trained nurses.

In regard to the treatment of tubercular invalids, it is as well for us to remember that there has been an evolution in the West as well as in the East regarding the use of pure air and wholesome food in treating consumption, while in the use of pure air we have had the advantage, as quality as well as quantity should be considered. Outdoor air is not of the same quality in all climates, and in my experience a patient will derive more benefit from four hours spent in the dry, sunny air of Colorado, than from eight hours spent in the damp and cloudy climate of some parts of the East. In a dry climate patients can be kept day and night outdoors with benefit and without risk.

I firmly believe that the truth regarding climate will prevail, and that the great sanatoriums of the future will be built where scientific facts show the best results can be obtained. The sanatoria now established by the Government at Fort Bayard, New Mexico, and at Fort Stanton, New Mexico, will in time prove the marked advantage of sanatoria methods, and the best climatic cure combined.

THE HOME TREATMENT OF PULMONARY TUBERCULOSIS.

DISCUSSION ON HOME TREATMENT *v.* CLIMATIC TREATMENT OF PULMONARY TUBERCULOSIS.

BY DR. ARNOLD C. KLEBS.
CHICAGO.

———

THE selection of an appropriate locality for the treatment of our tuberculous patients is one of the most difficult problems to solve. We have very few definite facts at our disposal to guide our choice. Many drugs and therapeutic measures have been recommended as possessing specific effect on the process of the disease, and just as many different climates find enthusiastic supporters.

When one reads the history of the treatment of the tuberculosis, one finds that at one time or other almost any combination of known atmospheric conditions was considered to constitute a climate, which had protective or curative qualities for consumptives.

Regions with warm temperatures were preferred, and the hordes of consumptives populated southern resorts. Then it was found that heat rather favoured the progress of the disease, and that cold arrested it. Madeira was brought into fashion, and the insular climates with their even temperatures and their absence of atmospheric changes were considered of the greatest value. Sea voyages found their advocates on the same logical grounds.

New " immune zones " with peculiar atmospheric conditions

were discovered, high altitudes and deserts with their dry air, and these conditions were made responsible for the alleged curative value. In this way every atmospheric element has passed scrutiny in its effect on the disease, and temperature, humidity of atmosphere and soil, barometric pressure, sunshine in varying degrees, were thought to possess some special effect on the disease.

It cannot be denied that any one of these climates, just as any one of the drugs recommended, can and has a favourable influence on some cases, but we have absolutely no fact or statistics at our disposal to prove that there is any one climate or drug that exerts a specific effect on all cases. Just in this multiplicity and variety of recommended agents lies the object lesson, that in spite of our intimate acquaintance with the cause of the disease, the bacillus tuberculosis, we know very little about the disease itself. As a matter of fact, it always seems to me that the discovery of the bacillus, although of eminent interest and importance in a preventative direction, has not furthered, but rather retarded the progress in the treatment of the disease. Climatological, physical, and medicinal methods ever since that time were chiefly directed against the bacillus, and the body was only considered in the second place. The aseptic atmosphere of high altitudes, the germ-destroying power of sunlight, the antibacterial effect of dry air, all accentuated in the recommendation of climates, show this tendency, not to speak of medicinal specifics, which almost all are antiseptics. And still the bacillus enjoys triumphantly the most prominent position in the bacterial world to the detriment of suffering humanity. Certain cases die, and probably always will die, but others with apparently good chances for recovery or arrest, slowly decline under one-sided therapeutic efforts, and it matters but little if the medicine employed is climate, hydrotherapy, or a so-called specific drug. The fight against the disease has formed as many distinct sects of therapeutists as there are therapeutic measures, and it would consume considerable time only to name them. Only in recent years more attention has been paid to the *vis medicatrix Naturæ* and her support through therapy, but also here we again meet with sectarian tendencies; one sees the *vis medicatrix* increased with the increase of the number of red blood corpuscles in high altitudes; another through the stimulating influence of ozone; another through intense insolation; another through prolonged exposure to the air; again another through overfeeding, and so on. And while we have to admit that in every one of these agents we have a valuable curative agent, the one-sided application can, and does, retard best possible results. It is a strange fact to note how many excellent observers and thorough physicians have found a stumbling block in this problem, and how many by the over-enthusiastic, though perfectly honest advocacy of their favourite prescription, have exposed themselves to the suspicion of charlatanism and quackery.

The reason for this somewhat chaotic condition lies probably in two directions. First, as already alluded to, in our very limited knowledge of the true cause of the disease. The easily demonstrable ubiquity of the bacillus, at least in civilised human surroundings, forcibly brings before us the fact that not more people fall sick with the disease. The discovery of tuberculosis in individuals succumbed to some other disease, without any suspicious symptoms through their lifetime, proves beyond doubt that the bacillus alone does not produce the disease, because disease without symptoms is, clinically speaking, not disease. And so in our dilemna we have to insert into our formula an unknown quantity, and we call it predisposition, being unable to define it in any definite and satisfactory manner. Herein is where we lack in knowledge, and here probably a great many problems expect their solution in the future.

To some extent we know what conditions produce a predisposition to the disease and favour its progress. Here no doubt heredity and climatic conditions are of importance, but in no way can they rank with the influence of social conditions.

The importance of heredity lies especially in the exposure of children with little resistance to the possibility of infection in their daily contact with the sick parent. It must also be admitted that climatic conditions will, in their effect on the human body, exert a modifying influence, which becomes manifest in a predisposition to certain endemic and epidemic diseases. Also do we know that the climatic elements, as sunshine, temperature, humidity, atmospheric pressure, &c., have a distinct relation to the prevalence of certain diseases. So, for instance, Ruheman has shown on the hand of excellent statistics, that the disappearance of the sun for 1·79 hour (1 hr. 50 min.), costs one death from respiratory disease above the average. On the other hand, and especially in the case of pulmonary tuberculosis, its almost absolute independence from local climatic conditions is proven without doubt.

The foci of the greatest prevalence of the disease correspond to the most densely populated districts, the cities, and "immune" zones we have only there where modern civilisation has not reached. So the increase of the disease, the more frequent production of predisposed individuals, can be traced to social conditions, which produce overcrowding in cities and towns within unhygienic and unsanitary surroundings, the tendency rather to protect from than to harden against atmospheric changes. The distribution from house to house is quite typical for tuberculosis. All these points are of eminent importance from both a preventative as well as therapeutic standpoint.

In advocating the home treatment of the disease, I can best do so in endeavouring first to show the disadvantages of a treatment in distant regions.

In the great majority of our patients the expense of a longer journey has to be taken seriously into account. This extra expense from already small means, the patient will try to reduce on arrival by the selection of the cheapest possible boarding-places. And if we add to this the long journey, with its discomforts in itself, the rapid transit from a low to a much higher

14

altitude, or from a cold to a much warmer climate, and the following necessary time for acclimatisation, with frequent, more or less severe disturbances, the psychical moments of home sickness, worry over expenses, &c., we have to expect many redeeming features in the new place to make up for it. Then the choice itself of an appropriate climate is most difficult, and only too often it happens that the patient is chased from one place to the other, often quite distinct from each other. In most instances, the physician who plans to send a patient away has only a very general knowledge of the different climates, and he selects the one most recommended, having very little or no knowledge of the accommodations a patient can find there. And this is of the utmost importance, and not even the most radical advocate of climatic treatment can deny it.

As a matter of fact, only in the very rarest instances can patients find in those health resorts accommodation suited for a pulmonary invalid. In the better places consumptives are not admitted, and the other boarding places—houses only few can afford to take—usually are thoroughly infected by former boarders, and unsanitary to a sometimes astonishing degree. Only in very few of these places proper food can be obtained, and the tales of woe I have heard in this respect from patients returned from abroad are often most pitiful. Arizona, New Mexico, and Colorado, where probably the plurality of wandering consumptives is mostly sent, are just the ones most poorly provided with good accommodations. Now if a patient has once overcome most or many of the disadvantages described, and has settled down, improving in body and spirits, a change in itself often does that, if he has become thoroughly acclimatised, then another danger for his future welfare is threatening —I mean the natural inducements he finds in his new surroundings, to overdo ; they climb mountains, ride horseback, in one word, " rough " it to the utmost, and I am sorry to say not unfrequently are encouraged in such practice by their medical advisers. Of course this can happen in any place, but I speak of it here because the incentive so to do is much greater in these health resorts. Another point, which physiologically to explain is extremely difficult, but nevertheless exists, is the practical impossibility of returning home for many patients. I have often seen, and no doubt you all have, patients who having made an apparent recovery in a distant resort, living in perfect comfort a life there no different from any other person, but showing all the signs of renewed activity, with doubled intensity of their former attack after a very short stay in their former home surroundings.

That there are undeniable advantages which we can produce for our patients only by a removal to another climate, our *confrères* from those regions will sufficiently emphasise, so that I need not dwell on them here. But to prove that climate in itself has to be a necessary adjunct to other therapeutic measures in the treatment of this disease, in a manner satisfactory to themselves as well as others, will be a difficult task. Here, on the other hand, we are able to observe from sanatorium statistics, that under proper management about 40 per cent. of cases from a mixed material can recover and remain well for a period of from one to ten years after dismissal from the institution, and this is not in climates with any very distinctive features. I refer to the statistics of Falkenstein and Hohenhonneff, where most cases are followed up for years after dismissal. That under the same *régime* in high altitudes not much better results can be accomplished, the Davos statistics of Dr. Turban clearly demonstrate. In a disease like this, of such pronounced chronic character, with such frequent remissions and exacerbations of activity, only observations over a series of years has value for the determination of the best therapeutic measures. This is a desideratum only too often neglected. Here we have facts before us which demand our attention, and the application of the lesson in the establishment of sanatoria everywhere is a most gratifying result. But not for years to come, if ever, can we provide accommodation for most of our tuberculous patients in sanatoriums. Still it is possible to apply the same principles in private practice. The difficulties are often very great, and to attempt to treat a patient in a city or larger town is almost impossible without having to make too great concessions. But we can find for the majority quarters in the suburbs, or still somewhat farther away, where a hygienic-dietetic *régime* can be carried out to perfection, where with appropriate shelters we can enable our patients to practically live out of doors in almost all kinds of weather, and as any one, who only tries it, will readily find out, to the distinct advantage of the patient. The supply of the proper kind of food is certainly facilitated, and at a considerably lower expense in most instances. And if we once come to it to have a corps of specially trained visiting nurses, we shall be able to supervise the details of the *régime* in a most satisfactory manner. That the larger cities are more apt to create such institutions hardly needs comment. Few cities have not in their surrounding country, localities of good climatic conditions; they do not have an abundance of sunshine, a dry atmosphere, a low barometric pressure, but they have air pure and uncontaminated, which we can, by appropriate measures, make available for our patients. Sudden changes, fogs, and rain, are more frequent perhaps, but when one has observed the effect of a prolonged " Frei-Luftkur " in all kinds of weather, one can dispense with the luxuries of more favoured regions. But of course it depends so much on the " how " it is done, and if well and thoroughly, the " where " is of secondary consideration. Pure air and wholesome food properly prepared, are the basic principles of the successful treatment of the disease. Both we can have in abundance near the places where most consumptives come from; to use them to the greatest advantage is the secret of success, and it needs only trying, the *rationale* for so doing being certainly given.

My condemnation of the " climatic " treatment must of needs seem very radical, but I am here speaking for the majority of patients which do not belong to the wealthier classes. I am also not speaking of those who wish and can make a permanent change of residence, neither am I blind to the benefit any change from the habitual surroundings exerts often on a patient's condition. Myself I send yearly numbers of patients away when I can satisfy myself they can find the same comforts abroad as at home.

My advocation of home treatment is based on the conviction that by its judicious application we can do for many of our patients a great deal more than by sending them away, and I do so especially in opposition to the practice of indiscriminately dispatching patients in all stages, "with little health and little wealth," without first considering the measure thoroughly and in every direction.

"Tuberculosis; therefore Creasote or Colorado," are much used watchwords which should be condemned wherever there is an occasion for it.

HOME TREATMENT *VERSUS* CLIMATIC TREATMENT OF PHTHISIS.

VINCENT Y. BOWDITCH, M.D.

BOSTON.

IN entering upon the discussion of the relative merits of home (sanatorium) and climatic treatment of phthisis, we are confronted not only by a certain vagueness in the terms used, but also by the lack thus far of evidence sufficiently reliable to warrant an absolutely fair·comparison. We have to rely up to the present, it seems to me, upon strong impressions made upon our minds from individual experience, rather than upon absolute data, the result of large collective experience.

We all know that up to the last few years there has been an astonishing lethargy in the medical world in regard to the sanatorium treatment of phthisis, a lethargy which has of very recent years been replaced by enthusiasm extending even to the laity, and to such a degree that those of us who have been preaching this gospel for some time, feel it often necessary to take almost a conservative ground, fearing that rash and unwarranted statements will only end by bringing discredit upon a system which thus far has been productive of better results than any other in the cure of phthisis. I need not reiterate before this Society my own position in regard to sanatorium treatment, for I have on several occasions had the pleasure of presenting to you the results obtained at the Sharon Sanitarium, near Boston. Of late my connection with the large State Sanatorium at Rutland, Massachusetts, would indicate my attitude on this question. My experience, however, is of course confined to a section of the United States which has always been considered a most unfavourable one for tubercular patients. The results obtained in these sanatoria certainly have justified us in materially changing our views as to the curability of phthisis, even in New England, under certain conditions. I have been deeply impressed, too, by the large percentage of not only those patients in whom the disease has been completely arrested, but with the gratifyingly large number who have had no apparent return of the disease, even when obliged, as in some cases, to return, against advice, to occupations unfavourable to health. Bearing these facts in mind, the following questions come to us :—

(1) How far is it necessary to send patients to distant climates to regain their health, provided they will submit themselves to a prolonged stay in a sanatorium near at home ?

(2) Will the percentage of cures in patients who receive treatment in home sanatoria be as large as those treated similarly in climates usually thought to be more favourable for cure than others ?

(3) Will the after-histories of " arrested " cases, including those " apparently cured," for instance, in a sanatorium in Massachusetts, show equally favourable results with those of patients who have been in a similar institution in Colorado, and who have remained in that region ?

At this juncture we are confronted by the fact of the singular lack of sanatoria thus far in certain western climates which are now considered to be the most favourable for consumptives. From the few which exist I know of no published and reliable statistics which would enable us to make fair comparisons, and, as I said at the outset, for our conclusions we are compelled thus far to rely upon general impressions rather than absolute data.

In answer to the first question, I can only say that it would be impossible for me to lay down the law absolutely for all cases. We know beyond the shadow of a doubt that the percentage of those who get well in unfavourable climates, when properly treated in sanatoria, is vastly better than when such cases are left to themselves at home, and yet I am perfectly certain that there are some cases which, not having done well even under sanatorium treatment in New England, have greatly improved when sent to Colorado for instance, or some other health resort. That the reverse is true I can also testify, for we have had cases at Rutland who have shown signs of going down hill in Colorado, but who have greatly improved upon their return to the hills of central Massachusetts. It would seem to me, therefore, equally foolish to say that it is no longer necessary to send patients to a distant climate, or that every patient must go far away to regain his health. Each case must be treated individually, and not as one of a class, and every attempt must be regarded always at first as experimental.

In answer to the second question, there can be no doubt in reasonable minds, it seems to me, that in following the old methods of merely sending patients away from home haphazard without special supervision, the chances of permanent cure are much greater if the patient selects a favourable climate, for instance like Colorado, New Mexico, or California, than if he stays without supervision in our changeable and harsh New England climate.

Sunshine and a dry porous soil are well known to be among the most important factors for health, and in the western regions just mentioned, these conditions are found in a remarkable degree, to say nothing of the altitude, which doubtless has its own favourable effect for various reasons, some of which can be obtained only by artificial means at a lower level.

Taking these facts into consideration then, and although greatly impressed by results which I have seen accomplished in most unfavourable climates, especially in New England, I am at present strongly of the belief that if sanatorium methods are adopted and thoroughly carried out in what are considered the most healthful climates, we shall accomplish even better results than in less favourable regions.

In regard to the third question, it would seem to me impossible with our present knowledge to answer it with any degree of precision, and we can only give our impressions gained from our experience in general.

In a paper read before this Society two years ago, I gave you the subsequent histories of cases of arrested phthisis,* which had been at the Sharon Sanitarium. Some of you will remember that the percentage of those who had remained well after a number of years was gratifyingly large, even when in some cases they had again taken up occupations not of the most hygienic nature.

It is too early yet to give satisfactory data upon this point at the Rutland Sanatorium, for not enough time has elapsed since the first arrested cases left the institution to make their subsequent histories of much value as yet. In our last annual report (1900), however, the following statement was made : —

" Of the thirty-five cases " arrested " at the time of discharge during the year 1898-1899, all are·alive, and with the exception of three cases, have not relapsed. Two of these relapsed cases have been readmitted. The recurrence of disease in these cases appears to be wholly due to lack of means and consequent inability to live under proper conditions. A large number, however, of the " arrested " cases, although advised to the contrary, returned to the former environments in which the disease originated, and have, contrary to our expectations, almost uniformly remained (to this date, October, 1900) free from abnormal symptoms of disease. A few with care have become even stronger and heavier than when they left the institution."

This is, to say the least, gratifying as far as it goes. The future alone must decide the matter when similar conditions prevail in the east and west, as far as the erection of sanatoria

* " Subsequent Histories of Arrested Cases of Phthisis treated at the Sharon Sanitarium, *Boston Med. and Surg. Journ.*, June 22, 1899.

is concerned. Here again my belief at present is that the latter will show superior results.

I trust that the foregoing remarks may not be so misconstrued that I shall be thought to have abated in the least in my desire to have sanatoria for consumptives erected wherever that disease may prevail. Such would be an entire misapprehension of my position. In every community there are many who, for various reasons, cannot go to distant resorts, and it is for these people especially, that we need large numbers of properly-equipped sanatoria throughout the country.

In a few words, then, my position in this discussion is as follows:—

(1) That from my own experience in New England, I am strongly in favour of the erection of sanatoria for the treatment and cure of consumption wherever the disease prevails.

(2) That as to the relative results to be obtained by this method in favourable or unfavourable climates, I do not think we are in a position to judge fairly at present.

(3) That I believe at present better results can in all probability be obtained by this form of treatment in the western regions like Colorado, New Mexico, California, and similar regions, than in the eastern sections of our country.

THE HOME TREATMENT OF TUBERCULOSIS *VERSUS* THE CLIMATIC TREATMENT.*

BY EDWARD O. OTIS, M.D.

BOSTON.

———

ALL treatment of pulmonary tuberculosis is in one sense climatic. Wherever you treat the disease certain climatic essentials are indispensable. These I consider to be first and foremost, pure air; next, freedom from dust and high winds; a fair amount at least, of sunshine; a reasonably dry soil, and freedom from sudden, great, and frequent variations of temperature. There are other climatic and regional conditions desirable and beneficial, but not essential, viz., altitude, dryness of the atmosphere, equability of temperature, continuous clear weather, absence of excessive heat or cold. Some, or all of these additional climatic conditions enhance, as we all recognise, the value of the climate *per se;* but when they have to be obtained by compelling the patient to be acclimated twice over, first to the new climate and then again reacclimated to the old, it is a debatable question whether the additional gain is worth the price paid. There are also various other sacrifices which have to be made for the gain, which I will mention presently.

If for example, the Colorado climate, and that of Rutland, Sharon, Saranac, or Lakewood, were equally accessible and equally easy of choice, I should say choose by all means Colorado, for it possesses a greater number of favourable

* Presented as a part of the discussion upon this subject at the American Climatological Association, May 31, at Niagara Falls.

climatic factors; but when we weigh the demands to be complied with, in order to obtain the Colorado climate, by the resident of the east or north, above those of the other near-at-home resorts, it is a question whether the additional climatic excellences are worth the additional cost.

Since we have arrived at a realising sense of the fundamental principles involved in the hygienic-dietetic treatment of pulmonary tuberculosis, the importance of climate, though great as it is, is now held, and with truth I believe, to be but one of the factors in the *ensemble* of the treatment. Formerly, as we know, climate was considered the predominating, nay, the sole factor. At one time it was a warm climate like Florida, and the exodus of patients was in that direction; at another a cold climate like Minnesota. Then the altitudes, and the rush of patients was to Colorado. The magic of climate as the totality of treatment, as I have said, now no longer holds sway, but any region whose climate permits the patients to continuously, or as nearly that as possible, remain out of doors in pure air, is a favourable one for the hygienic-dietetic treatment. Viewed in this light, the "home treatment," as here defined, is qualified to accomplish favourable results, and those already obtained in Europe and this country attest the soundness of this proposition.

In the home climate, moreover, there is the indubitable advantage of retaining the patient in the same climate in which he has previously passed his existence, and where he must live—in a large majority of cases at least—the remainder of it. Whatever risk there is in a double radical change of climate is obviated. Even so enthusiastic a partisan of the Colorado climate as Solly writes: "It is fair to assume that *about* 50 *per cent.* of the total number coming to Colorado can return to their homes to live in safety, provided of course, the danger to them in returning home is only climatic."

Furthermore, by treating the patient near his usual and accustomed residence, we take advantage of the psychic influence of familiar surroundings. A favourable mental attitude is no small factor in the cure of disease, as we all know. I recall the case of a patient whose improvement was more prompt and rapid from embracing the cult of " Christian Science," all through the hopeful mental attitude it placed him in, and the freedom from fear it produced. Proximity to friends and familiar scenes, if not abused, buoys up the spirits and strengthens the will ; nothing is more depressing than nostalgia.

Again, the pecuniary factor is a very important consideration with a large number of patients. The expense of a long journey and residence in a health resort, even if, by dint of sacrifice and exertion, it can be attained, is a source of more or less constant worry. " Here I am," says the patient, " spending all this money, and after all shall I recover ? If I do not recover within such a time I shall be obliged to return, because my money will be exhausted." How often have our Colorado *confrères* reiterated the statement that the most essential requisite in coming to this resort is a well-lined pocket book.

With the exception of Brehmer's and Dettweiler's experience, and that of a few others in sanatoria, it was not until a comparatively recent date that even phthisio-therapeutists assured themselves, or realised that pulmonary tuberculosis could be successfully treated in a home climate like that of England, Germany, or New England. The favourable experience of the last decade in these countries has been a revelation, I think, to us all, and an attestation of the truth that no excellence of climate will compensate for the disregard of a carefully-arranged plan of life, adapted to the individual patient, constantly insisted upon with authority, and supervised by the expert phthisio-therapeutist. If the strenuous life leads to moral victory and achievement, it none the less leads to success in the struggle against tuberculosis. Comparing sanatorium treatment at home with non-sanatorium treatment in a health resort, I doubt whether the additional climatic excellence compensates for the absence of the sanatorium *régime.* Try as he will, and be as faithful as he may, I do not believe it possible for the physician in a free resort to exercise that despotic power and personal influence over his patients which the physician in a closed resort is enabled to do. In the one case absolute power is possessed, in the other it is not. In either case a firm will and a sympathetic nature is essential on the side of the physician, but in the one case these attributes have full play, and in the other they do not.

It does not seem to me that we are yet in possession of sufficiently accurate and extended statistics of treatment, under the two different conditions here discussed, to judge, with any great precision, from the results obtained. The conditions, as to stages of the disease, class of patients, detail of treatment, &c., vary so greatly that comparison of results seems both impossible and unfair. For example, at Rutland, out of an almost unlimited number of applicants, only the very incipient and most hopeful cases are selected; and to compare results obtained under these ideal conditions with those of other sanatoria or free resorts, where cases of varying stages and differing degrees of prospective favourable issue are received, would be manifestly unjust and misleading.

Then again, before we are in a position to determine the end results, several years must elapse. Further, it seems to me that we must compare sanatorium results with sanatorium results, and open-resort results with open-resort results.

The statistics which have been used to show the advantages of the high altitude treatment over the home and sanatorium treatment, like the large number collected by Solly, and given in Hare's "System of Practical Therapeutics," and elsewhere, are those, it must be remembered, of ten years or more ago, before we thoroughly appreciated and employed, as we do to-day, the hygienic treatment of tuberculosis in all its strenuousness. The results we are obtaining to-day would, I believe, give a more favourable showing for the home treatment. Knoff†

† " Prophylaxis and Treatment of Pulmonary Tuberculosis," 1899.

is the authority for the statement that cures effected in our home climates have been more lasting and more assured than cures obtained in more genial climates away from home.   In this opinion concur Leyden, Gerhardt, Dettweiler, Walthers, and others.

If other things were equal, which, as I have pointed out, they are not, I am inclined to believe that a sanatorium favourably located in the Rockies, Alps, or other altitudes, conducted on the same lines as Dettweiler's, at Falkenstein, would, with the same class and stage of cases, produce better results than a sanatorium in our home climates.   Turban's elaborate report of results at Davos, published in 1900, appear to show this.

In conclusion, it must be a source of great congratulation to us all who are engaged in the treatment of tuberculosis, that the prospects of success in the home treatment appear so auspicious. It is the very small minority of the tuberculous who are able, or willing, to travel far afield for a resort in which to take the cure.   The majority, for one reason or another, must, if the hygienic cure is attempted at all, undertake it near home.

DISCUSSION UPON "CLIMATIC TREATMENT OF PULMONARY TUBERCULOSIS *VERSUS* HOME SANATORIA."

BY S. G. BONNEY, A.M., M.D.

DENVER, COLORADO.

IN attempting to discuss so broad a subject in a limited time, I will first define my position as an earnest advocate of the value of climate in the treatment of consumption. I am likewise heartily in support of a suitable *régime* of daily life and management, but believe this to bear to the preceding the relation chiefly of a most valuable adjunct. While each separately constitutes an exceedingly important factor in the effort to secure arrest, they are, nevertheless, mutually interdependent, with the best results only obtained through their conjoined effect.

By an appropriate system of daily life, I do not refer necessarily to the full interpretation of the closed treatment of tuberculosis as exhibited in sanatoria. Such institutions are of benefit by virtue of certain features of regimen and discipline, in addition to the relief from work, changed surroundings and open air existence. I believe that proper living, and obedience to detailed instructions, frequently can be insisted upon through the personal and interested attention of the medical adviser, even without the aid of special institutions. I am not, however, in sympathy with any effort to minimise the value of such resorts under certain conditions, and for properly selected cases. I recognise that even in unfavourable climates their field of usefulness is great, and perhaps even more so in health resorts, but must insist that life in a sanatorium is not always a *sine quâ non* for the observance of the strictest disciplinary system of regimen.

It is frequently admitted that State aid for consumptives, in the shape of home sanatoria for those in incipient stages, who are financially unable to seek climatic change, is a work of noble purpose, and attended by satisfying results. Of still greater value would be the erection of local hospitals for those hopelessly ill, on account of the excellent opportunities afforded for exercising proper prophylaxis and control. Such a class constitute a far greater source of danger to the community than many of the incipient cases, without expectoration and without bacilli, now often admitted to sanatoria. The latter, in an appropriate climate, are not too ill to engage in some occupation, if necessary, with a reasonable assurance of improvement.

It appears, then, that sanatorium *régime* without climate is obviously applicable to one class. Climatic influence, without an ideal manner of life, is likewise suited to the necessities of another. The essence of the present controversy relates to what shall be done for the enormous class who are able and anxious to avail themselves of every rational opportunity to recover from their disease. They appeal to their medical advisers to assist them, not merely in obtaining a degree of rest, but in securing *arrest* of an infectious process incident to their existing environment.

How can the logic of climatic truths be longer ignored? In the advocacy of home sanatoria, attempts are being made publicly to refute the favourable influence of climate. An undue enthusiasm throughout the country, awakened by the tardy recognition of the value of certain features of regimen, may be sufficient to delay the acceptance of the more comprehensive principles of management, at the expense of a considerable sacrifice of life.

The prevailing tendency to provide home sanatoria for all

15

classes, and to repudiate the established facts of climatic influence, cannot fail to prove in the end a most unfortunate delusion. It seems opportune at this time of local sanatoria agitation, to reassert and emphasise the intrinsic distinctive value of climate, reinforced by proper living, as the all-important factor in the treatment of disease.

The influence of climate itself, and that of sanatorium *régime*, should be studiously regarded without bias, prejudice, or preconceived ideas, in order to understand clearly the *rôle* played by each in the great tragedy of consumption. A final conclusion can only be reached from an impartial investigation of actual results obtained under approximately like conditions.

The advocates of home sanatoria base their claims for support upon their recorded results of improvement. Disclaiming any desire to reflect upon the actual worth of such institutions, the utility of which, for those unable to seek climatic change, has been accorded, it is nevertheless a matter of record that the heralded satisfactory results are very largely due to the fact that only the most incipient cases are admitted. Those more advanced, after a disastrous delay, are sent away from home to continue the struggle in a distant clime and against great odds.

A report of the work done and the results obtained for one year at a State hospital for consumptives in New England, states that out of 214 admissions, 35, or 16 per cent., were discharged as arrested. Of these 35 cases, 9 are reported as being at all times without bacilli, but with undoubted signs and symptoms, and 4 as without signs or bacilli, but with suspicious symptoms. Two were without sputum, but responded to the tuberculin test. Only 8 were described as having signs somewhat advanced. The average stay in the hospital of these cases was four and one-half months.

It is at once manifest that such cases belong to an entirely different category than the 71 per cent. of all cases previously reported by me as seeking climatic relief, with distinct evidence of advanced infection in each lung. The unanimity of recorded results, reported by various observers, to the effect that nearly three-fourths of these latter cases taken as they come, may be expected to improve in favourable climates, furnishes a standard for the purpose of comparison, as yet utterly unapproached by sanatorium *régime,* or by any special methods of treatment.

The good results of sanatorium management for early cases in unfavourable localities is fully admitted, but this shall not be construed as constituting an argument against the greatly increased benefits to be derived in an appropriate climate, and by a much larger class of cases, even in some instances despite limited opportunities for suitable *régime.* A considerable class are financially unable to observe a strict system of daily life either at home in closed sanatoria, or in health resorts, yet are permitted by virtue of pronounced climatic advantages to perform light work, at the same time securing a marked prolongation of life, and not infrequently an eventual arrest of the disease. Climate alone is certainly responsible for results obtained in such cases as these.

If a suitable regimen *without* the favourable influence of climate is capable of producing a perceptible improvement in very incipient cases, how much greater and more enduring results, and in how much greater number of cases, advanced though they be, may be obtained by precisely the *same manner* of life *plus* the beneficence of climate. Why should not a far more improved mode of life be enacted in an appropriate climate than in less favoured regions, by reason of added opportunities for outdoor air, on account of increased sunshine, warmth, dryness, and rarefaction? It would appear that only in such localities could the fullest conception of a proper method of living be satisfactorily conducted. If a system of regimen necessarily incomplete in moist, cloudy regions, is good, a wellnigh perfect adherence to its principles in a land of perpetual sunshine, invigorating air, inspiring scenery and blue sky is certainly better.

Again, are we not forced to consider the great infrequency with which consumption develops in certain climates, and is it not reasonable to expect invalids—other conditions of management being equal—to do far better under those climatic influences which have constantly sufficed to prevent the development of the disease, than when subjected to the same treacherous conditions which have operated directly in favour of its spread, and which will continue to be in force for all time.

Have not consumptives an inviolable right, provided their financial condition will permit, to expect their advisers to place them in the midst of a new environment, with opportunities for recreation and social advantages, facilities for industry and business enterprise, and possibilities of advancement and fortune incident to a new country, with its western stir and activity. The invalid is not thus cast into exile apart from family and friends, in some barren sanatorium, but at once in his own home is he surrounded by all the comforts of daily life, enjoying a suitable environment, although in the midst of an active civilisation. By degrees he is permitted to adapt himself to engage later in a useful and prosperous existence. Upon his recovery he is not compelled to go back again to previous conditions of danger, only to experience the dread return of his trouble, but finds a hearty welcome to the ranks of his fortunate predecessors, with abundant opportunities for the employment of the natural proclivities.

DISCUSSION.

Dr. S. A. FISK : The subject is so vast that I hardly know how to begin, but it strikes me that a sharp line of demarcation between the climatic and the home treatment is a question of the pocket-book. I think if any one of us were to choose for himself he would select the most favourable circumstances he could get, the best climate and the best home at the same time ; he would do everything that he could to build up his nutrition and at the same time provide an abundance of fresh dry air. He would not go to a good climate and starve himself or live in a damp room, on the other hand he would select, if he could, the best climate, and there endeavour to enjoy the best opportunities to regulate his life, seeking proper advice. He would not climb the mountains with an acute trouble; he would rest. I am glad to hear this question of rest emphasised. It is not a new thing at all, for some of us who have lived in the Rocky Mountains have insisted on the idea for years, and when Dr. Hance summarises what he has to say in the words food, fresh air and rest, I think he embodies what has been advocated in Colorado for some time, and I heartily approve of it. Personally I am very glad to see so much attention paid to home treatment: I believe in it, but it does not diminish my belief in climatic treatment at all. I would not neglect the one at the expense of the other. I would try to get both. Let me give a quotation: " These ought ye to have done and not to leave the other undone."

Dr. SOLLY: If I had my way every consumptive should first go into a sanatorium, not necessarily to remain there long, or even for treatment, but for observation. These patients come first under the observation of the family physician, who tells them they have a cold, or a bronchitis, and he allows them to drift on into a serious condition; then they go to a specialist who accurately diagnoses the trouble, but who does not know the man, which is the most unfortunate thing of all. If you would put your patients into sanatoria for a week or so before sending them away, then you could learn their tendencies and select the proper climate for them. There has been a great deal of talk about home-sickness, and no doubt a great many suffer from it. You remember the remark of the gentleman going to heaven who said, " It's all very well, but it isn't Boston." There are a number of patients to whom change is of great value if it only gets them away from their work, responsibilities, and business troubles.

Then the value of the sanatorium treatment as against the open-air treatment is seen in the evidence undoubtedly in favour of the former. The statistics show that, perhaps, better than they should, because they are mostly selected cases. Divided into classes, the first stage cases show better results in a sanatorium than do the open air cases in both climates. As regards the relative value of climate in sanatorium treatment, I made some studies last year, when for three or four months I was in Europe, and I am sure the results are better in the high than in the low climates.

As regards the changing from one climate to the other there is this to say, that there are many who cannot live anywhere else except in Colorado; for instance, if I was living in London to-day I would be dead! . . . . We meet patients living on the Atlantic sea coast and in England who have gotten well in Colorado, and if a patient gets well in a good climate he is well anywhere, but of course he has to adapt himself to the home climate again.

Dr. HART: I agree thoroughly with Dr. Klebs that no climate or drug is a specific for tuberculosis, but I consider climate an essential element in the treatment. The ideal home treatment is to be found in a climate that is favourable to the conditions of the patient. Fifteen miles from a city is not home treatment; it is merely seeking after climatic treatment. Health resorts are to some extent prohibiting the entrance of tuberculous patients, and I think the result will be more home treatment. Colorado is not closing its doors against the tuberculous.

Dr. EDSON : I agree very closely with Dr. Bowditch. It seems to me that in our discussions we are inclined to make the error that has been made too often in the past, of looking upon the climate as a specific and contrasting its effects with that of home treatment or creosote treatment. The attitude we should take with each patient is purely an individual one in which we give that patient the best opportunity for recovery that his disease and his social status will allow him. The best that he can get is what we must order, both as regards food, bed room, and quality of air. Many cannot obtain the best of all these, others are in such condition that they can obtain them by a little sacrifice, as by going to a sanatorium near home, and others who can afford the best should have it. The statistics of climatic resorts of ten to fifteen years ago belonged to a period prior to the full appreciation of the benefit of food and rest, but still those statistics do show better results than the treatment at home with the same neglect of rest and proper nutrition. Now, if a patient can obtain the best the advantages of climate still hold, and that climate which will give him the best opportunity to live in the air and sunshine gives him the best chance of recovery.

The PRESIDENT: The benefit of the discussion we are having this morning lies not alone in the attempt to discriminate between the treatment at home and the treatment in a climate away from home, but in the fact that as an association we are emphasising the importance of securing early proper treatment, which is the open air treatment with food and rest or exercise, according to the patient's condition, as determined by temperature and other points. If the average doctor were asked what he prescribed for his consumptives he would say tonics and cough mixtures, iron, strychnia, creosote, &c. Now, the important thing for us to emphasise is that it is not medicinal therapy that is needed but the proper hygienic management of the daily life.

Dr. BOWDITCH : I would like to have a statement put on record with reference to Rutland. Dr. Otis said that our cases were picked. That is true so far as we can do it, but to say that they are all incipient cases would not be correct. As a matter of fact the average duration of the disease previous to entrance is ten months. I have admitted some cases that had gone on even to the third stage, not as a rule, but where there seemed to be an opportunity to improve them. The results we have obtained are from all those that came in in the last year. Of the really incipient cases 80 per cent. were arrested.

Dr. OTIS : All I intended to convey by my remarks was that the conditions were remarkably favourable for securing good results, because, not necessarily the incipient cases, but the most favourable ones were selected.

Dr. MCGAHAN : I have been expecting our Boston friends to say something about what constitutes an ideal home treatment. As I understand there is a physician in Brooklyn who is treating his patients by having them sleep day and night on top of their houses. I think that is an ideal home treatment. When you come to testing places Dr. Fisk struck the key-note in saying that a man has to consult his pocket-book. There is no doubt we need good food and good air, but it is better to stay at home and get as much of these as we can, than to go to some health resort and be put into a cheap boarding-house. That, I think, is the worst thing that can happen to a patient. In my sanatorium at Aiken, all I hope to do for six months with these patients is to teach them how to take care of themselves. They come without the slightest idea of hygiene, and some of the hardest cases to handle have been doctors from the country. I had one such in a cottage, and it was with the greatest difficulty that I could keep him from having that house at a temperature of 75 degrees or over. Education is one of the most important features of our work. I can bear out Dr. Bowditch's statement that he does get a good many bad cases at Rutland. I have seen some this winter that he sent south for a warmer climate, and they had all been bad cases when he took them in.

Dr. FREMONT-SMITH: It may be of some interest if I state the results we have had in the treatment of tuberculosis in Florida. Between 1883 and 1893 a good many cases were sent there, and it was my privilege to observe these and note the results. Among the acute cases, those with temperature did badly if they remained, while some that were sent to other climates without the expectation of recovery got well. I remember a friend who went to California and lives there well now. The reason for not sending those patients to Florida I do not know, but certainly they do not do well. Cases of chronic fibroid phthisis will do well in Florida if they have no temperature. That is the classification I should make, perhaps, of the cases that might come to Florida.

Dr. CAMPBELL: In tuberculosis we have a wasting disease that has to be cured by improving nutrition. We can get this improved nutrition, to a degree, at home under proper regulations, but to a greater degree by a change of climate and surroundings that come with a residence away from home. I think our attention has been centred in those who are wealthy and are able to pay their fees in sanatoria as well as to make a change in their homes. There is another class who have not been given due consideration. Observing the labouring classes in Colorado, I have seen just as marked improvement in the poor who are labouring for their daily bread as in the wealthy who have all the luxuries; consequently I should advise the proper patients to go to Colorado even if they had to labour for their living.

Dr. GETCHELL: I want to bring out a point that has not been touched upon and that is the educative value of a sanatorium in any community. I speak of it here in the hope that it will influence legislation in some States In our State it has been of value not only to the patients but to the physicians and laity in the neighbourhood. Another point is that these sanatoria should be built by the State, and our experience is that it is exceedingly important that the initiative be taken and the institution founded and set to running under the proper conditions and influences. The people will take much more interest in such a public institution than in any private one, and its work will become better known, for there are annual reports of its condition, a visit from the Legislative Committee every year, and every year it is necessary to go before the Legislature for money, and then the matter is thoroughly discussed. These are advantages, but there are disadvantages which must be borne in mind, such as the attempt to use the institution for political purposes. The question is a much broader one than the treatment of a few con-sumptives. It is really the question of eradicating tuberculosis from the community.

Dr. KNIGHT: I have had a good deal of experience in the treatment of tuberculosis and I have had patients recover under all possible con-ditions, with and without treatment, at home and in better climates. One of the most remarkable cases of arrest of tuberculosis is that I have had under observation for nearly twenty years, occurred in a young girl of bad hereditary tendency, a hard-working teacher, living and working all the time at home. Undoubtedly there is something in climatic influences and we cannot give it up. It is a factor in cure and a powerful one for patients able to avail themselves of it. One reason for the pretty constant improve-ment in patients in sanatoria now is, I think, the conditions of rest and food. I remember very well that years ago in Bellevue Hospital consumptives improved, as a rule, after they came in, no matter whether advanced cases or not, and it was probably because they had rest and better food than they were accustomed to.

Dr. Minor said something that impressed me in regard to giving home treatment, that is, treatment not exactly at home, but away from home, yet perhaps near home. A patient will do a great deal better if you send him only five or ten miles from home, and put him under supervision, for it is almost impossible in the patient's own house to carry out such provisions as the doctor uses at Asheville, and others at other places. This is what is meant by many when they speak of "home treatment," i.e., treatment in a home climate, not necessarily in the patient's own home. It seems to me unfair to compare the results of sanatorium and so-called climatic treatment, because in the one case the patient is under constant observation and care, and in the other he is running wild even if in a good climate.

Dr. WHITNEY: I think the position taken by Dr. Knight is one of importance. We have watched from Denver with a great deal of interest, and without jealousy, the institution and development of the sanatorium plan of treatment, and I believe that as yet the whole question is *sub judice*. Those of us who come from Denver and have had the advantages of that climate may well be excused if we are still loyal to Colorado. Thirteen years ago I went to Colorado with bacilli, and since that time there has never been a month that I have not been engaged in active work. This would not have been possible in any institution, and I cannot but congratulate myself that I selected the sanatorium bounded by the Rocky Mountains and the Gulf of Mexico, instead of one confined within four walls. As emphasised by Dr. Knight, for a certain class of patients, no institutional treatment can ever supplant one which gives the patient the freedom of several States for purposes of business or amusement.

Dr. CURTIN : I have had considerable experience in sending patients away from home. I have visited the best health resorts and think that a great deal more can be accomplished by climate, but at the same time a great deal is to be accomplished at home. I have seen a great many cases recover entirely in the City of Philadelphia, which city is not considered to have a good climate for tuberculosis. One of the great difficulties is to get patients to follow directions at home, whereas if you have them away from family cares in a sanatorium you can much better control them. They have their trials and business cares at home which often prevents their being benefited to the fullest extent.

Dr. J. C. WILSON, of Philadelphia : These paper have been most interesting and important, and yet in certain respects I have been disappointed. I am sure there can be no contention as to the advantages of certain forms of climatic treatment in connection with other methods of personal hygiene, and there can be no question furthermore as regards the usefulness of organised systematic treatment, first as to the benefit of the individual, and second as to the laying down of rules that will influence the practice of physicians everywhere. I had hoped that there would be a little more discussion with regard to the management of individual cases in their homes. We have all met with cases that recover notwithstanding the fact that they live in unfavourable surroundings and continue to pursue their occupations. It is a question of social economics, and this association must draw the attention of the local governing bodies to the absolute necessity of developing plans for the treatment of tuberculosis in the localities where the disease occurs. Such institutions must be arranged in two general groups : First, those for the management of beginning cases, or at least, of cases in which there is a reasonable prospect of recovery ; and a second group, which comprises hospitals for the care of the hopeless cases and advanced consumptives. The incipient cases cannot be admitted to general hospitals, and if now and then a case of advanced phthisis finds its way into a general hospital it is apt to be shamefully neglected.

Dr. NEWTON : I am at present on a Committee in the State of New Jersey which is trying to induce the State to provide an institution of this kind, and the Chairman of the Legislative Committee said to us last year something like this, " Gentlemen, it is an incurable disease, the patients never get well, and what's the use of doing so much for them ? "

Dr. BALDWIN : In regard to the suggestion that has been made that well-to-do patients should be sent to the best climate they can afford, I think the gentlemen will agree with me that there are many such patients that will not go so far away as Colorado unless it is made plain to them that it is absolutely necessary to sell out their business and permanently change their residence. Therefore I would say that while no climate nor any other method of treatment is absolutely essential there is a demand for sanatoria in the best climates and also in those as near the patient's home as possible. I do not believe that statistics of sanatoria available at present are useful for comparing different altitudes, different sanatoria, or different climates. In order to get over the question as to whether it was best for this or that patient to go to a sanatorium I studied my records carefully and mentally concluded that two-fifths of my private patients would do better in a sanatorium; two-fifths for various reasons would be better outside; and of the remaining one-fifth I was in doubt. I seems to me that the keynote in the sanatorium question is to *individualise* according to the needs of each patient.

Dr. MINOR : I think this discussion shows the great necessity there always is in medicine of keeping the happy medium in our view. In every advance there are always those who run to the extremes. Everybody admits now that climate while of inestimable value is not a specific, and I was sorry to hear Dr. Bonney put climate before life and to have Dr. Solly put climate down as the first essential. I believe it is largely a question of money; the patient who can afford to leave home for a proper climate and is supervised carefully there and is willing to obey strict orders is wasting a precious opportunity in not going ; but a patient who cannot spend as a minimium say ten dollars a week, who is obliged to live in bad quarters on poor food, or who, if he goes, is his own doctor and regulates his own life, had far better stay at home.

Dr. HANCE : One thought occurred to me while listening to the discussion, and I agree with Dr. Whitney that the question is still *sub judice*, and that is, that if we the physicians were the patients we would all try to get to some good climate, and I think that puts the stamp of approval on climate as being one of the important things. When it comes to a question of ourselves whether we would go to the best climate when we had tuberculosis, we would every one answer yes.

Dr. ARNOLD C. KLEBS, of Chicago : I have very little to say except that I regret that this "fight" between adherents of home and climatic treatment has taken our attention away from Dr. Baldwin's very excellent paper. It is certainly a scheme that should be observed by every one for making his own prognosis of cases and before sending them away to some sanatorium. As regards the opinions expressed in favour of the different modes of treatment, it is most gratifying to note that we all agree to the chief importance of the basis principles: hygiene, diet, open air and the systematic carrying out of the *régime*, with due attention to the individuality of the patient and the state of his disease, and not pin down our faith to one element alone, may it be climate, medicinal preparations, or anything else.

CLINICAL ASPECTS OF SPA TREATMENT.

BY BEVERLEY ROBINSON, M.D.

NEW YORK.

IT is frequently affirmed by patients that they receive benefit from a particular spa treatment they can obtain in no other way. A short time ago a gentleman informed me that he was a sufferer from neurasthenia, that he had been to the hot springs of Virginia, that he had also spent some time at Aiken, South California, with the hope of being benefited, but he knew of only one place where he secured treatment which was helpful and curative, viz., at Divonne, in Switzerland, where the cold spinal douches made him feel like a new man. I advised him, as it was winter, to go to Lakewood, N.J., and see what the cold spinal douche as there given might accomplish for him. If it had been summer, I should have probably sent him to Sharon, or Richfield Springs, always supposing he could not go to Divonne, and could be persuaded to give one of these resorts a trial.

What is true of Divonne for the patient referred to, is true for other sufferers of Aix, Carlsbad, Homburg, Vichy, and foreign spas in general, not to speak of the well-known places at home, like Saratoga, Bedford, White Sulphur, Glenwood, and Avon Springs.

Many practical questions come to mind in view of these statements, which are frequently asked the general practitioner in regard to spas and their treatment. The questions are of climate, of waters, baths, scene, occupation, rest, food, exercise, massage, and electricity.

It is truly affirmed that there are natural springs in the United States, excelled by none elsewhere, and yet treatment is often unsatisfactory at these resorts. Take Saratoga as an example; is it not healthful and agreeable so far as summer climate is concerned, and are not the waters of Saratoga re-markable in their variety and curative effects, if *judiciously* used? Unfortunately, in the latter consideration, we find a problem difficult of solution.

The average American who goes to Saratoga even for a "cure," will not, or cannot, secure a suitable dietary *régime* while drinking the waters, nor will he rise and retire early, and walk a prescribed time each morning between his tumblerfuls of spring water. Later, is he satisfied to have his breakfast consist merely of a roll and cup of coffee; or are beefsteak, omelette, fish, griddle cakes, and maple sugar considered somewhat in-dispensable? to be followed with the enjoyment of a high-flavoured cigar, and his feet planted high up, as he sits on the piazza in a quiet, torpid condition. Later, perhaps, a cocktail precedes a too abundant lunch, followed at seven or eight o'clock in the evening by a dinner with sauces, sweets, and champagne. Later still, and again the patient seats himself on the piazza and listens to the orchestra. After a time he becomes tired of this recreation, and seeks the stuffy, ill-ventilated bil-liard or ball room, and finally retires at twelve or one o'clock.

Contrast the life briefly described, with that of a European spa, where the patient is under treatment. At these resorts the hours of sleep and exercise are rigorously enforced; so also the quantity and variety of food and drink; likewise the hours of rising and retiring. On the other hand, I have known more than one person who has endeavoured faithfully to carry out what his physician orders, at one of our health resorts, and it has proved almost impossible to do it, or if accomplished, there is no adequate return from it at all equivalent to a cure abroad.

Admitting that some of our spas equal those of Europe, and admitting that the same careful management of the patient becomes obligatory, could we obtain generally similar good results from spa treatment at home as we do abroad? I do not believe we could. Change of scene, of occupation, mental rest, are essential to many cures. The ocean trip, going and returning, is often invigorating and enjoyable. On board ship neither telegrams nor telephone messages are received. Hence, at times, untold satisfaction. Moreover, there is a subtlety for good in climate different from that we are accustomed to, just as there is remedial power in mineral waters, which mere chemical analysis cannot explain. Of them we may truly say, at times, as Dr. Samuel Wilks does of the "value of drugs": "Our knowledge of them has been mainly empirical, their mode of action being often unknown. I should still maintain, however, that our method of using them is unscientific, if we can say from long observation, that their administration is indicated in particular cases by special circumstances."

Besides, we must admit that occasionally we obtain practical results in the cure of disease, that neutralise completely all preconceived notions.

Another fact of considerable importance which I wish to emphasise, is that the mere use of mineral waters as baths, or for drinking or bath, is not essential in many instances, when compared with the value of guidance of the patient by the spa practitioner in other ways. Let this be well understood, and we shall have less self-medication, and thus the health of fewer people will be jeopardised.

When a patient arrives at a spa, let him put himself in the care of the best, most careful, conscientious practitioner he can secure; let him ignore all the kindly, officious health counsels given by friends, and let him not consider time and opportunity wasted, if his medical adviser tells him to abstain from other than most conservative treatment. And yet let him go regularly to see his physician, report his case, and follow his advice. Frequently it is highest wisdom to say, keep on just as you are doing; make no change; rather than to order some new drug or treatment, which would be useless or harmful.

Fortunately, at many European spas, there are able physicians who are willing tó guide patients wisely, and the latter, if they would merely heed their instructions, would obtain best results.

With respect to our own climatic resorts, there is in many instances a vacuum to be filled. Although I know of several spa practitioners who have good ability, and large and varied experience, owing to the fact that our resorts are relatively of new growth, and because an ambitious worker desires a city reputation, the best men, as 'a rule, seek our large centres of population. Except during the summer months, and for a few years, with a view mainly to the direct pecuniary return, the less popular resorts are poorly supplied with cultivated physicians, and even the best knowń can only boast of .a limited few. A change in this regard will, doubtless, come in time, but the time is not yet present. In time will come also, a true appreciation of the real value.of the spa physiciáns, not to change drugs or prescriptions already tried, but to be the wisest counsellor in the use of every curative agent to be found at the spa, *i.e.,* waters, baths, diet, exercise, massage, electricity, rest.

A difficult matter to adjudicate in a tactful way, is the following : Not infrequently a patient is sent by his family physician to a particular spa, and there directed to the care of a prominent local practitioner. The latter, after careful investigation of the case, may be forced to conclude that the patient has been misdirected, and that another spa was better suited to the cure of his ills ; or, indeed, he may be convinced that "no cure" is required. An embarrassing position for him! He should give his temporary patient the best advice ; he should also be loyal to the colleague who has honoured him, and not only by reason of courtesy and gratitude, but likewise for the ultimate good of the patient. Once let patients feel as though in one way or another, they are misguided or deceived, and confidence is restored with great difficulty. Again, the spa physician may recognise, and properly, that he is not necessarily the source of all wisdom, and he it is who may be in error as to diagnosis and treatment, while the family physician may be wholly correct. It becomes the spa physician, therefore, to be cautious in statement, and not pass judgment until he has had the time and opportunity sufficient to form an accurate and thorough conviction.

As I have intimated already, foreign spas possess an advantage over those at home, in that the reputation of some of their physicians has given additional fame to the spa itself. Not only have they grown grey in harness, but theirs has been a real growth, accompanied with valuable contributions to scientific or practical medicine, and not merely a passage of time, marked by no advances in either direction. Even men of this calibre may be led into error. Patients who really require very little in the way of treatment beyond regulation of diet, rest, exercise, sleep, are advised to do what is useless, or positively weakening and detrimental. In my judgment, there is little doubt that some patients have had their heart power impaired more or less permanently by excessive treatment.

In this connection Dr. Samuel Hyde writes: " There is ' an accumulated condition of depression ' which often follows too prolonged spa treatment, especially by baths of a temperature exceeding 90 degrees F., and this untoward result must always be considered and guarded against as far as possible. Conditions of heart weakness previously existing, may be exaggerated, or even others before absent may be developed " (vide *Journal of Balneology and Climatology*, vol. ii., p. 134). Therefore, wherever a well-trained and highly trustworthy assistant cannot be had, it is wiser to abandon treatment with baths and resistance movements," and to trust entirely to regulated walking exercise, pure fresh air, suitable diet, and drug tonics, not overlooking, of course, the psychical influences of expectancy, hope, and allayed anxiety and fear."—(Hyde.)

It is evident from the foregoing, how important it is to employ instructed and careful assistants, or bathers and manipulators, in spa treatment. Otherwise, even in well-selected cases, our results must be unsatisfactory. Of course the patient's physician must exercise close oversight, and direct the treatment personally, as much as possible. Still, in many instances he must rely considerably upon qualified assistants to do the right thing at the proper time, where some rapid or sudden change of symptoms or conditions occur, and until the physician can be consulted. Too active or too continuous treatment does real harm, and it is not infrequent later to have patients show signs of considerable physical depression during many weeks. The good results, after all, to be obtained from spa treatment, particularly by baths and exercises, depend largely upon the judgment and knowledge with which they are given. It is for this reason that I do not believe so much in the specific effects of certain spas in the treatment of special disorders, as I do in the manner in which the resident physicians make use of their opportunities. No doubt, for example, that the methods pursued by Schott and others, at Nauheim, are not wholly new; no doubt, also, that they have been of great use in certain cases, and finally and especially in showing well-trained physicians elsewhere, what may really be accomplished at the spas where they practise, and with waters quite different from the standpoint of chemical analysis and temperature. In other words, I am satisfied that as good results may be obtained elsewhere, if only the indications, so ably advocated by Schott, are carried out. This fact Schott himself, and to his great honour, has repeatedly emphasised.

In those cases where bad results have followed the treatment of grave forms of disease accurately made out, while it is much to be deplored, it does not not appear to me so regrettable as where the diagnosis is at best questionable, and where, of course, the benefits of any special course of treatment must be most problematical, as the cause and nature of the patient's disease are very obscure.

In the estimation of the value of spa treatment, much importance should be attached to the previous habits of the patient. If they have been correct, or nearly so, we shall not, I believe, get such good effects from treatment, even in well-selected cases, as we shall obtain where the habits have been improper or wrong, purely from a hygienic point of view; and this argument is readily understood without extending it. Of course this statement would not include certain gouty patients in whom periodical outbreaks, more or less continued, will occur, in my experience, despite all usual treatment at home, and can only be met efficiently, if at all, by a well-ordered spa treatment.

Spa physicians are apt to specialise too much. They regard every ailment from a narrow standpoint, and believe that every patient who comes to them is suited to the treatment at the resort where they are. In this belief resides oftentimes lamentable error. Where this source of error, however, is lacking, and there is a broad appreciation of the patient's condition, the physician may be willing, unfortunately, through desire for money, to keep patients coming to him who, he knows, do not require professional care. This stigma can be guarded against solely by recognition of high personal character in the spa physician as being of primary importance, even as it always is elsewhere. In one way or another, I have certainly known several patients who seemingly have been victims. This conviction would be calculated in the minds of physicians and patients at home, to bring the spa treatment into disrepute, and consequently is much to be deplored. In the matter of benefits from spa treatment, a wise and conservative judgment should be exercised. We should not attribute to it too great importance; we should not, on the other hand, undervalue its power for good. If we expect the impossible, of course we shall be disappointed, and disposed to criticise most unfairly. Take a chronic disease of long-standing, for example, should we expect in a few weeks of baths and other useful adjuncts of most rational treatment, a complete cure? Evidently not. . All we may properly hope for is amelioration; and in the *régime* adopted, we may afford an

16

object lesson to our patient which he will try to follow so far as may be indicated and possible upon his return home.

Again, there are many who are sent to a spa for a course of treatment, not because they have a well-defined, special disease to which we can give a particular name, but mainly because their whole system requires a change of life and *régime* in every way, and where " mere drugging " at home is sure to be of no material advantage, and may be even detrimental. Such patients are, unquestionably, more benefited by a spa treatment, rightly indicated and judiciously managed whilst there, than in any other known way. The mere regulation of their habits from day to day for several weeks, and their bringing back, as it were, to a physiological life, with plenty of fresh air and sunshine, moderate exercise, regulated diet, complete freedom from worry, whilst the emunctories of the economy are being stimulated to do good work through water drinking, baths, massage, resistant movements, &c., is productive of no end of good in appropriate cases.

In many of these instances, especially where the spa selected has been one whose effects, even in a moderate way, are slightly debilitating, owing to the effort made to get rid of worn-out, effete cells or retained excreta, an " after cure " is really essential. In the first place, if for no other reason, it is rational because it lengthens a vacation, which is at best none too long to accomplish the results we most desire, viz., the complete renewal or regeneration, as it were, of the fluids and tissues of the economy. In the second place, the site of the " after cure " is, or should be, some elevated mountain resort or sea-shore place, according to circumstances, which shall stimulate and invigorate the patient to that degree that he can return to his life's work later in the best physical condition attainable, and not break down soon again after the " cure," unless he gets it.

An " after cure " means in reality two things: (1) Perfect salubrity of environment; (2) careful and rational habits of daily life. Of course the best selection of a place for this so-called "after cure" will depend much upon the nature of the ailment and the condition of the patient, who has had a "cure."

In the selection of a place for the "after cure," the patient should not go immediately to a very high elevation, but should seek places first of lower altitude, and after these have been thoroughly tried, go to higher elevations if there is reasonable ground for so doing. Such action is, of course, based upon the idea that there may be cardiac depression after the spa treatment, and is pointed out by wise forethought, even though circulatory weakness is not always well defined at first, or even existant then or later.

In addition to the foregoing, I may add two considerations of moment. First, I would emphasise the importance of a patient who goes to a spa for treatment having a detailed history from his home physician of his physical examination and of his antecedent symptoms. Without these data much time and labour are lost, and independently of this, the spa physician is unable to obtain facts which may be compared with the preceding ones, and which are often essential, so as to appreciate accurately the march and evidences of impaired nutrition, or well-defined disease. Again, it is important here, as always in practice of medicine, for the spa physician to be in sympathetic touch with his patient, and by this I mean that he should become familiar with, or recognise, his personal peculiarity or susceptibility, so as to be able at a given moment, to shield or protect him from annoyance, discomfort, or positive injury; when without this transmitted or acquired knowledge he would be working in the dark.

This sort of information is doubtless more important with women, young and old, than with men; and yet even with many men we can do very little to help them even in their physical disabilities, unless we acquire a very considerable control over them mentally. All good, successful family practitioners recognise the important bearing of this statement. It is none the less valuable at times to the spa physician, if he really desires to be useful to his patients, and has a high ideal of his *rôle*.

The mental control of patients comes in part, at least, from the feeling that their own physician understands them, that he is familiar with their habits, peculiarities, and antecedents. ·It is desirable, therefore, if possible, other things being equal, to have medical advice from one's countryman. Few American physicians of reputation are found at foreign spas. Therefore, except in very rare instances, advice from this source cannot be had. It is not quite so true of English physicians, and I must confess I would be prone to recommend an Englishman to my patients rather than a German or Frenchman, if he were at all a man of equal value, on account of his nationality, and because I believe he would comprehend the average American better than the other two.

In all instances where we send patients to health resorts, we should bear in mind the importance of the condition of lungs, kidneys, liver, and skin. These organs are too often disregarded or overlooked in the counsels given to our patients, and yet we cannot too formally emphasise their importance.

I might continue in this way, but I feel I have said enough, especially in view of my great desire. I wish to open a discussion, which I trust may be fruitful of good to the city practitioner, to the resident spa physician, and above all to our patients.

SPA TREATMENT OF GOUT.

BY CHARLES C. RANSOM, M.D.

NEW YORK.

THE general principles involved in the treatment of gout are three, viz. : —

(1) The treatment of an acute paroxysm, with speedy relief of pain.

(2) The treatment of a sub-acute or chronic condition, with prevention of an acute attack, or of that condition known as goutiness, in which various irregular manifestations may appear from time to time, but in which an acute paroxysm rarely, if ever, occurs.

(3) The treatment of chronically affected joints, with removal of the uratic deposits and deformities, and restoration of their functions.

In the consideration of the spa treatment of gout, with which alone this paper has to do, the first of these principles may be entirely omitted from the discussion, as spa treatment of whatever form, is contraindicated in an acute attack.

The treatment of sub-acute or chronic gout.—In this form of gout, far more, perhaps, than in any other, is shown the influence of the gouty predisposition either inherited or acquired.

While it is impossible by any form of treatment to set aside this tendency to the occurrence of gout under circumstances favourable to its development, we can do much towards lessening the liability to its development, and when developed, we can by judicious care, almost always ameliorate the severity and frequency of its manifestations, and in many instances, get rid entirely of the symptom of the disease. How is this to be done ? And upon what theory as to the etiology of the disease do we base our plan of therapeutic action ?

While many theories have been advanced from time to time, as to the cause of this affection, none of them have stood the test of thorough investigation, and our treatment of this condition is now, as it has been since the days of Sydenham, purely empirical.

We have learned by experience that certain forms of treatment are better than others, and that by adopting certain measures we have obtained desired results, but why we get them, and in what manner our treatment acts, we are in no wise able positively to say.

The uric acid theory of gout, as set forth by Garrod in 1847, and modified by him at various times since, is, perhaps, the most popular and generally accepted theory of to-day, especially among practitioners of medicine in this country. But the observations of Garrod upon which he based his contentions, have not been confirmed by more recent investigators, and this theory, like all the others, is not borne out by facts.

Garrod contends as follows : —

(1) Uric acid is normally formed in the kidneys, and the onset of gout depends upon the absorption and retention of uric acid in the blood, due to partial failure in the uric acid excretory function of these organs.

(2) The separation of the urates from the blood, and deposition in the tissues, occurs when the blood is no longer able to dissolve the uric acid.

(a) Because the uric acid is in excess.

(b) Because the alkalescence of the blood is diminished.

With the exception of some experiments upon serpents, made by Zalensky, which, to my mind, are by no means conclusive, there are none that furnish proof that uric acid is formed in the kidneys, nor is there any evidence that the onset of gout is due to kidney failure. Ebstein says that while in primary articular gout the kidneys are only implicated after a longer or shorter period, there are many cases in which the kidneys do not become implicated up to the death of the patient, and he refers to a patient of Bramson's, a labourer who had suffered from gout for twenty years, who on autopsy showed absolute normal kidneys, though the gouty deposit was very extensive in the joints and tendons. Senator also holds the same views as Ebstein.

As to the excess of uric acid in the blood in gout, Magnus-Levy in ten observations in gout, found during and between the seizures, from 3 to 6 milligrammes of uric acid in 100 cc. of blood, about the normal amount, and no excess of uric acid during the gouty attack.

As to the alkalescence of the blood, Frankel and Benda examined three febrile cases of gout, and got normal values for the alkalescence of the blood. Magnus-Levy examined sixteen cases of gout during and between the seizures, and found no diminution in the alkalescence of the blood.

Garrod claims that the uric acid output in gout is diminished during the seizures. This contention is denied by Ffeffer, His, Magnus-Levy, and Futcher. These observers, by reliable methods, all find an excess of uric acid excretion during the seizure. My own observations confirm those of the latter. In a case of gout in which I made a daily estimate of the uric acid output by Gowland-Hopkin's method, for a period of fourteen days, during which time there was an acute exacerbation, I found the daily average output to be as follows: Before ·442 grammes; during, ·659 grammes; after, ·396 grammes.

Haig, who is also an enthusiastic advocate of the uric acid theory of gout, believes in the extreme toxicity of uric acid, formed or introduced into the system. The following observations which I have made during the past winter, in the laboratory of Dr. C. A. Herter, in New York, have made me very sceptical on this point, and while they are not conclusive, they are extremely suggestive. In two cases of chronic nephritis,

3 grammes of uric acid were given by the mouth in twenty-four
hours for three days in succession. A decided increase was
found in the urine during the time, but there was no systemic
disturbance. In one case of chronic nephritis, 3 grammes were
given in twenty-four hours for three days in succession, and on
the fourth day 6 grammes were given, without producing any
systemic disturbance. In four cases of chronic gout, a diet of
shad roe was given for five days, which caused a decided
increase in the excretion of uric acid in the urine, but no disturbance of the health. In animals I have also made some observations which tend to corroborate this view. In two rabbits,
two successive intravenous injections of 1 gramme each of uric
acid were made without systemic disturbance, though a large
part of the acid was recovered from the urine. In two dogs,
two successive intravenous injections of 2 grammes each of uric
acid were not followed by any disturbance, while the urine
showed a large increase. Taking into consideration the foregoing, together with the fact that many other diseases than gout
are always accompanied with an excessive output of uric acid, I
feel that at least we must look for some other substance than
uric acid as the cause of this disease. It is possible that we
may yet find some substance which may be considered the
materies morbi of this affection, and recent observations point to
the purin bases like adenine, which are intermediate between
nucleins and uric acid, as likely to furnish us with the toxic
principle.

At present, however, we must content ourselves with the
fact that we have to do with faulty metabolism, the cause of
which we can only surmise, and base our treatment upon those
general principles of hygiene, which experience has taught us
are best adapted for the relief of this condition. For this reason
the spa treatment, which is purely an hygienic one, based and
carried out upon thorough scientific principles, will seem to be
the proper method of procedure in these cases.

In ordering the spa treatment for our gouty patients, we

must bear in mind the fact that it is a complex treatment, made up of many factors, each of which has a decided bearing upon the successful issue of the whole. For purposes of discussion it will be advantageous to consider them separately under the various heads.

Hydrotherapy.—The bathing procedure itself, as regards temperature, duration and method of application of the waters, is, perhaps, one of the most important of these elements, and should be thoroughly understood. The effects obtained by bathing are due to the influence upon the organisms of thermal stimuli. In order to properly understand the bathing process, let us consider for a moment how the system is affected by the thermal stimuli.

The body temperature is maintained at a nearly constant standard by the generation in the interior of the body of animal heat. This production of heat is in proportion to the activity of the internal changes. These changes are especially indicated by the absorption of oxygen and the exhalation of carbonic acid. If the body is immersed in a cold bath there is an abstraction of heat at the surface, with a proportionate increase of heat production in the interior, to maintain the body standard. After the discontinuance of an abstraction of heat, not of excessive intensity or duration, during which the body temperature rose a little, a period follows when the temperature of the body becomes lower than it was before the bath (primary after-effect). To the stage of cooling succeeds a slight compensatory rise of the heat of the body (secondary after-effect). The primary after-effect is chiefly due to the relaxation of the capillaries and a cooling down of the blood, which thus flows rapidly through the cooled periphery. It is also in part due to a decrease in heat poduction, which thus compensates for the great increase in heat production which took place during the bath.

Immersion of the body in hot water increases the body temperature by the additional heat brought to the surface, and by checking the normal radiation of heat.

Baths of from 83·2 to 95 degrees, have no influence upon the healthy individual, either in the production or abstraction of heat, and they are called thermally indifferent baths. The thermally indifferent point will vary with different individuals, and in the same individual under different conditions, and will depend upon his sensibility, or susceptibility to impressions of heat and cold.

A thermally indifferent water applied to the skin by means of a spray or douche, produces a dilatation of the capillaries through stimulation of the sensory and vaso-motor nerves, and lowers the body temperature by allowing a greater amount of blood to flow through the colder periphery of the body. This loss of heat is compensated for by increased heat production. In such a stimulating bath there is a direct increase in the amount of oxygen consumed, and carbonic acid exhaled. In like manner, immersion in a hot bath for a short duration of time, lowers the body temperature. --

These various effects of temperature presuppose that the body at the time of the bath is in a normal condition, and that the air of the bathroom is at a temperature of from 60 to 70 degrees.

If the bath is taken when the temperature of the surface of the body is warmed, either by exercise or artificial means, the cutaneous circulation being thereby active and sensitive to impression, reaction will be quicker and more prompt, whereas if the skin is cold and inactive, reaction will be delayed, or may be entirely lacking.

It will thus be seen that in order to obtain the best results from the bath the condition of the circulation and the surface temperature should be taken into account in giving the bath.

It will be seen by the foregoing, that as the thermally indifferent point varies with different individuals, and in the same individual under different conditions, the temperature of the cold or hot bath is purely a relative thing, and in fixing the temperature of the bath it must be done solely in reference to the condition of the individual at the time of taking it, and his sensitiveness to thermal impressions, and cannot be regulated by the thermometer.

The intensity of the thermal stimuli will depend, then, not upon the temperature of the water used, but on the variation in temperature between the surface heat and the water used.

Immediately following the bath the skin will be in a more or less sensitive condition, from the effect of the thermal stimuli that have been employed.

The moisture upon the skin rapidly evaporates, and a distinct abstraction of heat will take place as a consequence of these conditions. In some instances when abstraction of heat is the end desired, this fact may be taken advantage of, but on the other hand, when we wish to have a tonic or sedative effect of the bath, and desire to obtain prompt reaction to favour that end, the patient must be protected by hot sheets or friction, or both, to reduce the heat radiation to a minimum, otherwise the results of the bath will be negatived, and a depression of the vital forces will be an invariable consequence.

The bath procedure, then, will consist really of three stages. The preparation stage, in which the body surface is put in a receptive condition. This may be accomplished by active exercise, to the degree of stimulating the cutaneous circulation and getting the body in a gentle glow. A bath following prolonged or severe exercise to the point of getting the body overheated, is always fraught with great danger, and must be sedulously avoided. Warming the skin with hot blankets or the hot air bath is another means of preparation; or, in the use of the douche bath, the skin may be most conveniently prepared, by beginning the process with warm water, continuing it until the skin is in a proper reactive condition, then using this temperature as a standard from which the water of the bath proper may be varied as desired.

The treatment stage, the second step in the bathing procedure, consists in the application of the thermal stimuli in such order and intensity, as to produce precise results, as regards heat production and abstraction, and the avoidance of subsequent reaction, which would interfere with, or nullify the effects desired.

The selection of a method for producing the thermal stimuli is purely a matter of choice, and will depend upon the condition of the patient, his vital energy and reactive power. The degree of temperature used, whether hot or cold, is selected with relation to the temperature of the preparation stage, and is based entirely upon the sensations of the patient, the intensity of the stimulus depending upon degree of variation.

In no therapeutic procedure is it so difficult to judge of the reactive power of a patient as in that by the bath. Individuals who seem robust, and in perfect physical condition, may have poor reaction to thermal stimuli, and in others who are delicate, sensitive, and apparently of deficient vital energy, the reaction to thermal stimuli will be prompt and profound.

In the reaction stage, the third step in the bathing process, our object is to retain or to intensify the effect of the thermal stimuli upon the nerves and circulation that has been produced by the bath, and thus to insure the precise result that has been the object of the treatment.

After the bath the patient should be immediately enveloped in a hot sheet, or bath robe, and stood upon a warm woollen blanket.

The drying can be done by friction outside of the covering. As soon as the body is dry, the damp sheet is removed and a warm one substituted. The patient is then put in bed, the feet wrapped in warm towels, and the body lightly covered, in which condition he rests for a varying period. From time to time the towels about the feet are changed if need be, to insure their warmth, and if the face is flushed, a cold compress may be laid upon the forehead.

The form of bath that is generally used in Richfield, for gout, is the immersion or tub bath. As the primary object is to increase the activity of the skin, and stimulate the circulation, a hot bath is usually given, varying in temperature from 98 to 102 degrees, and in duration from 8 to 12 minutes. From the foregoing, it will be seen that a bath of this kind will be highly stimulating, and on account of its short duration, does not tend to depress the patient by abstracting heat and lowering the vital energy.

In addition to the therapeutic effect of the bath *per se*, is the influence of the chemical ingredients contained in the waters.

The waters of Richfield hold in solution in small amounts, the sulphates of sodium, potassium, magnesium, and lime, but are exceedingly rich in sulphureted hydrogen gas, both in solution and free, and I am inclined to believe that their therapeutic value is due principally to the latter. There is no doubt that the chemical constituents of the waters enhance to a great degree the action of the bath, and this is doubtless due to their decidedly stimulating effect upon the glands generally, and especially upon the liver, kidneys, and skin. This effect of the mineral ingredients is shown very markedly in the general systemic disturbance that invariably occurs during the course of treatment by the baths.

After from four to six baths there is always a decided reaction, which manifests itself by a definite train of clinical phenomena. There is headache, loss of appetite, furred tongue, deranged bowels, and a feeling of lassitude and discomfort. If at this time the baths are discontinued for two or three days, these symptoms all disappear, and it is unusual for them to recur during the course of treatment.

The baths of Richfield are not contraindicated by diseases of the kidneys or heart, but on the contrary, they have a decidedly beneficial effect in these conditions, but of course unusual care must be exercised in adapting them to the needs of the individual.

The internal use of water is always of great value to the gouty, and those waters which can be taken in large quantities are to my mind of the greatest benefit.

The objection to taking the waters containing the sodium salts by gouty individuals, because of their tendency to render the deposits of urate of sodium less soluble, does not seem to me to be well founded. The *rôle* of the salts held in solution in mineral waters is probably not a direct one upon the uratic deposits, but a secondary one in their effect upon general metabolism, through their action in increasing the number of white blood cells.

His, in some experiments upon animals, found that by injection of sodium urate or biurate into the joints, he produced inflammation, with necrosis. Resolution was rapid, and considerable amounts of the uric acid were absorbed. The uric acid was taken away by the phagocytes. Uni- and polyneuclear leucocytes and the giant cells were concerned in the process.

Diet.—In no phase of the treatment of gout is there so great a diversity of opinion as in the matter of diet. I have frequently had patients say, " If I abstained from all the different foods that have been advised, I would have nothing left to eat."

Those who believe in the toxic effect of uric acid in the organism, withhold nitrogenised foods almost altogether, because in their use a larger amount of uric acid is introduced into the body.

Red meats are especially proscribed, and some go even so far as to withhold all proteid-holding foods, such as eggs, milk, and certain of the vegetables.

My observations in the use of nuclein-holding foods, such as shad roe, which produce in the body an excessive amount of uric acid, to which I have already referred, would show that we are not justified in believing that uric acid producing foods have any deleterious effect upon the gouty subject. On the other hand, there is no class of food stuff which gives so great an amount of energy as animal food, and which in the majority of gouty people is as easily digested. As these cases are, as a rule, lowered in tone and vital force, and almost invariably anæmic, it would seem that these foods, above all others, are best to use, and the result of my clinical experiences bears out the truth of this fact, as I invariably prescribe meat freely in the diet.

The carbohydrates, too, are supposed to have some ulterior effect upon the gouty individual, and are usually interdicted.

To determine what effect, if any, a diet consisting largely of carbohydrates would have upon the gouty subject, I gave for fourteen consecutive days an average daily amount of one and a half quarts of simple syrup, made from cane sugar, to four gouty patients, giving as high as two quarts a day in some instances.

The effect upon the gout was *nil*. There was no gastric disturbance induced, and the patients all gained in weight, and looked and felt better. The only other effect noticeable was a repugnance to fats, which the diet seemed to produce.

I would withhold carbohydrates only in those cases in which obesity is a prominent symptom, unless they should be contra-indicated for some individual reason.

Fats do not seem to have any especial influence in these patients, but may be used with good effect, particularly in those individuals in whom we reduce the carbohydrates to a minimum.

Some quite elaborate experiments have been made to show the influence of the various vegetable salts in rendering soluble the sodium urate in the blood of gouty subjects, but I must confess, they do not impress me as having any great practical value.

A mixed general diet, which contains a fair proportion of vegetable food, will, on the whole, be found to be the most rational and satisfactory diet in these cases. The choice of vegetables will depend upon the digestive capacity of the individual.

The diet in gout, then, must be adapted to each particular case, having in mind the general principle that it is to be simple, ample, wholesome, and withal nourishing.

Alcohol, when taken in excess, is decidedly pernicious, and

even in small amounts if continued for a long time, in most instances is probably injurious. He made some interesting observations, which are pertinent to this subject.: He finds that when acid sodium urate is injected into subcutaneous tissue, the capsule formed around the acid remains in an early stage of connective tissue formation. But if alcohol be given repeatedly to animals, in small doses, the capsule developes into true fully-formed fibrillary connective tissue, which is less liable to permit the removal of uric acid.

In elderly people, or in the feeble, whisky may be given in moderation, with excellent results.

Exercise.—In all gouty cases exercise is of the greatest value. Active out-of-door exercise is, of course, the best, but when for various reasons this cannot be taken, passive exercise in the form of massage and resistance movements, will be found a most valuable substitute. The amount of exercise, its form and the time of taking it, should always be specifically ordered, otherwise the best results will not be obtained, and positive harm may ensue.

Climate has, undoubtedly, a certain influence on the well-being of these people, and a dry inland region of moderate altitude will, in the majority of instances, be found the best. Sudden changes in temperature are harmful, and exposure of all kinds must be seduously guarded against.

In the selection of a spa, we should seek to have these conditions, if possible, and we should not forget the influence that a pleasant environment will give. The gouty patient is irritable and worrysome as a rule, and cheerful surroundings, with diversions which do not tax his energies, will add very materially to his comfort, and aid in the restoration to a normal condition of body and mind.

An advantage of the spa treatment that I have not yet mentioned, lies in the fact that we have the patient under much better control than at home. He goes to the springs for the express purpose of the cure, and his time and energies are given over to that alone, and if he is properly directed, he will be so occupied by his treatment, he will have but little time for retrospection and worry. He is away from the cares of business, and the thousand and one petty annoyances that wear upon him at home, so with the rest and out-of-door life, the change in itself has a powerful influence for good.

In the treatment of chronically affected joints, with removal of uratic deposits, the general treatment will be the same as that outlined above. In addition, there are various measures which we may employ to improve the local condition. Foremost among them is, perhaps, the local douche, either of hot water alone, or of hot and cold used alternately.

The method of applying the douche is as follows: A fairly good-sized solid stream is thrown with considerable force upon the affected part. The water which at first is as cold as it will come from the nozzle, is changed to hot after half a minute, and is made as hot as the patient can possibly bear it; this temperature is continued for a minute, when it is again changed to cold, the process being repeated for twenty to thirty minutes. The action is purely a local one, and is produced by the great stimulating effect of the repeated, alternating temperatures upon the circulation about the joint, thereby increasing tissue change, and favouring absorption. The stimulating effect is greatly enhanced by the force of the stream, and this should be limited only by the comfort of the patient.

Massage of the joint should be used in conjunction with the douche, and is best applied immediately after the latter, as the tissues then are in a relaxed condition and are more favourable to manipulation. Where the enlargements of the joints are due to inflammatory thickening, and the uratic deposit is in the early stage, vigorous movements may be made to overcome contractions, and break up slight adhesions, without danger of doing the joint harm, but if the joint is fixed by old uratic deposits which have already become calcareous, the manipulation of the part must be restricted to massage alone.

17

The hot-air treatment of such joints is in some instances of great service, and especially in those in which there is considerable pain and soreness, it seems to give greater relief than any other kind. Its effect upon the swelling is practically the same as that of the douche.

Of late static electricity has been used in these joint cases quite a little, and those who have had experience with it are very enthusiastic over its effects.

A most important feature in the successful treatment of joints is in having the treatment carried out under the direct observation of the physician. This is simple enough at the spa, and is one of the great advantages of spa treatment; but in town it is very difficult, if not impossible, to do this unless patients are treated in one's office.

If further experience with static electricity bears out the claims of its supporters as to the effect in restoring the joints, it will be to us who do a great deal of this work, a tremendous help, as it certainly possesses many advantages for office treatment over any other

---

DISCUSSION.

Dr. QUIMBY: Dr. Ransom has spoken of the difficulty of fixing the diet in gout and the need of meat. I recognise this need, but it has seemed to me that the trouble comes not from either form of food by itself but from the combination. Meat is not objectionable because of the uric acid which may be formed from it, but because, in these conditions of defective oxygenation the starches are cared for first, and the proteids not being taken up remain in part in the intestine, where they furnish the elements for infective toxæmia. It will often be found that, if we remove the meat foods entirely from the diet for a month or so, meantime thoroughly clearing out the intestine, we can then come back to a meat diet in moderation without ill effects.

Dr. FISK: Let me call the attention of the Association to the two table waters, the Shasta Springs and the Idan-há— to be found on the Pacific slope.

Dr. WALKER: The question of diet in rheumatic and gouty patients is an individual one. I have always felt it necessary to remove the sugars more than any other articles of food, and I think one reason they are objectionable is that they are so apt to be taken between meals. In lady patients especially it is frequently important to remove all sweets on account of this habit of nibbling at the candy box. Murchison, and later Fothergill, seem to me to have struck the key-note of the method of dieting gouty cases, in their showing that the sugars and starches, with their greed of oxygen and ease of consuming all there is of this element available, rob the albuminates which are slower to oxygenate and make the latter appear to be the offending cause. Whereas the removal of the sugars and starches or their limitation corrects the difficulty more surely than that of the albuminates. Often all that is needed is to diminish the quantity without otherwise modifying the dietary.

Dr. HARVEY : I think the effect of water in these cases is certainly very useful on the outside, but a goodly quantity is also necessary on the inside, for a general washing out by drinking quarts of water. I have one patient who has been put through this course several times with benefit. He pours it in until he cannot hold any more, sometimes taking nearly a gallon of water. With this washing I have found that a diet that is simple, and in order to be certain that it will be so, I prescribe milk, meat, and bread and butter only, is very beneficial. The cooking of the food is a point that is not generally sufficiently attended to.

Dr. HEFFRON : It seems to me it will be practically impossible for any body of physicians to agree on any one line of diet in this class of cases, for the simple reason that the people who develop this trouble do not belong to any one type. We have them all the way from the thin and wiry, and the thin and poorly nourished, to the excessively fat, whether they be florid or anæmic. I thoroughly agree with Dr. Ransom's position. Luff, in his recent work on gout, makes the statement that if there is any reason why nitrogenous food should be excluded, the source from which it is obtained, whether from the animal or the vegetable kingdom, is of little or less importance. It is usually true, however, that most physicians exclude red meats, so-called "butcher's meat," while they allow fowls, &c. I have no knowledge of any investigations which show that the meat of one animal differs essentially from that of another, except in the length of fibre and the necessarily different ease of disintegration. The position the doctor takes in regard to carbohydrates is, I think, correct ; for if sugar is digested there is no reason why it should not be given, but if it undergoes fermentation in the stomach it should be excluded from the dietary. It seems to me the blood condition is one of the most important to be considered in this connection, and a careful examination should be made as to the relative proportion of the corpuscles, the hæmoglobin, &c., and the diet regulated accordingly.

I would like to speak also of the regulation of the quantity of fluid to be ingested by the individual. We make a mistake sometimes in encouraging individuals that are anæmic to drink large quantities of water. If there is any disturbance of the circulation it is a matter of embarrassment to the heart to have an increased volume of blood to propel. I believe that in these cases with acute exacerbation, particularly where we have arterial sclerosis and where exercise is impracticable, we can get an enormous amount of good from the systematic inhalation of oxygen. If simply applied to the patient's mouth, of course the effect is nothing, but if it be deeply inhaled and retained as long as possible in the lungs, and if it be repeated systematically and sufficiently often, you will get positive evidence of its efficacy as a curative remedy.

Dr. NEWTON : No discussion of dietetics would be complete without warning the gentlemen of a thing we often lose sight of, namely, that in most of these cases of lithæmia, the kind of food makes less difference than its quantity makes. Whatever they eat they should not use too much of it. How to fit the diet to the patient is often one of the most puzzling things in medicine.

I cannot help alluding to my experience while attending physician to the Essex County, N.J., Penitentiary. The refractory prisoners were punished by solitary confinement for five days, on an exclusive diet of bread and water. The effect on the general health was, so far as I can recall, good in every instance.

Dr. CURTIN : I would like to say a few words on the subject of diet and heart disease. I think the majority of people, especially those leading sedentary lives, are apt to eat too much. I am in the habit of giving them but one hearty meal a day and that in the middle of the day, making them take a light breakfast and supper. I have seen a number of these cases that had been undergoing treatment for obesity. The heart in these cases seemed to suffer materially for the want of proper nourishment, and muscular weakness occurred with serious and in four cases fatal results. People differ in their ability to digest different articles. In treating heart disease I think it is a very important matter to study the peculiarities of each patient and be governed by these. The great benefit derived from foreign resorts in the treatment of gout and heart disease are that such patients going from the United States are very willing to place themselves under the physician, who strictly regulates their diet, exercise and rest. In this country they generally go to a resort, commit all sorts of indiscretions and expect the water to cure them, and as a consequence they come away unimproved and disappointed. The sanatoria in this country should be regulated by careful resident physicians, so that every patient going there should place themselves under the physician's care for proper directions and follow them strictly. We may then expect better results in the United States than we have had in the past.

Dr. HANCE: The question of diet has been chiefly under discussion, but Dr. Ransom spoke also of the spa treatment. At Lakewood we have no distinct spa treatment, but we have hydrotherapy, and I think the point Dr. Curtin just mentioned should be insisted upon, namely, that the patient should be definitely instructed to put himself under the care of the physician, because the change is such that not one prescription in fifty given at home is the proper one for the patient to follow when he arrives at the place where the treatment is to be given. During the past season at the Lakewood I have had that illustrated more clearly than at any other time, inasmuch as two of the prescriptions given by men who are daily making use of hydrotherapeutic measures with the same sort of plant we use would, if carried out, have caused the patient to faint in the bath. Some of our patients are gouty, most of them very slightly so, but I have found it absolutely essential to treat the patient liberally and not put them on anti-gout diet at once lest they should be weakened and injured by the baths. I recall a recent patient to whom, although the food produced gouty symptoms, I had to give a full diet until the baths had improved the acute condition, and then gradually restricted the diet.

I would like to ask Dr. Ransom, in reference to preparatory baths, if he does not find it necessary in all cases to lead gradually up to the stronger baths.

The PRESIDENT: I frankly confess that the more I hear on the subject of diet, the hazier my notions become. It has settled down in my practice to this, that the diet for the individual is the one which he can best digest, and that is the thing I try to ascertain in studying the particular patient.

It seems to me the uric acid theory has been shown to be practically a fallacy, and we must find something else, and in this line I should like to suggest to Dr. Reed that if he has not already become familiar with the investigations made in regard to the part played by oxalic acid in the production of so-called lithæmia, he will find something interesting in it. One of our Chicago physicians has done some interesting work in that connection. Oxaluria has been shown to be almost universally present in these cases and in many of them there is indicanuria.

Dr. RANSOM: The remarks which have been made in relation to the diet in gout, coincide entirely with my own ideas. The anti-gout diet that Dr. Quimby spoke of is the one that should be given in all these patients, because an anti-gout diet is a diet that is adapted to the needs of the individual. The fact that there was no ill effect felt by any of the five cases of gout in whom I produced an excessive amount of uric acid by feeding them on shad roe, makes me feel that uric acid boldin foods are not necessarily deleterious to gouty patients. The same may be said of carbohydrates, any of the foods may be used provided they do not disturb the digestion of the individual. The point I wished to make was that there is no single class of food-stuffs which of themselves are productive of gout.

The great difficulty in the treatment of patients at the Springs in this country is lack of control and the tendency of patients to follow out treatment without proper medical supervision. This is almost entirely due to the men who send their patients to the Springs.

If, instead of saying go to Richfield and take treatment, you would say "go to Dr. so-and-so and let him put you under treatment," much of the difficulty would be removed, for it is fair to suppose that the medical men at these places who have them in charge and who have spent years in observing and studying the effects of the waters, are better fitted to carry on the treatment than any one else. Then, too, in order to get proper results it is necessary to see the patient from time to time during a course of baths. It is impossible for instance for Dr. Hance to give a prescription to a patient on the first day he sees him that will suit his needs throughout his stay. He will probably change it half a dozen times to meet the changes in the patient's condition, and to successfully treat him he must see him almost from day to day.

It is my habit to begin with the weaker baths, which cannot possibly do harm, and increase them gradually.

Dr. HINSDALE : I would like to ask whether the Doctor considers the medicinal effect of the bath due to the solid or gaseous constituents of the water.

Dr. RANSOM : The amount of solid constituents in the waters at Richfield is so small that the part they play cannot be of great importance, the amount of sulphuretted hydrogen both free and combined is, however, very great, and it is to this constituent probably that most of the effect comes. There is in these waters, common with all natural mineral waters, an effect which cannot be ascribed to any known chemical body, which also contributes very largely to the therapeutic value of the baths.

Dr. REED : In grouping these papers I fear we have lost something in the discussion, for I find that some of the main points of my paper have been overlooked, for instance, the effect of exercise and hydriatic treatment on the arterioles. In regard to the diet, the truth was hit very nearly by Dr. Newton, when he said that the great fault has been in the excess of foods of all kinds. It is very true that often if patients take only a small quantity of food, they will not suffer no matter what kind of food they use. Sometimes, however, it does make a great deal of difference what kind of food is chosen, and I cannot agree with Dr. Ransom that in general a meat diet or a sugar diet would be healthful. I think that one reason why Dr. Ransom has come to this conclusion is that he has at the same time given his patients the hot bath treatment and on this account they could bear a large amount of meat and sugar, perhaps when they could not begin to bear it under other conditions.

Dr. RANSOM : These experiments I made were not at Richfield but in the hospital in New York, last winter, and the patients were not given hot baths or any other kind. They were men between 45 and 50 years of age, living on hospital diet and under treatment for gout.

Dr. REED : How long were the experiments carried on ?

Dr. RANSOM : Fourteen days.

Dr. REED : I think that would hardly be long enough to be conclusive ; however, the majority of investigators in this line have agreed that a largely nitrogenous diet does in the end increase gout.

SOME ANALOGOUS EUROPEAN AND AMERICAN MINERAL SPRINGS.

BY GUY HINSDALE, M.D.

PHILADELPHIA.

———

AMERICA possesses a vast number of mineral springs. The majority have not been analysed or even named. In the Yellowstone National Park there are 2,000 springs and 100 geysers, and in a single county of Kentucky there are said to be 2,000 springs. Attempts have been made by Dr. A. C. Peale, of the U.S. Geological Survey, to tabulate the springs in the United States, and he has classified 2,822 spring localities and 8,843 individual springs.* More recently Dr. James K. Crook has published detailed information in his work, " The Mineral Waters of the United States and their Therapeutic Uses."†

In this work the springs are described in groups by States, with analyses appended where available and definite information given as to elevation, climate, access, and accommodation. Over 25,000,000 gallons of natural American mineral waters are sold annually in the United States at a valuation of about $5,000,000. Only about $1,500 worth is exported. On the other hand, the importations of natural mineral waters reach about 3,000,000 gallons yearly, valued at $500,000. As American springs are more fully investigated, and as better accommodations for hydrotherapeutic treatment are provided at American mineral spring resorts, it is gradually being

---

* Bulletin No. 32, U.S. Geological Survey, 1886, Washington, D.C.
† Lea, Bros. and Co., Philadelphia, 1899, 588 pp.

recognised that we have in America the counterparts of nearly all the springs of Europe. The accessories of bathing establishments, *régime*, and the tone of European Spas, are of a much higher grade in Europe, but in time we trust that these deficiencies can be remedied.

We have ventured to indicate some of the American analogues of European mineral waters. The list is far from being satisfactory, but serves in a measure to show that a comparison can be made.

ANALOGOUS EUROPEAN AND AMERICAN SPRINGS

Achsel-Mannstein, Bavaria	Mt. Clemens, Michigan.
Aix-la-Chapelle	Hot Springs, Arkansas; Beck's Hot Sulphur Springs, Utah.
Aix-les-Bains	Hot Springs, Virginia.
Apenta	Pagosa Hot Springs, Colorado.
Apollinaris	Idanha Spring, Idaho; Manitou Soda Springs, Colorado; Napa Soda Springs, California; Shasta Springs, California; a Spring at Mill Creek, Livingstone, Montana.
Bocklet, near Kissingen, Bavaria	Cooper's Well, Hinds Co., Miss.; Bedford Chalybeate, Pennsylvania; Napa Soda, Iron Spring, California.
Carlsbad, Bohemia, Sprudel	Springdale Seltzer, Pagosa Hot Springs, Royal Gorge Hot Springs, Idaho Hot Springs, Colorado; Bedford Magnesia Spring, Pennsylvania (partly); American Carlsbad, Washington Co., Illinois.
Carlsbad, Bohemia, Mud Baths	Las Vegas Hot Springs, New Mexico; Klamath Hot Springs, California; Mudlavia, near Attica, Indiana.
Contrexeville, France ...	Geyser, Saratoga.
Duerkheim...	Deer Lick, Glen Springs, New York.
Eilsen	Massena Springs, St. Lawrence Co., N.Y.
Ems •	Healing Springs, Virginia; Ojo Caliente, New Mexico; Enna Soda Springs, California; Hot Springs, North Carolina.
Franzensbad, Neuquelle ...	Buffalo Lithia and Nye Lithia, Virginia.
Friedreichschall	Champion and Congress, Saratoga; Crab Orchard, Kentucky; Royal Gorge Hot Springs, Colorado.

Wildbad-Gastein, Switzerland	Hudson Hot Springs, New Mexico; Las Vegas Hot Springs, New Mexico; Hunter's Hot Springs, Montana; Ferris Hot Springs, Montana; Boulder Hot Springs, Montana; Hot Springs, Virginia; Castle Creek Hot Springs, Arizona.
Geisshubler, Bohemia ...	Sweet Springs, West Virginia.
Hunjadi Janos, Hungary...	Park's Spring, Caswell Co., North Carolina. Castalian Mineral Springs, California.
Homburg	Salubria Spring, Glen Springs, New York.
Jaxfelt	Neptune Spring, Glen Springs, New York.
Kissengen	Sheboygan Mineral Well, Wisconsin; Lower Blue Lick Springs, Kentucky.
Kreutznach, Edisonquelle	Sheboygan Mineral Wells, Wisconsin; Climax Springs, Camden Co., Missouri; Spring Lake Well, Michigan; Deer Lick, Glen Springs, New York.
Levico	Thompson's Bromine-Arsenic, North Carolina.
La Bourboule, France ...	Thompson's Bromine-Arsenic, North Carolina.
Marienbad, Rudolfsquelle.	
Nauheim	Neptune Spring, Glen Springs, New York; Massanetta Springs, Virginia.
Pyrmont, Waldeck, Germany	Rock Enon Springs, Virginia; Rawley Springs, Virginia.
Pullna	Elgin Spring, Addison Co., Vermont.
Rehme	Neptune Spring, Glen Springs, New York.
Salles, Savoy	Salt Sulphur, Wisconsin.
San Moritz, Old Source ...	Springdale Seltzer Springs, Colorado.
Seltzer, Nassau, Germany	Azule Springs, Santa Clara Co., California.
Seidlitz	Elgin Springs, Addison Co., Vermont.
Schlangenbad	Hot Springs, Virginia (Healing Spring).
Schwalbach	New Almaden Vichy Spring, California.
Tunbridge Wells, England	Bedford Springs, Penna.
Vichy, France, Grand Grille	Geyser, Saratoga, New York; Ukiah Vichy Spring, Mendocino Co., Congress, California; Vichy Spring, Saratoga, N.Y.; Ojo Caliente, New Mexico.
Wiesbaden...	Blue Lick, Kentucky; Lubec, Maine; Salt Spring, near Alba, Pennsylvania; Steamboat Springs, Colorado; Wagon Wheel Gap, Colorado; South Park, Colorado.
None in Europe	Oak Orchard, New York, Chalybeate with free Sulphuric Acid; Texas Sour Springs; Matchless Mineral Wells, Butler Co., Alabama; Tuscarora Springs, Canada; Thermal Acid, Inyo Co., California.

A CASE OF PULMONARY OSTEO-ARTHROPATHY.

BY RICHARD COLE NEWTON, M.D., AND ELIZABETH MERCELIS, M.D.

MONTCLAIR, NEW JERSEY.

J. T. came into the Mountainside Hospital, Montclair, on July 28, 1900, suffering from a large abscess in the right axilla.

Family History.—The members of his father's family suffered from cough and shortness of breath, and died, as a rule, of some lung trouble. His paternal grandfather had the clubbed finger tips and " big nails." His father, who was an asthmatic, died of cholera at 36. He did not have the " big nails." His mother is living at 56, and enjoys fair health. She is subject to rheumatism; has not enlarged finger tips. His sister died at 2 years, of unknown cause. His brother is living at 27, and is in good health. He has the " big nails." (See fig. 1 which is from a photograph of the patient's brother.) The brother appears to be a fairly well-nourished young man, and the enlarged nails can be discerned in the picture. Patient says that his ancestors have always been sober and industrious. No history of intemperance or nervous or mental disease obtainable. The patient's wife is living at 27. She is in the old country. They have had four children, of whom three are dead. One was drowned at 2½ years; one died at 7 days, of unknown cause; one at 6 months of " jaundice "; and one, a girl, is living at 4, and is reported to be healthy. Patient says that all of his children had the big nails. He shows a photo-

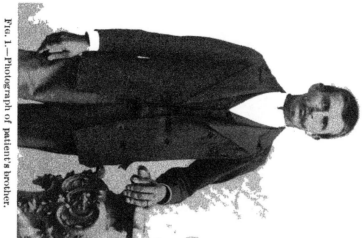

Fig. 1.—Photograph of patient's brother.

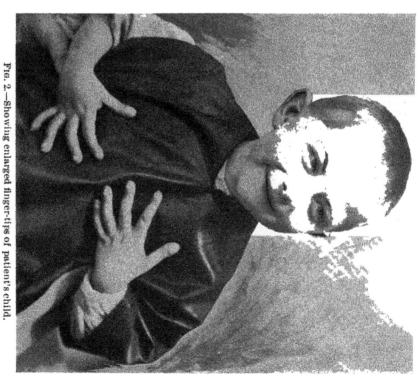

Fig. 2.—Showing enlarged finger-tips of patient's child.

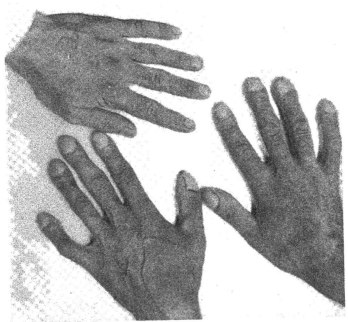

FIG. 3.—Picture of patient's hands compared with a normal hand.

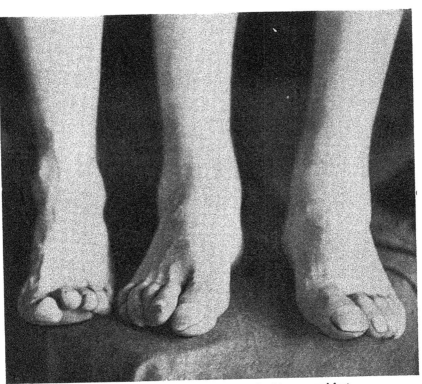

FIG. 4.—Picture of patient's feet compared with a normal foot.

graph of his little daughter, which represents a well-appearing child, with enlarged finger tips and clubbed nails.*

Previous History.—Our patient denies rheumatism or intemperance in himself or wife. Cannot remember ever having received a severe injury, or having undergone a shock, either bodily or mental. When 13 years old he suffered from frontal headache, which ceased without treatment. At 14, had' the mumps. Does not remember having suffered from any other infectious disease. He has always coughed on rising in the morning. In 1888, he contracted a venereal ulcer, of which the cicatrix can be seen on the dorsum of the penis, near the corona. The edges of the cicatrix are somewhat dim and ill defined. A small, hard ridge, however, runs through it. Patient says that the ulcer healed in three weeks, and no secondary symptoms appeared. He saw a doctor for the trouble only twice. He took some medicine, and used an ointment. The treatment only lasted two weeks. At 19 years of age he was examined for the Hungarian army, and was rejected for " weak chest." He says that he was examined four times for military service, and always rejected. He denies gonorrhœa and any urinary or bladder trouble. He says that his general health and vigour have improved of late years.†

Present Condition.—On admission to the hospital the patient's condition was as follows :..J. T., married ; aged 33 ; Hungarian labourer ; seeks treatment for a very large axillary abscess. This was freely incised, discharging a large quantity of pus. A superficial examination of the chest reveals nothing abnormal. Urinary examination negative. The enormous size of the ends of the fingers and toes and the nails was noted

---

* It is much to be regretted that this photograph is so small and indistinct that it seems impossible to reproduce it in such a way as to demonstrate the enlarged nails.

† We are indebted to Dr. Carl Buttner, of Orange, without whose courteous interest and knowledge of the Hungarian language this history could not have been obtained.

(see figs. 2, 3, 4, and 6), as well as the enlargement of the distal extremities of the bones of the forearms and legs, and the condyles of the femora. The man was emaciated, with a sallow and somewhat pigmented skin. He was clumsy in his movements. His intelligence was fair. Spleen and liver not perceptibly enlarged. Bowels sluggish, and appetite good. Owing to the size of his abscess, and the pain which motion gave the patient, the chest and abdomen were not thoroughly examined until some time after his admission to the hospital. His blood, however, was examined by one of us, and revealed nothing except moderate anæmia, and the leucocytosis, which would be expected with a large abscess. The pus from the abscess was also examined for tubercle bacilli, but none were found. As the patient did not raise anything when he coughed, no mucus from the throat could be obtained for examination.

The blood count on August 4, 1900, revealed:—

Red corpuscles	4,752,000
White corpuscles	13,400
Hæmoglobin	77 per cent.

Differential count of leucocytes:—

Small mononuclear	7·94 per cent.
Large mononuclear and transitory ...	12·35 ,,
Polymorphonuclear	78·80
Eösinophiles	·30
Myelocytes...	·60
	99·99 ,,

Red corpuscles of average size and shape. No nucleated reds, poikilocytes, micro- or macrocytes. No malarial organisms in fresh or dried specimens.

The healing of the abscess was markedly tardy. Twice or three times the cavity was opened, more or less grumous material scraped out, and fresh drainage tubes inserted. As he complained a good deal of weakness, and was troubled with profuse sweats, he was put upon a course of quinine and aromatic sulphuric acid.

On September 22 he was discharged from the hospital, the abscess being only partly healed. On November 18 he was seen again, and submitted to careful examination, and the following weights and measures recorded. The abscess had left a sinus, which extended through the anterior axillary wall. The man, however, was able to work, and was supporting himself by his labour. He could move his arm quite freely. For the first time his chest was carefully examined. This was well shaped, and the results of inspection and palpation were negative on auscultation and percussion. The heart and lungs appeared normal, except a little bronchitis, probably subacute, most marked at right apex posteriorly, where only a few fine râles were heard. Pulse of good rhythm and tension. No sclerosis of the arteries observed, and no excessive abdominal respiration. There was a slight dorsal and dorso-lumbar curvature of the spine. Abdomen not pendulous. Facies not enlarged or elongated. Zygomata, inferior maxilla, nose, chin, tongue, lips, and teeth, normal in size and appearance. Teeth showed moderate Rigg's disease in lower jaw, otherwise their shape, position, and general condition were good. The sterno-cleido-mastoid muscles were large and prominent. The thyroid body was not palpable. The larynx seemed broader than normal (was 7 cm in width). The intraclavicular space was well marked. The thymus gland was not palpable. The body muscles were small. Skin soft, and apparently healthy. Some increase of pigment noted at waistband of trousers, collar of shirt, and in the groins and axillæ. The skin of the hands was soft; no fleshy pads observed. No tumours or warty growths on the neck or elsewhere. No hyperæsthesia nor anæsthesia detected in any part of the body. The special senses were normally acute. Knee-jerks normal. Genital organs well formed and healthy, but rather small. A rather large scar, apparently from a glandular abscess, was noted in the left Scarpa's space near the saphenous opening. No definite history of the causation of the scar could be obtained, nor did the man remember whether or not it had any connection with the venereal ulcer previously spoken of.

The temperature in the mouth was normal, that of the axilla 97⅘ degrees, and of the palm 95⅓ degrees. The man's height was 5 feet 9 inches (1·75 metres); weight 157·5 lbs. (71·44 kilos.). The circumference of the right wrist was 18 cm.; of the left 17½ cm.; the right metacarpo-phalangeal circumference 2½ cm.; left metacarpo-phalangeal circumference 21½ cm.; length of right hand 21 cm.; left hand 22 cm.; circumference of right thumb at base of nail 7½ cm., and left thumb the same.

						Right hand		Left hand
Circumference of first finger at base of nail					...	6 cm.	...	6 cm.
,,	,, second ,,	,,	,,		...	6·5 cm.	...	6·8 cm.
,,	,, third ,,	,,	,,		...	6·5 cm.	...	6·3 cm.
,,	,, fourth ,,	,,	,,		...	5·8 cm.	...	5·5 cm.
,,	,, first ,,	,, middle phalanx			...	5·5 cm.	...	5·4 cm.
,,	,, second ,,	,,	,,		...	5·8 cm.	...	6 cm.
,,	,, third ,,	,,	,,		...	5·5 cm.	...	5·4 cm.
,,	,, fourth ,,	,,	,,		...	5 cm.	...	5·3 cm.

Measurements of diameters of finger nails in centimetres: --

			Right			Left	
		Trans.		Long		Trans.	Long
Thumb	... ...	2·7	...	2·5	...	2·7	... 2·7
First finger ...	... ...	2·2	...	2·4	...	2·2	... 2·2
Second ,,	... ...	2·5	...	2·5	...	2·5	... 2·3
Third ,,	... ...	2·5	...	2·5	...	2·5	... 2·3
Fourth ,,	... ...	2	...	2	...	2	... 2·7

Little fingers of both hands are somewhat flexed and adducted at the middle phalangeal joints. These joints are somewhat enlarged. No warts or protuberances noted on the hands.

The following measurements of the feet and legs were taken :—

Circumference of right leg at 15 cm. above the sole				...	...	25·5 cm.
,,	,,	,,	thickest part of ankle	...	...	...	25·5 cm.
,,	,,	,,	above tips of malleoli	...	...	..	30 cm.
,,	,,	,,	at calf ...	..	...	..	37·5 cm.

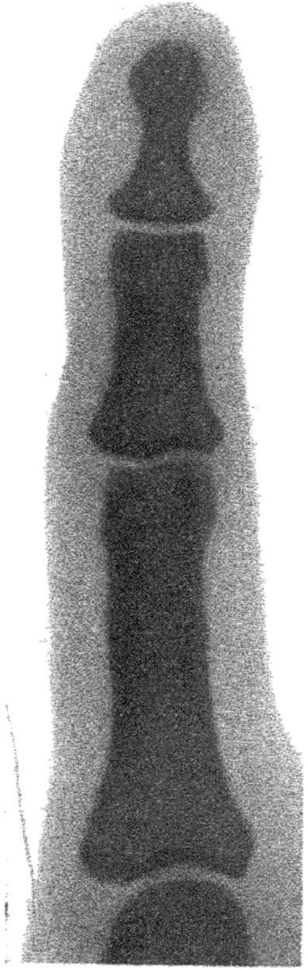

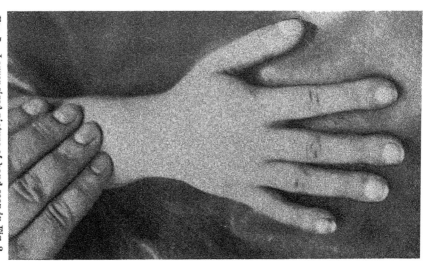

FIG. 5.—Skiagraph of index-finger of a case of osteo-arthropathy.

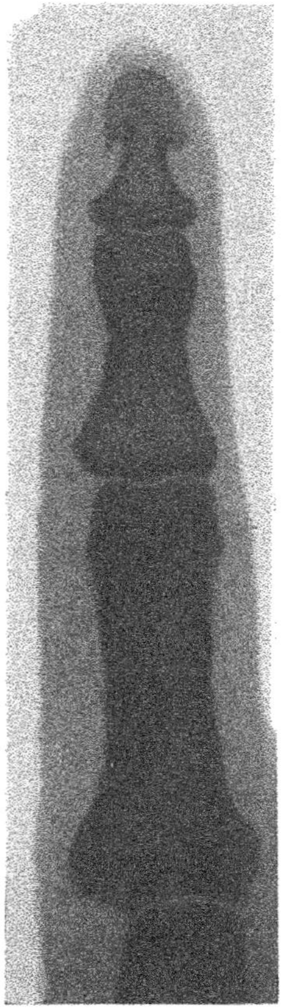

FIG. 6.—Skiagraph of index-finger of a case of phthisis.

FIG. 7.—Larger-sized picture of hand seen in Fig. 2.

An enlargement (exostosis) of right tibia (see fig. 7) externally, seems to be continuous with the fibula.‡ Both right malleoli were enlarged and thickened. The anterior portion of the foot between these two points was enlarged by (apparently) an increase in the thickness of the bones. The foot was thick and chunky, but not deformed.

Circumference of Right Foot

Around metatarso-phalangeal joints at great toe	26 cm.
Circumference of right great toe at base of nail	11 cm.
Length of right great toe	8 cm.
Transverse diameter of great toe nail	4 cm.
Length of right foot	27·5 cm.

Left Foot and Leg

Circumference of left leg 15 cm. above sole	25·5 cm.
,, ,, ,, malleoli	30 cm.
,, ,, metatarso-phalangeal joint of great toe	26 cm.
,, ,, left great toe at base of nail	10·5 cm.
Length of left great toe	8·2 cm.
Transverse diameter of great toe nail	3·7 cm.
Longitudinal diameter of great toe nail	3 cm.
Length of left foot	26·5 cm.

An enlargement of the left shin bone similar to that in the right leg was present, but not so marked.

The eye grounds were kindly examined for us by Dr. Wilton D. Garrett, of East Orange, who pronounced them both practically normal. Vision fair. No pressure symptoms were present. No scotomata ; no choked discs.

On November 17, one of us again made a blood count, and found the following improved condition :—

Hæmoglobin	90 per cent.
Red corpuscles	5,496,006
White corpuscles	5,330

Differential count of leucocytes :—

Small mononuclear	28·4 per cent.	
Large mononuclear and transitory ...	13·2	,,
Polymorphonuclear	55·6	,,
Eösinophiles	2·8	,,

‡ Two skiagraphs intended to represent this phenomenon have turned out too indistinct for use.

No microcytes, no macrocytes, no poikilocytes.

December 5 urine examined chemically, quantitatively, and microscopically, and found to be normal. The man's condition was gradually impróving, and by the latter part of December, the sinus in the right anterior axillary wall had completely closeu.

The fingers and toes remained the same. It should have been stated that the base of the nail is raised above the level of the knuckle, so that its outline can be discerned beneath the skin. It is movable, and has the peculiar semi-fluctuating property spoken of in the literature. The texture of the nail seemed healthy, although some tendency to split or fissure longitudinally was noted. The nails were not at all painful upon manipulation. There were marked transverse striæ, especially of the thumb nails, and the curvature was both lateral and longitudinal (Parrot beak clubbing). If one exerted pressure on either the tip or the base of the nail, the latter would rock up and down as though only fastened at the centre. The man himself declares that his finger and toe tips and nails have always been in the same proportion to his hands and feet that they are now, and that they have never pained him, nor prevented him from work. He does not seem to be aware of the enlargement of the distal extremities of his long bones, nor of his spinal curvature, and can give no history of these phenomena. It is only fair to add that he is not a man of much intelligence, although his story has been told to a number of questioners without marked variation. He can write legibly, and is making good progress in acquiring the English language. His assertion that his brother and child have the large nails is proved by the photographs which he shows us. Unfortunately we have no similar corroboration of the interesting statement that both are now, and always have been, in good health.§

§ Our thanks are due to Dr. Harvey, of Orange, for several excellent skiagraphs, and to Dr. Halsey, of Montclair, for some photographs of this patient's hands and feet. Dr. Harvey has also put us under obligation by two careful physical examinations of the chest.

So far as we can learn, there have been up to this time, seven cases of pulmonary osteo-arthropathy reported in America, one by Packard, one by N. S. Davis, Jr., four by W. S. Thayer, and one by Hasbrouck. Ours makes the eighth. Thayer in 1898 placed the total number of undoubted cases so far reported in this country and abroad at fifty-five. Of these twenty came to the autopsy table, and in eleven was the condition of the bones satisfactorily recorded. In all these there was an ossifying periostitis, limited almost entirely to the diaphyses of the long bones of the hands, feet, arms, and legs, and most marked at their distal extremities. Once the skull was thickened. The ribs and the rest of the skeleton seem to have been unaffected. Of the affected bones the periosteum is thickened, and new bone is in some cases laid on more or less regularly in layers; in others in an irregular and warty manner. Many erosions of the joint cartilages were noted together with an excess of fluid in the joints. The skin is practically unaffected. Dr. Thayer continues: "The clubbing of the fingers does not depend upon bony changes, the terminal phalanges having been always unchanged." (See accompanying skiagraph of the hand in our case, fig. 4. Fig. 7 represents a phthisical hand, and fig. 8 a working man's hand. These are merely for comparison.) We also call attention to the practically unaltered condition of the bones of the hand, as shown in the skiagraph. These slight increases of bony tissue, being so much less than those observed in other cases, lead us to infer that the morbid process in our case has ceased, or practically so, before extensive deformities have occurred. The change underlying the clubbed fingers would seem to have been in the main vascular. Freytag described a dilatation of the papillary processes, but no other cutaneous alteration. No sclerosis of the corium, nor of the subcutaneous tissues were noted.

As to the etiology of the condition, all the theories so far advanced have this in common, that they fail utterly to account for the extreme rarity of the so-called disease. Thayer and

18

others compare the process to amyloid degeneration, which in certain unexplained conditions, follows or accompanies protracted suppuration, and may occur in syphilis, and sometimes without assignable cause. In like manner clubbed fingers may accompany or follow a number of conditions, generally suppurative diseases of the bronchi, lungs, or pleuræ, and may occur in heart disease and in healthy people, from no discernable cause. Godlee and others have recorded such cases. However, when these are accompanied, as in our case, by spinal curvature and enlargements of the extremities of the long bones, it is a case of so-called pulmonary osteo-arthropathy. This in our patient, at least, seems to have an hereditary or family history, and in his person it seems to accompany, or be dependent upon, a tendency (constitutional or acquired) to prolonged suppuration (observe that an axillary abscess took five months to heal). This is in accord with the opinion of some of the best authorities, that suppuration has an etiological relation to the condition. Yet in J. T.'s case it can hardly be in consequence of suppuration in his own body, since he is especially clear on the point that he was born with the big fingers, and that in his children and his brother they were congenital, and apparently permanent, and have always been in the same proportion to the hands and feet that they are at present. Of course the statement of an Hungarian peasant must be taken with some reserve, but, as said before, cross-examination has not broken down or impaired the man's testimony.

Dr. Thayer states the antecedent disease known to have been present in the 55 cases as follows: Pulmonary tuberculosis, 9 cases; empyema, 9 cases; pleurisy, 5 cases; bronchitis, with or without bronchiectasis, 14 cases; sarcoma of lung, 2 cases; abscess of lung, 2 cases; carcinoma of pleura with effusion, 1 case; acute pneumonia, 1 case; total, 43 cases.

Of the remaining 12 cases the antecedent condition was: Syphilis, 3 cases; valvular heart disease, 3 cases; chronic diarrhœa, 2 cases; spinal caries, 1 case; unknown causes, 3 cases; total, 12.

We must admit that with a family history of pulmonary disease on the father's side, and with a chance that J. T. acquired syphilis thirteen years ago, added to the fact that his children seem to have been short-lived, and his rejection for the Hungarian army, he cannot be said to be free from constitutional dyscrasiæ. But—and this to our mind is the most striking thing in the peculiar condition we are considering—why are not more cases of osteo-arthropathy observed among the millions of people who have tubercular and syphilitic histories? We cannot avoid the conclusion that this condition must depend upon an etiological factor, which has so far escaped detection, and it may be nutritional or regional, like goitre. So many members of J. T.'s family having had the enlarged nails, leads us to suspect that there is some condition of climate, soil, or drinking water, to which this family was subjected, which led to the development of the condition amongst them.

The observations of Legrain, quoted by Walters, which do not seem to have attracted a great deal of notice, are to our minds, at least, interesting, and worthy of study in a condition which may be said to have baffled all inquirers into its etiology. Legrain says that the bones in osteo-arthropathy have an undue proportion of magnesia with diminution of the lime, and he attributes this to the drinking waters, especially in the desert of Sahara, where he had observed a number of cases which he asserts were unconnected with any bronchial or pulmonary lesion. He further claims to have strengthened this assumption by some experiments upon animals. It is known that feeding hens upon phosphorus will produce a condition resembling pulmonary osteo-arthropathy. Whether this occurs from the introduction of a toxin into the system, or from an interference with nutrition, has, so far as we know, not been determined. According to our view, a vicious or defective nutrition would be as likely to be the determining cause of this peculiar condition as any other. But we must admit that it shares in the objection, which we have advanced against the other theories, to wit, it fails to explain the extreme rarity of the condition.

We will not tire you by giving the detailed differential diagnosis between acromegaly and osteo-arthropathy, which we believe is sufficiently well known. We earnestly hope that the present meagre knowledge of the pathology of the latter condition (for we are strongly inclined to call it a condition and not a disease) will shortly be so reinforced and amplified, that the etiology will no longer remain so much of a mystery.

In closing, we join with others in deploring the unfortunate clumsy name which the condition has received, based upon the premature assumption that there is always an antecedent pulmonary disease. Dropping the word pulmonary from the title, and calling the condition osteo-arthropathy, would, in our opinion, be a decided improvement, as at least not misleading, albeit rather vague.

We append a bibliography, which is supplementary to that of Walters. Walters' extended to 1895, and ours gives what references we have been able to obtain from that year to 1901.

BIBLIOGRAPHY.

JANUARY, 1895—MARCH, 1901.

Springthorpe, *Brit. Med. Journ.*, 1895, vol. i., pp. 125-7.

Walters, *St. Thomas' Hosp. Rep.*, 1895, vol. xxiv., pp. 50, 105.

Davis, *Journ. Am. Med. Assoc.*, 1895, xxiv., p. 845.

Walters, *Brit. Med. Journ.*, 1896, vol. i., p. 329.

Lockwood, *Trans. Cl. Soc. London*, 1896, vol. xxx., p. 133.

Thayer, *N.Y. Med. Journ.*, 1896, p. 33.

Thorburn and Westmacott, *Path. Soc. Trans.*, 1896, p. 177.

Godlee, *N.Y. Med. Record*, 1896, December 12, p. 87 ; *Brit. Med. Journ.*, 1896, July 11, pp. 57, 116, 1417.

Fournier, *J.B.C., Rev. de Med.*, 1897, xvii., 221.

Massalongo, *Il Policlinico*, 1897, p. 572.

Teleky, *Weiner Klin. Wochen.*, 1897, No. 6.

Thayer, *Phila. Med. Journ.*, 1898, vol. ii., p. 955.

Hasbrouck, *N.Y. Med. Journ.*, 1898, pp. 67, 655.

Sonneville, *Echo Med. du Nord.*, 1898, vol. ii., p. 610.

O'Carroll, *Trans. Royal Acad. Med., Ireland*, 1898, vol. xvi., p. 318.

Whitman, *Pediatrics, N.Y. and Lond.*, 1899, vol. vii., p. 154.

Gasne, *Rev. Neurol.*, 1900, vol. vii, p. 539 ; or *N. Iconog de la Salpetrière*, 1900, vol. xiii., p. 449.

ON THE FEASIBILITY AND MANAGEMENT OF A HYGIENIC CURE OF PULMONARY TUBERCULOSIS OUTSIDE OF CLOSED SANATORIA.*

BY CHARLES L. MINOR, M.D.

ASHVILLE, N.C.

———

THE profession has so generally accepted, in theory, if not in practice, the hygienic open-air treatment of pulmonary tuberculosis, that before this audience I need not champion its claims, but to those coming in daily contact with this disease, it is very evident that with a large part of the medical public its acceptance has been one of faith without works, and that there is a crying need of making its features familiar not only to the specialist, but to the general practitioner, so that an early diagnosis being presupposed as a *sine quâ non* of success, the tubercular patient shall be able to obtain, both in our health resorts and outside them in their homes, that minute care and oversight which are essential to a cure.

Every one before me to-day can, I doubt not, recall cases where people with hectic in their cheeks and every evidence of advanced trouble, have been sent off for their health with no better instruction than to live out of doors, eat heartily, and take plenty of exercise, and who, in a faithful attempt to carry out these nebulous and often dangerous instructions, were losing what little chance of recovery they ever had.

It is sad enough to see the heedless and disobedient doing

* Read at the Annual Meeting of the American Climatological Association, at Niagara, January, 1901.

badly through their own wilfulness, but to see those who desire to do right, and have the necessary seriousness of purpose and determination, if rightly instructed, to recover, thus neglected by their physicians, is much worse.

If we search for reasons why the tubercular are so often neglected they are not far to seek.

Pulmonary tuberculosis is a chronic disease, and chronic diseases are unfortunately unpopular with the profession. If there is any disease which demands of the doctor patient, persistent effort, and attention to even trivial details, it is this, and the results, though excellent in properly selected cases, are slow. Yet taken early and handled faithfully, there is no disease which better repays the time and effort expended on it, and to-day there is no chronic disease which is so curable and yields such brilliant results, and those who will give the care and time to their tubercular cases that they do to their typhoids and pneumonias, will find them as absorbing in their interest, and as hopeful in their outcome, as any they have ever handled.

Coming to details, the causes of this neglect are various; in part the fault of the doctor, in part of the patient. Of the former I might note a lack of interest in a disease which is too generally supposed to be incurable, a want of familiarity with the details of the treatment, or of time to attend to them, and often a deficiency in the teaching faculty.

Of the latter, the chief are a want of sufficient intelligence or earnestness to grasp and carry out the objects of the treatment, an unwillingness to obey instructions faithfully, or a lack of means to obtain that minimum of comforts without which, save with State aid, the tubercular poor cannot hope to recover.

Granted that my contentions are right, it is most important to spread among the profession a knowledge of the hygienic method and a live faith in its possibilities; the truths taught by its founders and verified by so much experience must become common property, and should be taught in our medical schools, and applied in every-day practice.

Granted that this method is to-day the best and most rational, if not the only method of treating phthisis, then for the poor, or for those of very moderate means, the only hope lies in the opening of such institutions by the States and Cities, a movement admirably begun in this country by Dr. Trudeau, at his Adirondack Cottage Sanatorium. Only by State aid can the poor ever get the necessary elements for such a treatment, and I regret that it is not possible in this country to have such a compulsory workman's insurance as has in Germany led to the opening of so many sanatoria for the poor.

Object of the Paper.—But when in writing on the subject of the hygienic and dietetic treatment, sanatorium doctors and others assume, as they do so generally, that it is impossible outside such institutions to get satisfactory results with any certainty, I must lodge a protest, for it is feasible to get the best results, the most implicit obedience, the closest supervision of the patients' lives, in carefully selected private houses, and I feel that it is time to contradict assertions which, if not denied, would be finally accepted as facts. Were these exclusive claims admitted, their effect on phthisio-therapy would be harmful, and only tend to discourage the general adoption of the method in private practice as impracticable outside special institutions, and since it is evident that there are not, nor are likely ever to be, enough such establishments for the well-to-do to supply the demands of all the tubercular in easy circumstances, those who could not be accommodated would be in a sorry plight.

If by treatment in open resorts is meant the sending of patients to some place where, as so often happens, they are turned over to their unguided care of themselves, and allowed to follow every whim and neglect every precaution, and living as they choose, throw away all their chances, then, of course, sanatoria, with their supervised life, are essential; but if instead of comparing the results in sanatorium patients with those in people thus neglected, they are compared with cases outside of sanatoria, but properly supervised, I believe their assertions

cannot be supported, and it is to a study of this question that
this paper is devoted.

Here let me say that I am not combating, and would never
combat, the general spread of properly managed sanatoria.   No
one recognises more fully than I the great good they have
accomplished, but I believe that enthusiasm over the results
they have yielded has blinded their advocates to the general
applicability of the methods there used, and their infinite value
in general practice.   To apply them outside such institutions
will, I am willing to admit, demand more work on the doctor's
part to get equal results, as well as intelligence in the patient;
but these granted—and neither are too much to ask—it is not
only feasible, but in many cases, especially with American
patients, to be preferred to a sanatorium, which, despite its many
advantages, has certain inherent faults more felt in this country
than in Germany, where the temper of the people better fits
them for sanatorium life.   Indeed, it is, I believe, partly because
all statistics have been gathered from Germany in this matter,
that the view of the indispensability of sanatoria for the successful treatment of tuberculosis pulmonum has gained such
ground.

Definition of a Sanatorium.—Before going further, to avoid
misconception, let me state that in this paper I will confine
the use of the term sanatorium for tuberculosis to institutions
like the original ones of Brehmer and Dettweiler, or that of
Dr. Trudeau, in this country, where the outdoor rest treatment,
combined with hygiene and diet, is the chief reliance, and where
other methods are used only experimentally or as adjuncts, or,
to quote Walters,† an authority, " establishments for the open-
air treatment of presumably curable cases of consumption,
by hygiene and educational methods."

Requisites for a Sanatorium.—In adapting it then for use
in private practice, it is wise to see what are the advantages

† Walters, " Sanatoria for Consumptives." London, 1899.

claimed for sanatoria by their most ardent advocates, and to see whether these conditions cannot be had outside their walls.

According to Penzoldt,‡ the advantages which a well-arranged and managed sanatorium must combine are in general the following: Favourable protected location in a pure atmosphere near mountains and woods, with ample grounds; hygienic construction of the buildings as to location of rooms, ventilation, heating, &c.; good facilities for the open-air rest cure (pavilions, verandahs, balconies); absolute cleanliness, especially as to expectoration; good cooking and good milk; management by a capable, energetic doctor, especially experienced in phthisio-therapy, with absolute authority over the patients; enough trained assistant physicians, sufficient practised attendants; removal from their daily surroundings, with a lightening of the sadness of separation by a kind welcome; proper amusements, and the impossibility of all excesses, and the greatest possible avoidance of intercurrent diseases."

Quoting again, Walters§ says: " Sanatorium treatment is based on a careful regulation of each patient's daily life in all its hygienic and medical details. He is gradually trained to stand a life in the fresh air in all weathers, while his tendency to chill is removed by simple hydropathic applications and other common-sense precautions. The nature and amount of his daily exercises are regulated according to the weather, and to his momentary state of health, in an ascending scale, beginning with absolute rest in bed. His food ranges from fever diet to a rich and varied though digestible dietary.

" Strict precautions are taken to prevent all risks of infection, while the training he receives is useful not only to himself but to the whole community after his departure from the sanatorium. A resident medical and nursing staff assist in carrying out these daily measures, and are immediately available in cases

‡ Penzoldt, " Anstaetsbehand, der Lungen Tuberculose," vol. iii., p. 333, of Penzoldt " Stintzing Handbuch Therapie Innere Krank "

§ Walters, " Sanatoria for Consumptives," p. 11. London, 1899.

of hæmoptysis, &c. . . . They have to prevent imprudences in some cases, to encourage to perseverance in others ; to strictly enforce all the essential rules, while they allow sufficient personal liberty in less important matters to prevent the irksomeness of restraint ; to suggest harmless and beneficial forms of recreation, while they discourage those likely to do mischief. Mind has a great influence over bodily health, and the stimulus of hope and the encouragement which results from steady progress and sympathetic attention, will count for much in curing the patient."

Reviewing these desiderata as stated by the foremost authorities, it will be evident to those who have treated this disease, that while certain of them can be more easily attained in a closed institution, all the essential ones can be attained outside them in private houses, only granted sufficient interest in and attention to the matter on the doctor's part. Certain patients will, owing to their nature, do better in closed sanatoria, others far better outside, but under close supervision, and I believe that the majority of American patients will belong to the latter class, as a majority of the German ones do to the former. If the trouble is taken to make a study of the locality from the hygienic point of view, doctors will not find it hard to get houses with proper location, southern exposure, good construction, and proper porches, many of the best known sanatoria being only ordinary houses turned to the new use. All our health resorts, and many suburban localities, offer proper facilities for the open-air treatment in pure air, mountains, open country, fields, woods, and shady footpaths, away from roads, and a little study of the gradients and distances will enable the doctor to plan out his patient's exercise with accuracy and effect.

Proper cooking, while in my experience the most difficult of these desiderata to obtain, can with sufficient care always be had not only if the patient is in his own house, but when he is in a properly selected boarding house. The landlady of the house can be readily made to realise that it is to her interest to keep the best possible table, and that if she fail in this the patients will be placed elsewhere.

Properly supervised milk supplies are daily, I am glad to say, more common, and veterinarily tested herds are to be found at all our resorts, while the houses where one's patients stay will be kept clean, and the sputum disposal closely watched, if their owners are made to feel that their patronage will suffer if it is wanting.

Home-sickness is not less evident in than out of sanatoria, and if the cases are well located, can be soon removed if they are interested in their own cases, and occupied with the work of getting well.

The chief point, however, on which is based the statement that the method cannot be carried out successfully outside such institutions, is the fact that the doctor cannot at all times be with the patient, who therefore, it is claimed, cannot be protected from imprudences or disobedience.

An experience covering several years has, however, shown me that if proper precautions are taken, and the patient properly taught in the beginning, if proper records are kept, of which I will speak more fully later on, and if the proper relation between the patient and the doctor has been established, and the confidence of the former won, and his co-operation assured, this difficulty will not be felt, and an amply close watch be kept over him without the constant presence of a mentor, which is very trying to many people.

Excesses in exercise, amusements, diet, &c., will be easily avoided if our teaching faculty and control of our patients is what it should be. If we cannot get their confidence and co-operation, cannot teach them or control them, we would fail even if with our patients every moment; with these we can safely trust them out of our sight for a considerable length of time, knowing that they have been taught what to do and what to avoid, and can be trusted to obey us and keep a close record of everything they do.

Application in Private Practice.—Turning now to the application of the method outside of a sanatorium, there are certain variations dependent on whether we are to carry it out in the patient's home, or with the added assistance of a special climate.

Where pecuniary reasons prevent the patient from seeking one of the latter, excellent results can be had, though with greater difficulty, in the patient's home, if the case be not too advanced, but anyone who has seen the remarkable gains that can be gotten in our resorts, even in severe cases, cannot doubt that climate can greatly improve the results to be gotten by hygiene and diet, and will enable us to obtain cures not otherwise possible.

If, however, one has to choose between treating patients in narrow circumstances in their own homes or sending them to a resort where their poverty will not enable them to get the necessary conditions of quarters, diet, and care, which are so essential, by all means let them stay at home; by changing their houses, moving to the top floor, using the roof as an outdoor sun-parlour, and spending the utmost possible part of their time there, by economising in every other way in order to be able to spend freely for good food and cookery, much can be done, provided always that their work can be relinquished, rest taken, and their lives properly supervised.

Study of Locality.—While in our cities the house of the patient cannot be well controlled, in a health resort the doctor's first duty is to make a careful study of all the local conditions, and to familiarise himself with the houses fitted for his patient's use. Their topography must be studied, so as to get sunny, protected exposures, with good drainage; the location and advantages of the various ones should be well known, and the housekeeper informed of the essentials which her house must offer. The kindliness, ability, and willingness to accept suggestions of the landlady are most important, perfect location and drainage not compensating for a poor table or a cheerless, untidy house.

Locating Patients.—It is most important that the patient agree to locate himself in accordance with the doctor's advice ; strange to say, they generally seem to think that this is a matter of no medical importance, and are apt first to settle themselves in some badly located house, in the centre of the town, before consulting him.

I need hardly say that it is essential that the thickly settled, central parts of the town, or even village, be avoided, and the patients placed in the outskirts, and that the house chosen shall have either its own lawn and trees, or be surrounded by country.

In locating a patient, the company he will be thrown with needs the doctor's attention ; agreeable companions have a good effect on the course of the case, and the doctor should try to see that congenial ones are obtained.

Personally, I am satisfied that no patient can be properly followed in the average large hotel ; the temptations are too great ; the local conditions cannot be properly controlled ; there is too much noise and excitement, and early hours are not possible. They must, therefore, either have their own home, or be placed in some properly run house, where a good land-lady keeps things in proper shape, where there is amusement without over-excitement, where the table and other conditions can be controlled.

The doctor will find a list of such houses as he approves of as to location and management most needful and useful, and while the physician does not live under the roof, they offer for all practical purposes the condition which sanatorium doctors demand.

Whether a patient will be best in his own cottage or in such a properly kept house, is a question which must be answered separately for each case, and depends largely on the temperament of the patient. Some—possibly a majority—do best under their own roof, if the family or friends who accompany him are judicious and sensible, but I find that a large number are better off in a well-run house with other people, and away from their families. To some the presence of others all engaged in the same pursuit is an encouragement and aid, to others it is depressing ; to some the absence of their own family is not felt, and is rather an assistance than a hindrance, while to others the presence of their dear ones is indispensable.

Here, as everywhere else in medicine, each case must be studied on its own merits, and no hard and fast rule can be made.

Arrangement of Quarters.—When the location has been settled, the doctor should himself inspect the room or house, and show the patient how to arrange it in accordance with the rules of hygiene ; the ignorance of even educated people in these matters is deplorable, and left to themselves they will almost surely make mistakes.

Room.—The room should, of course, face south, south-east, or south-west, and should have 2,000 to 3,000 cubic feet of air space, though sometimes, if there are plenty of windows and an open fireplace, less can be tolerated. It had best be rectangular, as irregularly-shaped rooms ventilate badly, and the ceiling must never be too low. An open fireplace, as much as a ventilator as a heater, is invaluable, and save in the, very coldest climates, such a fireplace will be sufficient for warming purposes. Where more heat is needed, hot water should be chosen, and in no case should a hot air furnace flue open into the bedroom of the pulmonary patient ; its bad effects will have been noted by all who have seen much phthisis.

There should at least be two windows, and where they can be had, French windows which open like double doors, and allow full ventilation, should be chosen. Where possible, the cracks in the floor should be filled with some good composition, that given by Petit‖ being good, while painted or kalsomined

‖ Leon Petit, "Le Phthisique et son Traitment Hygienique," p. 55. Paris, 1895.

walls, which can be washed or renewed frequently, are far better than papered ones.

Some writers, pushing their fear of contagion to unnecessary extremes, as I believe, would banish all pictures and ornaments from the room as possible places of dust lodgment and bacillary storehouses. While it is true that the patient's room is rarely used save as a sleeping place, its cheerfulness is an important factor in the case, especially if the patient be confined to bed, and while thick hangings cutting off light and air, nailed down carpets, and needless flummery are to be forbidden, it is not necessary to convert the room into a species of cell, with four bare walls, a bed and a chair ; and an intelligent patient of decent habits can safely be allowed pictures on his walls, attractive furniture in sufficient but not superfluous amount, and pretty removable rugs, which can be steamed or sunned frequently ; while light, washable window curtains, which can go to the laundry, add to the homelikeness of the room and its cheerfulness, and therefore improve it.

Single beds alone should be allowed, preferably of iron or brass ; the persistence of the use of double beds, those relics of an unhygienic age, is a painful commentary on the ignorance of the public on sanitary matters. Mattresses should be firm, never soft, and of hair, and the bed-covers should be light but warm ; the best are woollen blankets and cotton sheets ; the popular comforters of cotton wadding are heavy, and cannot be cleaned, and linen sheets allow of chilling. The bed-head should never be allowed to be in a corner, as it is well known¶ that air does not circulate there properly ; and the bed had best be well out in the room, yet not in a direct draught from constantly open windows. A living room is generally not needed, but where raw, damp days are common, may be at times useful ; it should never be so attractive as to tempt to indoor life. When used, they should be kept between 58 and 68 degrees F.

¶ Kruger, " Der Werth der Ventilation." Strasburg, 1899.

Porch.—An absolutely necessary adjunct is a good wide porch, or a good summer house in the yard, well protected from winds, and with southern exposure. If it opens from the patient's room, so that the bed can be rolled out on it, it will, during the febrile period, be advantageous, as allowing the bed to be placed out doors. Glazing, save on the most exposed side, where it is necessary, turns a porch from a fresh air rest-place, to a sweat box, and robs it of its usefulness. In cities where porches are often wanting, they can be extemporised by the carpenter at no very great expense.

Cooking and Diet.—To nothing need more attention be given than the cooking and housekeeping; the food need not be elaborate, but must be good, nourishing, and tempting, and in generous amount, but very rich food or many made dishes are not desirable. The proportion of good red meat must be far larger than would be necessary for well people, and there must be plenty of good milk available, veterinarily tested where feasible.

Outside sanatoria, and even in them, judging from the literature, the doctor will find that the greatest difficulty is apt to lie in procuring a proper table, but with care and the co-operation of the housekeeper, it can be overcome. In the more hopeful early cases the diet does not give much trouble, for in no disease is so much freedom in diet permissible, but when dyspepsia or anorexia are present it becomes our hardest problem, and will tax all our ingenuity.

Granted no especial gastric trouble, a generous diet, with insistence on red meat daily, milk freely, but not to disgust, plenty of butter, cream, and animal fats, with plenty of green vegetables, but a limitation of starches—not from any harm in them, but because being filling, they lessen the desire for more nourishing food, and are bulky—is what we will generally find best. Careful cooking of the meats is most needful, and I have found that great assistance from a good meat grinder, which yields a fine meat pulp free of fibre, which can be made into

19

patties and broiled till the outside alone is brown. Such patties are generally liked, and easily eaten, and have a high nutritive value. After trying various arrangements of the meals, I have found most satisfaction from three regular meals a day, supplemented by nourishment on waking, at 11 a.m., 4 p.m., and at bed-time, this consisting generally of milk and a cracker, and raw egg, or any other easily digested food, care only being taken that the patient does not take enough to destroy his appetite for the next meal. In some cases milk, especially at bed-time, does not agree, but generally the lack of agreement is in the patient's mind rather than his stomach, and with care can be educated away. Dilution with Vichy, disguising it by adding a little digestible cocoa or coffee, &c., will generally be enough. Certainly the tubercular who really cannot take milk are sorely handicapped in their efforts at recovery. Where milk cannot be tolerated, tropon, plasmon, somatose, peptonoids, panopeptone, raw eggs, scraped beef, chicken soup, &c., can be used, and even where milk is taken these can be added to it with advantage ; and thus a familiarity with the various prepared foods and concentrated nutrients on the market is of value to the doctor. I rarely push milk beyond 1½ or 2 quarts in a day (six to eight glasses), save where no other food is taken.

Anorexia is probably the commonest difficulty one has to meet in tuberculosis, and there is little one can say on the subject. Where outdoor life after a fair trial does not remove it, as it very generally does, the prognosis is made far more serious. Penzoldt's suggestion that a poor appetite can be greatly assisted by using soft foods that need no chewing, cold food rather than hot, and liquids rather than solids, will appeal to those who know from personal experience what anorexia really is ; certainly no drug has in my hands proved of any but temporary benefit.

Outdoor life, variety and daintiness in the food, and at times frequent small meals, rather than the usual three large ones, are our best simple measures. Febrile cases generally regain an appetite as the fever falls under the influence of outdoor rest; where fever persists, liquid diet has to be resorted to. Lavage, as advocated by De Bove, may be useful for certain cases; when resorted to it is generally too late to expect anything from it but the pain to the patient from the tube, and a slight prolongation of a life he is anxious to give up.

Intestinal indigestion and myasthenia gastrica are common and troublesome digestive conditions in the tubercular; their treatment cannot be gone into here, but for the sake of the patient's nutrition they need to be closely cared for.

Family Surroundings.—The control of the patient's family is often a great difficulty. At times a wife, sister, or sensible husband will be of great assistance; more generally they hinder the progress of the case, and our patients are better without them, if well located in a pleasant house. Where the patient is in his own house, and their presence cannot be avoided, they have to be taught to be a help, and not, as they so often are, a hindrance. Too often they are either so depressed as to discourage the patient, or are so little aware of the seriousness of the case, as to be constantly tempting him to over-exertion or imprudence.

Study of the Case.—After these matters of location, quarters, surroundings, diet, &c., are settled, the patient's physical and mental condition next demand attention, and on the first few week's intercourse with him, on the correctness of our estimate of his character, on the impression we make on him, and on his belief in our earnestness and our interest in his case, fully as much as on our history-taking and physical examination, depends largely our success with him, and no pains should be spared at this time to familiarise ourselves with his nature, and win his confidence. Such time and pains are never wasted, and our first few interviews should never be hurried, or give the impression that we are not interested in the case; and indeed, studied rightly, every case becomes deeply interesting.

Character-study ought to be of interest to every physician.

and in tuberculosis is more important than in almost any other disease. The patient's psychological attitude towards his disease, his family relations and idiosyncrasies, must be known if possible, as on them often hinges our treatment; but this is a matter that need hardly be mentioned to any intelligent doctor. A good history is a good foundation on which to base treatment, and is too often neglected. There are many questions in phthisiology which only the study of carefully-taken histories can settle, but I believe such histories are not as yet as carefully taken as they should be. In seeking for heredity, close enough search is not always made. Previous possible exposure to infection in the home, school, or business, ought to be closely inquired after. If looked for, it will often be found that a history of childhood cervical adenitis or otorrhœa can be gotten, and the supposedly recent infection referred back to childhood. Close search for unnoted prodromata, years before the patient thought himself sick, persistent dyspepsias, anæmias, nervous prostrations, and different departures from the normal, which the patient would never pay attention to, and which the doctor has to search for closely to elicit, will, I believe, tend to show a longer duration of the incubative period than is often credited, and point to a preponderance of childhood infections which lie latent, only to manifest themselves in later life, when conditions depressing vitality occur.

It is almost needless to note that the physical examination which follows must be of the most searching and accurate nature known to modern scientific medicine. No modesty or hurry should prevent an examination of the skin, and the keeping of a chart of the findings, which can be filed away with the rest of the card indexed history, and at each re-examination will be found far better for reference than our unassisted memory.

Such re-examinations, I believe, save when intercurrent trouble makes them more frequent, need not be oftener than once a month; the progress of tuberculosis is too gradual to make more frequent ones desirable.   Of course all these things are routine matters with all careful men, but all men are not careful, and were these things more generally attended to results would be better.

Truth Telling.—After the examination, a frank and free talk with the patient must follow, and while many writers on the subject have declaimed against the common sin of conceal·ing the truth, and calming fears by subterfuges, it seems not to have been heeded, either from a mistaken kind-heartedness, or from a misconception of its effects on the patient.

As has been well said, " Why should the patient who is told he is suffering from an apical catarrh, and who otherwise feels well and strong, take care of himself?   How shall we bring him to observe the hundreds of cautions and rules, to give up so many favourite habits and pleasures for months and years? How shall we induce him, following our advice, to temporarily give up his calling, to separate himself from home and family, to sacrifice money and time, if we do not honestly explain to him the seriousness of the case."[*]

Of course no one would advise a blunt and brutal revelation of the whole unvarnished truth without proper explanations and preparation, but even this, much as it would shock him, is less bad than the mistaken kindness that so often leads doctors to conceal facts, a proper realisation of which is so essential to the patient's recovery.   Let it never be forgotten that the patient is to be our partner and co-worker on his own case, and that a partnership in which one member is ignorant of the course of the business is sure to end in failure.   Of course in hopeless cases concealment of the bitter truth is needed, and with nervous and timid people time must be taken to educate them to understand the situation before the whole truth is revealed, but gone about tactfully, it will never be found hard to accomplish, and even the most rebellious will thank you for it in the long run.

* Cornet, " Die Tuberculose ; Nothnagle's System," p. 478.

In this connection, I would dwell on the advantage of making a distinction in talking with the patient, and clinically, between pulmonary tuberculosis and consumption. While the latter, which should be applied only to advanced cases with much destruction, and generally with mixed infection, is a hopeless disease, and so recognised by the public, the former, which should be reserved for uncomplicated first and even second stage cases, is one of the most curable of chronic diseases, and if the patient is taught this, taught that yearly many recover from it without even knowing that they had it, as shown by many autopsies, taught that his recovery lies largely in his own hands, and depends very much on his own good sense, that you are to be his teacher, to show him how to live wisely, and that he must help in the treatment, and not be a passive subject, he will thank you for your frankness, where, had you concealed the truth from him in a cruelly mistaken kind-heartedness, he would, when in the inevitable course of events the truth was forced home on him, hate you for it. In all teaching—but never more than here—one finds that it is necessary, if the pupil is really to learn, to give the reasons for the facts one imparts, if these facts are to be real and living, and not the mere dry bones of knowledge. Only thus will you get willing and intelligent obedience.

Explicit Directions.—After having talked with the patient, and told him the facts in the case, show him carefully exactly what he must do, how he must live, and let him distinctly understand that you will require of him an absolute obedience, and tolerate no insubordination. Written orders, covering every detail, should be given him for reference, and let him know that whatever is not explicitly allowed is implicitly forbidden.

Especially should his orders as to sputum disposal be carefully given, and the danger to himself, not less than to others, of their neglect made clear, for in sputum disposal all now admit lies the key to the eradication of this disease. But even after he has your written orders, it will not do to take for granted that he will obey; most men are fools about themselves, sick men more than others, and if you are to properly watch the case, you will need a detailed information about his life which he cannot give you satisfactorily even twelve hours after the event.

Record Keeping.—Realising this, I have adopted the use of a record book, ruled and printed properly for the purpose, in which the patient records not only his temperature and pulse, but everything he does, how he feels, his hours of outdoor rest, the exact amount and nature of his exercise, his cough and expectoration, his spirits, appetite, digestion, &c.; nothing should be omitted which happens to him during the day. This plan I have, after a long trial, found most satisfactory, and can heartily recommend it. It teaches the patient to study his own case, and though many will say that this is harmful and depressing, *it is what the tubercular patient must do if he is to master his disease,* as all the best authorities are agreed. It helps him to avoid imprudences, and makes him think twice before he acts once, and keeps you in close and intimate contact with the case. It rarely makes the patient nervous, and in such cases I of course always stop it, but I always closely question him on this point, and it is not often that this is necessary; on the contrary, most take a lively interest in keeping it, and I have often had them tell me that it helps them greatly in obeying orders, and is a help and encouragement to them. I use in conjunction with this, with great advantage, a specially arranged graphic temperature chart, which I have no trouble in teaching them to keep, and which I have ruled with horizontal red lines at 99.5 and 97.5 F., to denote the limits within which the temperature must stay if exercise is to be allowed, and with black lines at 98 and 98.8 F., to show the range within which, subject, of course, to special indications, free exercise is permitted. From this they can see at a glance, after instruction, when to stop exercise and when to increase it between the times when I see them, while the almost unfailing effect of outdoor rest in reducing temperature is shown so clearly and convincingly by the falling curve, that aside from keeping me posted as no written list of temperatures could, it greatly encourages the patient. Without a temperature record I do not believe a tubercular case can—certainly in the earlier period of the treatment—be properly studied. On the nature of the fever curves depends the treatment, and it cannot be intelligently directed without it.

A knowledge of his life is equally needful, and without these adjuncts I would find great, and I fear, insuperable difficulty, in following my cases as closely as they need, and in carrying on this method outside a sanatorium, and would feel like a captain in trying to navigate his vessel without a compass.

Temperature Study.—With these record blanks and a careful diet list, I send him to his quarters to carry out a week of rest, during which he keeps a two-hourly temperature and pulse record during the day-time, beginning with one before rising in the morning, and ending with one at bed-time. If exercise were allowed during this week, the record would be materially affected by it, hence even in mild cases I insist on this week being spent quietly. A study of this record after the first week in connection with the history and physical findings, enables one to form a prognosis, and to plan out the future treatment, and make any changes in the general orders needed. As soon as one is familiar with the case the record is made four hourly, or even thrice a day; and finally thrice a day is amply sufficient to keep one informed of the temperature; but at first for a month or more, at times, the two-hourly record I believe most important. In severe cases it is not wise to allow the patient to know his own temperature, and I have it taken by others, but all cases with any outlook will finally reach a point when the temperature is steady and not very high, when they can be trusted to know it, while those where this does not occur are generally those who have little or no prospect of recovery. In connection with the subject of temperature I would note that it is necessary to be sure the thermometer the patient uses is reliable; the records yielded by the cheap thermometers often sold by druggists to laymen, are absolutely unreliable, and a thermometer with no error greater than at the most two-tenths of a degree F. must be used. Then, too, many patients will keep the thermometer in the mouth too short a time. Some experimentation on the subject has convinced me that the so-called rapid registering thermometers are not nearly as rapid as is claimed, and that it is wise to keep any thermometer in the mouth and properly under the tongue for a full five minutes, while some even after that time will register a further rise up to as much as ten minutes. These are small points, but it is often in small points that lies the difference between success and failure.

Nursing.—In all but severe cases I find that one can dispense with a trained nurse if only a servant be within call to attend to the wants of the patient, but in the early treatment of active cases which have not yet begun to gain, and need every assistance to enable them to start up hill, they have been of great use, and indispensable; but a nurse to properly care for this class of patient, needs even more tact than is demanded for ordinary nursing, and the maximum of patience.

In bringing a bedridden case slowly back to health, tempting his appetite by delicately served dainties, increasing his nourishment by oil rubs, &c., and doing the thousand and one little things which a good nurse understands, no affectionate relative, however willing, can take her place. In less severe cases, however, where the patients are able to care for themselves largely, and where they are outdoors all day, they can be dispensed with easily, especially if there is an attendant at hand to answer the patients' calls, and bring them their nourishment.

Necessary Paraphernalia.—Before beginning the cure, the patient must provide himself with certain necessary adjuncts, which cannot be conveniently dispensed with. These are a proper reclining chair, satisfactory wraps for outdoors, proper underclothing, a good sputum cup and flask, and arrangements for simple hydrotherapy. The choice of these should not be left to the judgment of the patient, and the doctor had best specify just the articles needed, else unsuitable ones will often be gotten.

Reclining Chair.—Both the customary sea chair and the wicker reclining chairs made for the purpose, are unsatisfactory, as they do not allow of a perfectly horizontal position, such as is needed in febrile cases, nor permit of a change of position, which is demanded if the chair is not to be fatiguing. To lie all day with the back at an angle of 30 or 40 degrees is not really resting, keeps certain muscles constantly on the strain, and can be most tiring. I therefore insist on a chair, of which several are on the market at various prices, which will allow of all positions, from the perfectly horizontal to the upright. By using such a chair, I find I can lessen the number of those who, on account of fever, have to be kept in bed in their rooms, it being easy to wrap patients in blankets, and putting them recumbent in such a chair, wheel them outdoors, where they can spend the day as comfortably as if in bed.

Wraps.—In the matter of wraps, the common blanket, unless very carefully adjusted and frequently watched, leaves too many openings for the air, so I always advise one of the various blanket bags or steamer rugs made in bag form, and in which the patient sits, and by buttoning up the robe in front, is enclosed on all sides from the weather. For those who suffer from cold feet, a hot bottle in the foot of the bag is useful; for those who are upright, a couple of hot bricks in a wooden box, in which the feet can be kept, serve to overcome the difficulty. However, it is surprising how quickly the patients get accustomed to the cold, and do not mind it at all.

Underclothing.—As to the underclothing, despite the commercially exploited claims of various new systems, wool remains the most desirable for winter use, and since Rubner's work, rests on a firm scientific basis. Its weight should never be excessive, and the necks should be cut high, though here one runs counter to the predilections of the fair sex, and will often have trouble in enforcing this point. In summer, any garment not allowing a too rapid chilling of the surface will do, although the very lightest grade of thin wool is still the best.

Sputum Cups.—A sputum cup is, of course, essential, and for use at home, I know nothing at once so good and so cheap as the common square tin frame and cover, holding a folded pasteboard container, which can be burned after use, though it could be improved by impregnating the paper with paraffin to render it water-tight, and to facilitate its burning. It is light, its opening is amply large—a fault in many other popular receivers—the flaps folding inward prevent the contents from being disagreeably in evidence, or from running out if upset, while the tin lid makes it inaccessible to flies, a most important point, I am satisfied. Save for ambulant cases, it is in every way superior to the glass hand spittoon and the pocket flasks of the Dettweiler model, whose openings are, as all who have used them must admit, far too small for cleanly use. Of course in ambulant cases the flask is at present the best thing we have, but it is to be hoped that when American ingenuity turns itself to the matter a better one will be evolved. While it is true that generally before the case has reached the ambulant stage the expectoration has entirely ceased, the flask should always be at hand in case the need of it arises. Two methods of sputum disposal are so unfortunately popular, and so very bad, that I would stop to note them here. I refer to expectoration into cloths, which are later burned or thrown into the fire. The cloths are an easy means of soiling the hands or the pockets, while those who spit into a fireplace are liable to have parts of the sputum strike in some cool corner, or fall through into the ashes, where it can escape incineration, and be later blown around. All instructions as to sputum disposal need to be very specific, and infractions should be never excused.

Hydrotherapy.—Simple but very satisfactory hydrotherapy can be carried out with such common articles as a tin, hat tub, salt, a bath thermometer, and rough towels, as I have elsewhere† explained, and so I need not dwell on them here. Cases which are too sick to bathe themselves generally need a nurse, who can give such treatment as the doctor orders.

Frequency of Visits.—In caring for cases outside of sanatoria, the question of how often it is necessary to see one's patients is of importance ; the advocates of sanatoria claim that without seeing a case many times a day it is impossible to get the necessary oversight of it, or to compel the needed obedience, but from practical experience, I am satisfied that with such records as I have described, and having won his confidence and co-operation, you can keep fully in touch with every detail of your patient's life, and control him completely, while seeing him, according to the severity of the case, or his lightmindedness, from once to four times a week. The more intelligent the patient, the less frequently will he need to be seen, and generally one or two visits a week are sufficient. If you have taught him to realise the seriousness of the case, have explained the aims of the treatment, and convinced him of its hopefulness, you will get an obedience more minute than he would yield to any other adviser, whether spiritual or legal, and will have no fault to find with his carrying out your orders. As has been said, the heedless and headstrong have to be seen oftener than the intelligent and docile, but it is not often that patients are so intractable and lightminded as to persist in disobedience after careful warning, and such had best be given up, as no results can be hoped for from them.

Amount of Rest.—One or two week's study of the case while at absolute rest will enable you to decide the amounts of rest and exercise needed, and as a general rule, unless the temperature passes 102 degrees F., it is best from the first to carry on the rest treatment, not in bed in the room, as so many advocate, but on a cot or reclining chair outdoors. " Bed," as I have said elsewhere,‡ " does a violence to the feelings and hopes

† *New York Medical Journal,* January 14, 21, 1899.
‡ *Loc. cit.*

which can be ill tolerated, and often turns the balance to the wrong side . . . and robs him of what little strength he still has," and my experience since I wrote this has only confirmed me in the opinion, that while recumbent rest is essential, bed is generally undesirable, and to be avoided where possible. A patient kept flat, with every muscle relaxed, loses his fever as quickly out of doors as in bed in his room, and misses the depressing effect of being confined to his room and bed.   When the temperature does not pass 100·5 degrees F. I begin to allow sitting up, but never consider exercise till the temperature for a week has not exceeded 99·5 degrees F., and am even then careful of it save as a further lowering of the curve and the absence of any bad effects permit further increase.   Of course there are exceptions to every rule, and at times in certain patients who cannot stand absolute quiet exceptions have to be made, individualising being more important in the treatment of phthisis than in any other trouble.

It is remarkable how quickly outdoor rest will reduce fever and pulse rate, and increase strength even in very severe cases. When a month of it shows no effect the prognosis becomes serious.   To cite an instance, which, while remarkable, is by no means exceptional, of what rest can do, I would report briefly the case of a gentleman under my care in the winter of 1890-1, who on arrival had an active tubercular broncho-pneumonia of the upper half of the left lung, around a large cavity, and an active tubercular bronchitis of the upper one-third of the right. There were numerous tubercle bacilli and streptococci in the abundant purulent sputum, and both sugar and albumen in the abundant urine. The temperature in the afternoon was 103 to 104 F.; his pulse 120; his respiration from 35 to 40; and the able practitioner who had sent him had told him the hopelessness of his case, but allowed him, at his own desire, to try what the mountains could do for him.   Absolute rest, first in bed and then flat on his back outdoors, with strict regulation of his diet, life, &c., rapidly reduced the fever and other symptoms, and improved the signs. He began to hope, and to think he might recover, and made real gains.

When six months after his arrival he went home, the activity of the process in the lung had been checked, the cavity was dry, the mixed infection had long ceased, and the tubercle bacilli were much fewer; the sugar and albumen had left the urine; the temperature had not been above 98˙8 F. for six weeks or more, nor over 99˙5 F. for three months. There was an 18 lbs. gain in weight; the pulse averaged 72 to 96; the respiration 24. The appetite was good, and the strength good enough to permit of walks of one or two miles without bad effect, and his spirits were excellent. Of course such a case could not be cured in the proper sense of the term, but there had been a marked arrest for such a severe trouble in so short a time, which could only be ascribed to the systemised outdoor rest and the care of his life, while he had acquired such a comprehension of his trouble, and such a knowledge of how to handle himself, as should be of infinite value to him in the future course of his case.

Exercise.—The question of exercise for these patients needs the closest attention, for, according as it is wisely or foolishly used, it can become a blessing or a curse. Exercise is best measured by time, not distance, at first, for it is thus far more easily graduated, and no mistakes can be made when the watch is made the judge. As to the kind of exercise to begin with, save for the very weak, who had best begin with massage, walking is to be preferred to driving as a commencing exercise, with rare exceptions. I begin with a short stroll on a level, of from two to five minutes' duration, increasing gradually by from one to five minutes daily, up to an hour, or even more, according to the indications given by pulse and temperature, and sense of fatigue, and promptly returning to the chair if these show a bad effect, or during any increase of symptoms, or with women during the period. Used in this way and choosing for our patients gradually increasing inclines, exercise is as beneficial later on as rest is earlier in the trouble, and those who like the French school, forbid its use until the temperature is normal, are, I believe, pushing a good idea too far and throwing away an invaluable aid. In the beginning all exercise should be taken in the morning hours, save in those few cases where the maximum temperature rise is at that time, and afternoon exercise had best be reserved till later. In the beginning all walks should be chosen for the patients, not left to their unassisted judgment; and here a familiarity with all the paths and roads in the neighbourhood on the physician's part is necessary. When the patient can walk for an hour or over, he can be left to choose his own paths if he has been well instructed.

Driving.—As a general rule drives are more tiring than walks at first, and had best not be allowed till walking has been tried. There is more temptation in driving to overdo and go beyond one's strength before it is realised. Riding, in convalescent cases with little or no rise at all, is excellent, as Alonzo Clark long ago taught, and before him, Sydenham, but it is too violent to be used where signs of activity are present.

Pulmonary Gymnastics.—Pulmonary gymnastics have lately been opposed by some, who claim that since we put a tubercular joint at rest, it is irrational to exercise a tubercular lung, but a considerable experience with them has convinced me that this view is fallacious. When we recall that the occupations that narrow the thorax notably favour the incidence of phthisis, that the advancing disease is always accompanied by a steadily contracting chest, and that improving cases show, with few exceptions, a gradual thoracic re-expansion, I cannot think that we are going against nature in using this method in properly chosen cases, and regard the tendency to discourage its use as a backward step in phthisio-therapy. When signs of activity are nearly gone, as shown by the disappearance of râles, when the temperature does not go above 99·5 degrees F., and the pulse begins to slow, I have found it an invaluable aid, and believe that it combats the peripheral atelectasis, which prepares the way for further spread of the trouble. If an open functioning alveolus, well aerated, offers a stronger resistance to the advancing process than an inactive one, then pulmonary gymnastics, which I have elsewhere described in detail, and need not dwell upon here, are certainly of value, for that they increase the thoracic perimeter is easily shown by systematically kept lead tape tracings; that they markedly increase ease of breathing and expansion is proven by the patient's feelings, and by the tape measure; that they increase vital capacity, undoubtedly by opening up collapsed alveoli, is attested by the spirometer; and when they are used with discretion, neither the pulse, temperature, symptoms, or physical signs are harmfully affected, as any one can convince himself who will give them a judicious and fair trial.

Amusements.—Both as a great help and a serious hindrance, accordingly as they are used or abused, the patient's amusements demand close attention, whether in or out of a sanatorium.

For those still carrying out a strict rest cure, and kept horizontal, there are few available, but with the lowering of the fever, which is generally soon noted, the semi-upright position is allowed, and then simple games, such as solitaire, dominoes, checkers, and for the ladies light fancy work are permissible. Any game or occupation demanding mental concentration or excitement has to be forbidden, for mental tire is nearly as bad as physical. For this reason, chess playing, studying, or even letter writing in many cases, especially if they be business letters, cannot be allowed. When the patient begins to walk, the walk will be found a pleasant amusement, which can later be diversified by botanising, geologising, sketching, &c., if not followed too eagerly. Active games should be reserved for the most convalescent, and there are not many that can be recommended unreservedly. Tennis, rowing, skating, and the coasting that is so popular in the Alpine resorts, are all too violent, and are not to be thought of. Riding and driving I have already referred to. Golf, if wisely restricted, is an ideal sport for the tubercular, being easily dosed from a little mild physical exertion up to the most active allowable. That all indoor night entertainments are to be forbidden goes without saying— the theatre above all—for not only is the psychical excitement bad, but the long sitting in a crowded, hot, and draughty room, and the exit amidst clouds of dust into a cold street, is most harmful for such people. Dancing must be totally given up, not simply during the cure, but I believe for ever, for it combines excitement and over-exertion in a hot, dusty atmosphere. In nothing more than in our control of his amusements will our hold on our patient show itself, and there is no better test of that control than the willingness on his part to give up some favourite amusement at the doctor's orders. Of course the close restriction of their amusements will, with the light-minded, meet with much opposition, and it is often the rock on which treatment splits, but the earnest will, if they understand the reasons, not fail to obey.

Worries.—Having spoken of his amusements, let me here refer to the worries that can, and often do, harm our patients. Frequently set-backs that we are at a loss to understand will be found to result from some family trouble, some business worry, or some other anxiety, and such must be looked for, and, if possible, guarded against. Indeed, this is one of the advantages of removing the patient to a climatic resort, where family worries and business affairs are left behind. The family, if alone, should be taught to keep from the sick one all such things, and watched lest they trouble him with matters they should have kept to themselves.

I have under my care a very impressionable young lady, who has several times given proof of the bad effect of mental worry on the course of the disease, and who has had two serious set-backs that could only be ascribed to severe disappointments in

20

the inability of a dear friend to come to her. Such impression-ability is by no means rare, and must be reckoned with. In America, our typical nervous business man, who can never drop his affairs, who takes them to bed with him at night, and thinks of them all day, is a great problem for the phthisio-therapeutist; and I congratulate the colleague who can so dominate this type of patient as to make him put his business behind him, and devote himself with all the ardour he formerly put into it to his restoration to health.

Among the worries that trouble the patient, one is very often spoken of that I do not find as serious as is often supposed after the first week or so—I refer to homesickness. While all feel it at first, the large majority become interested in their own cure and lose it entirely. In a few, especially with the Irish, I have found it severe, persistent, and troublesome, and in such cases the patient may have to go home either for a short stay or permanently. I have seen Irishmen struck by it as by some acute infection, and have seen their *morale* go entirely to pieces under it. Strange to say, I have found men much more subject to it than women, who can more quickly establish a homelike atmosphere about them than the stronger sex. If they are occupied earnestly with getting well, and not allowed aimlessly to loaf around doing nothing definite, it will not often give trouble.

Hardening the Body.—That most important detail, the hardening of the patient's body to withstand changes of weather, draughts and chilling, and to make him less sus-ceptible to catching cold, is accomplished best by the combined effects of the constant outdoor life and hydrotherapeutics.

Medicinal Treatment.—The medicinal treatment is, I believe, more and more recognised as best when it is purely symptomatic, and though at first patients seem to expect a series of prescriptions, and are disappointed if they do not get them, they soon cease to look for them, save where definite indications call for them.

Time Needed for a Cure.—The length of time that should be devoted to a hygienic and dietetic cure, cannot of course be even approximately stated. A cure will naturally be much quicker at a climatic resort than in the patient's home, but wherever it is carried out it is wise to be cautious in applying the term " case cured " rather than " process arrested " to the final note on the case.

The collection of reliable statistics on the results of phthisio-therapy would be greatly facilitated if the profession were more cautious in the use of the term cured, for while pulmonary tuberculosis is perfectly curable, a long period of observation should follow discharge before we can feel justified in regarding any case as cured, and the most minute examination by an experienced physical diagnostician should always be presupposed.

As to the time devoted to the cure, the more incipient cases will often, after a three to six months' stay, have so well learned the lessons of hygienic and sensible living that they have been taught, that they can be trusted to return to favourable country localities near their homes, there to complete, under the family physician's eye, the cure begun in the resort, whose position should in this matter resemble that of the University, which educates its students, and then sends them forth trained, to carry out by themselves their further education, and fulfil successfully their calling in life.

Of course no exact period can be set, for many patients not six months nor a year spent wisely in a health resort, under skilled supervision, will produce that absolute quiescence of the trouble which is generally spoken of as a cure, but speaking generally, I would risk the statement that as an average six months to a year in a resort, followed by two years of great care at home (and a lifetime of common sense thereafter), will generally be successful, while in our cities the time must be much prolonged.

That such a cure carried out outside a sanatorium need be

any slower or less successful than one within their precincts,
I from my experience cannot admit, but I would repeat that it
will demand much hard work on the part of the doctor, and the
ability to win his patient's confidence, and to control him, and
surely these are things that the majority of our profession have
not been wanting in.

Day's Routine.—Before closing, I would give a brief sketch
of the day's routine in an average case, treated according to this
plan. An hour before rising the servant closes the windows,
and in winter lights the fire, that the room may be comfortably
warm by rising time. The room being warmed to about 55 or
65 degrees, the patient, who, if he wakes early, has previously
drunk his warm milk, takes his morning cool salt bath, lasting
but a few seconds, and after a brisk rub dresses, and where
they are in his orders, goes through his pulmonary gymnastics.
Breakfast, which, like all other meals, should be very regular,
and enlivened by conversation, being over, he goes to the
porch and his reclining chair, and this, save for a few exceptions, chiefly among the aged, whatever the weather. He
wraps himself warmly to be weather proof, and has at hand
such light literature as is allowed. Conversation with others
should be encouraged if there be no laryngitis, but symptom
talking should be prohibited. According to the case, more or
less of the morning is spent recumbent, and a regulated portion
given to exercise in specified ways, from a few minutes to an
hour or more.

During the morning, and also in the afternoon, such nourishment as has been ordered between meals is brought out and
eaten, and in cases where digestion is troublesome, a rest on
their backs or their beds, away from company, for the half hour
preceding meals is advisable. The afternoon is like the morning, but exercise when first allowed comes in the morning rather
than the afternoon hour. After supper, if there be artificial
light, the porch is again used till bed time. It is most undesirable for patients to sit all the evening in close parlours, and if

they cannot use the porch they had best sit in their own rooms, where they can have a few visitors for amusement, and where ventilation is more easily controlled. Bed is always early ; nine in winter, and ten in summer is the best hour. Before bed, such gymnastics as are ordered are gone through with. In cases where it is called for, alcohol or vinegar rubs, &c., are given, and such symptomatic remedies for cough, sweats, sleeplessness, or. the like, are taken, and the last thing before bed a glass of hot milk is drunk and the teeth cleaned to prevent mouth fer. mentation.

As the health returns more and more to the normal this regimen is gradually relaxed and fuller liberty is allowed until the patient leads an ordinary out door life, and is turned over largely to his own care of himself.

The doctor at his visit, which till the temperature is sufficiently lowered is at the patient's house, and not the office, scans the record carefully and minutely, investigates the diet, corrects errors, keeps a sharp look-out for defects in the table and housekeeping, interviewing the housekeeper if necessary, indicates any faults in the carrying out of his orders, encourages faithful attention to them, and reproves neglect, watches the patient's mental attitude and physical state, encouraging, controlling, warning or stimulating as the case may be ; and those who will try it can soon convince themselves that in this way the supervision which some claim is only to be had in sanatoria, can be most satisfactorily obtained in private practice.

If I have taken your time to-day to describe closely the way one can successfully carry out the hygienic and dietetic treatment outside of a sanatorium, and have contended that it was feasible and desirable so to treat a large number of cases, and that in no respect need the results fall behind those gotten in these institutions, I have been impelled to do so, not to belittle the splendid efforts they are making to solve this great problem, but by the belief that doctors practising outside sanatoria do not rightly appreciate the method, or think they cannot apply it in private practice, while those within them are too prone to think that there alone good results can be gotten.

If the general treatment of pulmonary tuberculosis is to improve, the general practitioner, into whose hands such cases first come, should realise that they are curable and hopeful. Hopelessness is still too much the keynote in the treatment of this trouble, and the teachings of those whose results long since disproved this have too often fallen on deaf ears.

When I recall the consumptive ward of my old hospital, the long line of beds filled with doomed mortals, the small amount of window space and sunlight, the limited quantity of fresh air and of outdoor life, I do not wonder that I then thought, as still do so many, that the treatment of consumption was the saddest and most hopeless task that ever the medical man was called on to undertake. I can still hear the dismal coughing that every night ran through the ward like a contagion, can still see the hectic in their cheeks, and the suffering in their eyes; but " times change, and we change with them," and now with the light of experience of this incomparable method, I feel that the hopelessness which overhung that ward is a thing of the past; that following in the footsteps of Bennett and Brehmer and Dettweiler, we have reached the time when to these poor mortals healing shall come, and men after having followed for ages the *ignis fatuus* of medicinal treatment, have begun to realise that in the cultivation of the " *vis medicatrix naturæ*," in the building up of the system by food and air, rest, and exercise, till it is capable of repelling the invader, lies the solution of the great tuberculosis problem, which for centuries has baffled the medical skill of the world.

If the new gospel is anything, it is a gospel of common sense and of hope; and now, with all the world aroused to the seriousness of the problem, and learning the efficacy of the remedy that has lain unnoticed at her doors so long, the day begins to dawn when this scourge of humanity, held in check in its beginning by a scientific prophylaxis, detected in its incipiency by an acute and early diagnosis, and cured in all but its most advanced cases, which through this very diagnosis will get fewer and fewer, by a rational therapeusis will cease to be the "white plague," at whose name men's faces now pale, and yearly millions will be saved to civilisation who heretofore had been doomed to hopelessness and death.

BIBLIOGRAPHY.

Weber, "Chronic Pulmonary Phthisis," Croonian Lectures. London, 1885.

Walters, "Sanatoria for Consumptives." London, 1899.

Harris and Beale, "The Treatment of Consumption." London.

Ziemssen, "The Etiology, Symptomatology and Treatment of Pulmonary Tuberculosis." Trans. from *Klinische Vortrage*, 1888.

Penzoldt, "Behandlung Tuberculose," in Penzoldt's "Stintzing Handbuch Therapie," vol. iii. Jenner, 1898.

Cornet, "Die Tuberculose ; Nothnagel's Spec. Path. und Therap., Wien, 1899.

Dettweiler, "Behandlung Lungenschwindsucht." Berlin, 1880.

Wolff, "Moderne Behandlung Lungenschwindsucht." Berlin, 1894.

Brehmer, "Die Therap. der Chr. Lungenschwind." Wiesbaden, 1887.

"Bericht über den Congress zur bekampf. der Tuberculose." Berlin, 1899.

Leon Petit, "Le Phthisique et son Traitment Hygienique." Paris, 1895.

Daremborg, "Traitment de la Phthisique Pulmon." Paris, 1893.

Chuqut, "Le Hygiene des Tuberculeux." Paris, 1899.

Bath, "Therapeutique de la Tuberculose." Paris, 1896.

Lauth, "Traitment de la Tuberc. par l'Altitude." Paris, 1896.

"Congress pour l'Etude de la Tuberc." Paris, 1899.

STATISTICAL NOTE CONCERNING THE CONTAGIOUSNESS OF TUBERCULOSIS PULMONALIS.

BY E. L. SHURLY, M.D.

DETROIT, MICH.

I INTENDED to present to you data deduced from cases coming under my personal observation in private practice during the last five years, but have been unable to do so. I will, however, offer as an apology the following facts derived from my notes of 130 adult cases, all of which have come under my observation during 1898.

In formulating the data I have been careful to exclude consideration of cases which were too imperfectly known to warrant their use as evidence. I have formulated the data under the following headings, viz., Exposure, Previous Disease, Heredity, Previous Condition, and the Presence or Absence of Tubercle Bacilli.

Under Exposure are those cases which were known to have been especially exposed.

Under Previous Disease are noted those cases whose clinical history shows the disease or diseases mentioned to have been just antecedent to the development of the pulmonary affection.

Under Heredity no note of predisposition farther back than grandparents has been considered.

Under Previous Condition, only that part of the domestic history of the patient has been considered which for a considerable period antedated the development of the disease.

The notes regarding the presence or absence of tubercle

bacilli are undoubtedly far from perfect, for in some of the cases reported as negative, tubercle bacilli were found in the sputum at a later period, and *vice versâ*.

The diagnosis of all these cases was determined from the commonly accepted signs and symptoms belonging to the clinical history of this disease—exclusive of the tuberculin test. All case notes bearing uncertain diagnostic stamp have been excluded from this category, so that the 130 cases here summarised, represent unmistakably the several conditions and forms denominated tuberculosis or phthisis pulmonalis.

Concerning exposure, the recording and presentation of any data under the head of Exposure would seem, to radically inclined minds, a work of supererogation, as such persons believe that all cases of tuberculosis pulmonalis are tuberculosis from "start to finish," and that all cases of tuberculosis necessarily arise from communicability of one sort or another by the agency of tubercle bacilli. The 130 cases upon which these remarks are based, all came under observation during the year 1898, in private practice, and certainly would seem, by their clinical history, to throw some doubt upon the truth of the specious and widespread theory just mentioned. The analysis of these (130 cases) for some unaccountable reason shows that the question of particular exposure was not recorded in 9 cases. This is to be regretted, but I may say that it is my habit always to inquire closely upon this point by direct and cross examination of not only the patient, but the patient's friends and family physician, so that it is fair to infer that these 9 patients were not especially exposed. It is recorded of the whole number (130) that 9 were particularly exposed as follows :—

CASE 24.—The patient had nursed and taken care of a sister who died of tuberculosis. Others members of the household, to the number of five are yet healthy.

CASE 43.—Patient had nursed her husband who was ill with tuberculosis for eight years. She had large lymphatic glands in the neck for years, and previous to the development of tuberculosis had acute lobar pneumonia.

CASE 47.—Patient had lost two sisters, the whole family living in the same house, three and four years respectively before the development of the pulmonary tuberculosis. This patient had also a diastolic cardiac murmur.

CASE 49.—Patient was associated more or less with a younger brother, who died four years before the development of the disease, which was preceded by chronic diarrhœa.

CASE 67.—Patient lost two sisters, aged 4 years and 18 months respectively, living in the same house. He was a commercial traveller, who was away from home a greater part of the time. His family history was bad.

CASE 77.—Patient was with a brother the greater part of the time for five weeks, and was also living in the house where the mother died a few years previously.

CASE 114.—Patient lived in the same house, and took more or less care of a brother who died four months previous to the onset of her sickness. Other members of the family were never affected, and this patient recovered.

CASE 115.—The father of the patient died six years before and the brother three months previous to the onset of the symptoms. All lived in the same house. Three of the other members of the family have not been affected.

CASE 116.—This patient two years ago roomed with a companion for six months who had first pleuritis and then pulmonary tuberculosis. Since that time (a year ago) the patient saw her companion but a few times. This patient has apparently recovered.

The following 12 cases (16, 38, 69, 71, 73, 75, 83, 93, 94, 116, 129, and 130) might through careless observation be considered as having originated from communicability or contagion, but a rigid examination of all the circumstances surrounding their origin and development will serve at once to eliminate the contagious or communicable factor in their etiology; for instance : —

CASE 16.—Was supposed without doubt to have originated

from living in a boarding-house, where two cases of tuberculosis had existed for several months, but a detailed investigation showed that this patient (16) was an intemperate sailor, and cousin of the two subjects (who were cousins also), occupying the same house, and, furthermore, that he had been treated two years previously in Chicago for severe cough, &c., which was then diagnosed as tuberculosis.

CASE 38.—Was at first supposed by the family physician and the writer to have originated from the ingestion of tuberculous milk. Indeed, it was considered a clear case until subsequent investigation showed that the cow whose milk this patient drank freely for four months was not tuberculous. It was with considerable difficulty that this fact was ascertained, because the farmer had traded her off to another farmer, who, in turn, discovered that the cow was suffering from some intestinal worms. This sage granger finally administered remedies to the cow which brought about her complete recovery. I might say parenthetically that I was told, but not authoritatively, that the former suspicious condemnation of the animal rested upon the optical acumen and supposed dexterity of a young and ardent devotee of the microscope.

CASE 69.—Patient lost a father and a sister, but was not with them to any extent during her illness because a resident in another city.

CASE 71.—This patient's father was aged 71, and has had a cough for many years; undoubtedly a case of chronic bronchitis. The brother of the patient was taken sick, and died in the West, being away from home during the whole period.

CASE 73.—Patient lost several aunts and cousins, but was never associated with them to any extent.

CASE 75.—Patient lost three sisters, one four years, one two years before his illness (the family consisting of parents and two brothers, all of whom still occupy the house, and are well). This patient had a psoas abscess from injury, followed by empyema and then tuberculosis.

CASE 83.—Patient lost father, mother, and brother. The father and mother died during his early life—eighteen years ago, and a brother was taken ill and died, although in another city.

CASE 93.—Patient lost two sisters, but it was ascertained that each of these sisters was married, and had been taken sick and died in their own homes.

CASE 94.—Patient was associated more or less with a brother, who had a cough for two years. They were in the same store, and lived in the same house, but did not room together. It was found from friends of the family that both these young men were exposed during a fishing trip to very great hardship and wetting, and that both suffered from broncho-pneumonia at the same time.

CASE 129.—At the time of the record this patient had a married sister living in another city, who was said to be suffering from tuberculosis, but the patient had seldom been in her company since they had grown up. This is one of the cases in which syphilis undoubtedly played an important part in the etiology.

CASE 130.—Patient lost a sister of general tuberculosis two years before the development of her illness. This patient, however, has been at home very little, having lived with an, aunt and at a boarding-school most of the time.

Regarding previous disease, it is noted that 16 of these cases have been almost immediately preceded by acute pneumonia, 22 by influenza or *la grippe*, 12 by hemoptysis with little or no antecedent cough, 1 by appendicitis; several of them, it is noted, have had occupations which exposed them to metal, flour, or other dust; 25 have been preceded by acute or chronic laryngitis or bronchitis, 11 by pleuritis, 9 by parturition, 2 by chronic uterine disease, 2 by measles, 1 by diabetes, 7 by syphilis (secondary or tertiary), 3 by rheumatism, 3 by typhoid fever, 1 by empyema of antrum, 1 by suppurative otitis; 7 are recorded as having had large lymphatic glands; 3 were preceded by severe dyspepsia and diarrhœa, 1 by psoas abscess,

1 by remittent fever, 4 by anæmia, and 1 by physical exhaustion. In 10 cases marked intemperance in the use of alcololic liquors was noted.

Regardıng family history, 65 cases are recorded as having good or fair family history ; of the other 65 cases the parents in 31 cases were affected. In 42 cases brothers and sisters were affected, and in 58 cases some distant relative had been affected also. With regard to the previous condition of these patients long· before the development of the disease in question, it is reported that 76 were well and healthy, while 54 were noted as being delicate, never very well, &c.

Concerning the presence or absence of tubercle bacilli in these (130) cases, it is noted that the bacillus was present in 65, absent in 52 cases, and in 13 cases the result of the examination was considered doubtful. In 6 cases it is noted that no particular disease immediately preceded the development of pulmonary disorder. In 20 cases 2 or 3 co-existing diseased conditions are recorded.

In conclusion, allow me to state that I am not unconscious of the relative inaccuracy which usually belongs to statistical knowledge, but in presenting this fragment, which I hope to be soon able to multiply, I feel confident of having in a reasonable measure avoided bias and error. If this be so, then we have presented by this series of data the following facts, that of 121 cases (eliminating the 9 doubtful ones) there is a possibility of 9 only having originated through ordinary natural communicability ; while upon further analysis there is a possibility that 5 only so originated, and further, that of the whole number (130), at least 112 were immediately preceded by some acute or subacute disease.

DISCUSSION.

Dr. CASSELBERRY : Single instances, of course, count for but little, but this one was so convincing to me that I will relate it. A man of powerful physique, six feet or more in height, and weighing over 190 lbs., applied for examination and stated that he believed he had tuberculosis. My first impulse was to laugh him out of it, but an examination showed that it was only too true. He said he and his wife lived on a farm in North Dakota, several miles from any other habitation, and he had always been in good health until recently. Two years before they had taken into the household a niece who came from the East with advanced tuberculosis, and she died there about one year ago. They had all lived in the same room, and no care had been taken in regard to disposal of sputum. The disease steadily developed in the man and he died within two years thereafter.

The PRESIDENT : I think, none of us can doubt the possibility of the communicable nature of tuberculosis. It is only a question of how often it occurs and of the many cases in which tuberculosis develops with the history of some antecedent disease. It is a question whether they are not inoculations in some manner that possibly could not be traced, because we are all disposed to the disease every day of our lives.

Dr. FISK : Those of us who practise in Colorado often come across men who work in the mines, free from any apparent contagion, who die of rapid acute tuberculosis ; and I wish to remind you that Dr. Conan Doyle has called attention to the fact that when a man falls below par morally he is likely to be carried off by drink, and when he falls below par physically he is apt to be carried off by tuberculosis. They are the scavengers of mankind.

Dr. SHURLY : We have not the time now to take up the discussion of immunity. My principle object in bringing this paper forward was to awaken the gentlemen who are better posted and have had a larger experience than I have, to an all-round consideration of this important question. Of course we cannot doubt that there are cases that arise in some way through personal communication, but to make the wholesale statement that all cases arise in that way is begging the question and refusing the light of experience ! It would be absurd if you saw a man with a burned finger to say that he burned it by ignited gas and to insist upon it, when he might have burned it in any one of a number of other ways. It is going too far against our clinical experience to assert that this disease is contagious and communicable in the same way as small-pox, or diphtheria, or other such infectious diseases.

One reason why I seem to speak so feelingly is because I have been engaged in a controversy over this question with the Michigan State Board of Health. The Secretary of our State Board, a very worthy member of this Society, is thoroughly convinced that the disease is very contagious, " worse than a wild tiger running loose in the streets," so to speak. Believing this, he is tempted to coerce the profession of our State into the support of that position. I would like to see the profession of the United States decide whether this contagious belief is based upon fact or upon theoretical generalisations. Although I am considered somewhat of a heretic on this question, it is not from choice I assure you. I am willing to say that a certain disease arises from the tubercle bacillus, but I would like to know where that bacillus comes from.

THE INFLUENCE OF CLIMATE UPON NERVOUS DISEASES, CONSIDERED FROM A PHYSIOLOGICAL STANDPOINT.

BY F. SAVARY PEARCE, M.D.

PHILADELPHIA.

THAT a more accurate understanding of the effect of meteorological conditions in a given place and at different altitudes is needed, since these do most positively affect the human economy, however difficult of determination is their mode of action, every physiologist and scientific physician realises. The effect of continued sameness of atmospheric pressure, moisture, winds, and of the chemical products carried in the air, becomes a more or less natural condition in the environment of the individual living in a particular locality. Thus, through continued ages, the different races are undoubtedly modified, mentally, morally, and physically, by the climate in which they reside, so that the effects of environment on a particular race are much regulated by climatic conditions, *e.g.*, the stunted people upon the plateau of Thibet and our robust Western cow-boy living in the lower open plains. Thus conditions of stature and the proportional brain power, associated with physical strength and agility, are important facts in the evolution of high types, so that the happy mean between the extremes of dwarfism and giantism, always abnormal states, is left for our sifting to determine, if possible, the scientific relation of the individual to his environment in health or disease. We contend that it is just here, where failure to inter-

pret the cause and the result resident in climatological condi_
tions of the earth, must be got through a study of a large
number of racial and individual statistics. Not until such
extended observations *are* made, will the study of climatology
be truly of scientific benefit to mankind.

It shall be the endeavour in this paper to collate the physiological and physical effects known to exist, or to result respectively from certain diseases of the nervous system, which we
shall urge as a basis for study. And, even back of this, the
whole process of modification of the nervous system through
climatological influences must, it seems to me, be placed upon
a nutritional basis, therefore, as to the effect upon blood
pressure allowing more or less healthy circulation, to the carrying off of waste products through the proper metabolism of the
nerve centres, and, finally, to the elimination of waste products
in proper amount, so that there should be no imbalance whatever in the healthy organism.

The effects of decreased atmospheric pressure permitting a
freer circulation in the surface of the body is, to my mind, an
important physiological and physical fact for us to use as a
basis for studying the effects of altitude upon disease, knowing
the pathological nature of the malady (as tabes); secondly, the
effect of placing the body in a vacuum jar under decreased atmospheric pressure produces the same results, in a measure, as
those experienced in the ascent of a mountain; and thirdly, the
beneficial influence of massage in hurrying the blood stream
to the surface, which therefore produces better nutrition, as
shown by experiments of Mitchell—these are all three important observations, which lead to the same conclusion,
namely, that reduced atmospheric pressure causing a *vis a
fronte*, as it were, is similar in its results upon the human body
to the *vis a tergo* produced by the manipulator during massage.

In the *Archives des sciences physiques et naturelles* for
December, 1900, M. Jaquet takes a different view of the effects
of altitude upon nutrition, and concludes that the chief, if not

the only, factor in the action of altitudes, is diminution of pressure, which acts by chemical modification of the blood. He says that the temperature is without evident effect upon the blood, and that light plays no more active part. This author contends that the diminution of pressure obtained through laboratory experimentation in placing the body under lessened atmospheric pressure, is *exactly* similar in results to that in the case of a person ascending a high mountain. His contention is that more nitrogen is admitted to the blood through the atmosphere under such lowered atmospheric pressure. The writer, while admitting this, feels perfectly sure that nutrition is also bettered by the fact that the nitrogen of the proteid foods already existing in the blood is given freer circulation to the periphery of the body, and that thereby better nutrition is transmitted to the tissues ; so that, probably, we have therefore a double mode of chemical action in regard to the same element, nitrogen : First, that coming in excess from the atmosphere at lowered pressure ; secondly, the freer circulation, as indicated, of the nitrogen produced from within. We also feel certain, from clinical experience at least, that purity of the air and the intenser sunlight of the heights do much to improve bodily metabolism, and are, therefore, active adjutants. The effect of winds alone seems to me to act in the following fashion : not from any chemical change produced in the body, but by reflex action upon the peripheral nervous system causing increased excitability of the general bodily functions.

Hence in *neurasthenia*, where we have a typical condition of irritable weakness prevailing, high winds are to be avoided, and altitudes above 2,000 feet should be eschewed, for the reason that we hasten metabolic processes too rapidly by such means, and therefore tend to the physiological overwork of the central nervous system. This is also witnessed to by the palpitation of the heart occurring in nervous or well people at heights, and due, undoubtedly, to the lessened peripheral pressure. I have considered elsewhere the effects of climat-

21

ology on neurasthenia, concerning which the foregoing paragraph is now given in possible explanation of the facts recorded in that paper.*

Hysterical subjects will generally be found to do badly at great altitudes, for the same reason of increased excitability caused by over activity in the superficial circulation; and insomnia in them will be more pronounced at heights, due, perhaps, to the increased vigour of circulation in the membranes of the brain† (vaso-motor tone). Climates in which there is continual prevalence of fogs, with low atmospheric pressure, are also bad for the neurasthenic and hysterical, for the same reason of reduced pressure, as well as of the psychic depression upon the individual and the liability to "catching cold" in this moist atmosphere.

Melancholia, on the other hand, needs great increase of circulation and metabolism to effect proper functioning of the body in the carrying to and from the tissues products for assimilation, and in a better combustion of by-products, with an equally free elimination of the waste matter of catabolism. I have seen subjects of melancholia greatly improved by going to the mountains, where the climatic conditions were not different from those of lowlands, other than in obtaining reduced atmospheric pressure, in the purer air, and in the intenser sunlight—a trio of meteorological states, active, to my mind, in the order given. High winds will be stimulating to the melancholic or to the hypochondriacal patient, and will tend to benefit him; so also with the graver forms of insanity of these types. It may not be expecting too much to hope that, some day, municipal aid will be given to sanatoria where the subjects of exaltation of the mental aberration may be sent to lesser altitudes for benefit; and those with excitation of the depressive emotions may be sent to altitudes perhaps several thousand feet above sea-level.

* "Climatology of Neurasthenia," *Medical News*, January 26, 1901.
† *Philadelphia Medical Journal*, May 25, 1901.

Chorea is a disease most surely made worse by high winds and increase of altitude beyond a happy mean of a few hundred feet, and is ill affected for the reason already given. Thus, while the freer interchange of nitrogen gas from the atmosphere to the blood is desirable in many cases in internal medicine, as in phthisis, still, as pointed out in this paper, among *nervous* diseases, where the central nervous system is at fault, we do have types of cases in which it is better to be conservative in the use of this very valuable chemical element for the proper nutrition of the body.

Insomnia.—I wish to lay special stress on that annoying symptom, insomnia, as influenced by circulation, besides the neurone motility theory, which would also account for sleeplessness. If we consider that the dendrites are in particular activity in such cases, we must still, it seems to me, go back to the old theory of hyperæmia being the original etiological factor in any case, and this would also uphold the neuronic theory, since excess of blood would tend to greater tonicity of the neurones, and thus a retraction of the protoplasmic mass such as is necessitated for the production of sleep would not so readily occur. That palsy of the vaso-motor system is the fundamental condition permitting persisting insomnia, we must admit. So that whatever will tend to restore vaso-motor tone to the sympathetic nervous system must be good treatment for sleeplessness. The effect of the warm bath given at night will be explained, as to its action for good in insomnia, by the fact that the blood-vessels of the extremities are thus dilated, permitting of a better equalisation of blood pressure and of relief to the congested meninges ; so, too, the other hydrotherapeutic procedure of the cold douche to the spine in the morning, which produces reaction to the nervous system, favours an equilibration of circulation. The use of massage is also well known to influence insomnia favourably. If these measures, together with a reasonable use of the milder hypnotic drugs, do not avail, my experience has been that of a change of scene, and particularly of latitude and altitude, will be the paramount measure for affording relief to the sufferer.

There is nothing better than the quiet *ensemble* of a sea voyage in these cases, not a little of the benefit of which arises from the soothing effect of the salt air, as well as from its influence upon metabolism; and, finally, from the low level and consequent great atmospheric pressure, which tends to prevent the circulation in the periphery of the body, and consequently in the great sinuses of the brain. If the patient is at the sea-shore, the ill effects of high winds from week to week have been made evident by my own cases, in which previous benefit had resulted from this descent from the mountainous country. This is shown in the instance of B. H., a man, aged 57 years, from the interior of Pennsylvania, who improved as to the insomnia immediately upon his return from Atlantic City, in April, 1901, where high winds were prevailing. This man immediately began to rest well at night on returning to Philadelphia. There was no psychic element in the case as to this symptom, I should declare, because of the fact that the patient persisted in going to the shore for a week, and was not at all fond of the Quaker City.

In an experience with *idiopathic epilepsy*, I have found that patients living at a great altitude are very apt to be benefited by coming to the sea-level; a patient under my own care, a young woman from the mountain district of Luzerne county, Pa., it occurs to me, was helped in the reduction of her attacks by coming to Philadelphia; taking into account, also, the benefit frequently occurring by mere change alone, in this enigmatic disease.

Organic Diseases of the Nervous System.—In these affections we cannot hope for great benefit from any climatic conditions in the alleviation of the pathological state, but the insidious action of a properly maintained circulation in these disabled individuals must have great weight in favourably affecting, or not, the underlying organic change. Many of the harassing symptoms, as the pain of tabes, for example, are frequently, to my mind, due to the impeded circulation about the sensory tracts or nerve roots. This can be in some measure helped in other ways than by the mechanical means at our disposal, *e.g.*, massage ; as by placing the patient in a condition of dry atmosphere, and especially where there are currents of air actively moving, and thus favouring circulation as well as influencing other reflex action by the winds stimulating the sensory nerve, and, therefore, the insensible, though ever acting, afferent impulse. The change of altitude is again important in diseases of the *central* nervous system. A case in question, one of specific disease of the cord coming under the care of Dr. S. Weir Mitchell, which I had the opportunity to study and report, was greatly benefited, as to pain paroxysms, by passing to an altitude of 6,000 feet, whither the patient went as a ranchman in the far West, from the low damp country of southern California. An ataxic patient of my own I have seen benefited by a sojourn in the mountains in Colorado, the particular relief being to his pain and in the general upbuilding of the system, due, I take it, to a hastening of the peripheral circulation, since his cardiac action was always weak, and drugs given to stimulate the heart invariably produced præcordial distress, while nitroglycerine caused an annoying cyanosis.

In *chronic peripheral neuritis*, the patient does better in a dry climate with little or no wind, and at a lesser altitude, where the tendency would be to favour the blood current towards the interior of the body.

In a general way, then, it may be said, we know very little about the effect of climate upon organic changes in the nervous system; but, reasoning by analogy, it would seem that the foregoing statements might be correct, from a physical and physiological point of view, as to conditions tending toward possible betterment, at least, of some of the symptoms. I propose to make record of cases in future, particularly as to this whole subject, feeling amply repaid for the meagre personal observation which it has been my privilege to note. Erythromelalgia would be a typical example to my mind, as would Raynaud's disease, and also conditions of morbid blushing, where a great altitude would be distinctly harmful to the patient. In fact, I have seen an instance of the latter distressing malady in a case treated electrically for Dr. John H. Musser, in which the man was made distinctly worse by a trip to the inland country of New Brunswick.

CONCLUSIONS.

The influence of climate upon nervous disease is the open sesame for fruitful study. Functional diseases are more particularly affected by climate. Organic diseases, it will no doubt be found, are especially influenced by meteorological conditions as yet not definitely-known to the physician, but in each type, the few gleanings of clinical facts at our command seem to place the said therapeutic climatic results as principally dependent on states of atmospheric pressure and the consequent nutritional improvement produced thereby. The great altitudes favour circulation of the blood in the periphery of the body, and assist nutrition, both by aiding the absorption of nitrogen from the air at low barometric pressure, and also by producing a much more active circulation of the blood, and therefore of its proteids containing nitrogen received from food products of digestion, thus doubly fortifying nutrition in some cases, as neurasthenia; therefore the trophic function may advance too rapidly by the patient's ascending great heights. So that a great altitude is not good for the neurasthenic, who must appropriate nutriments slowly on account of the weakened central nervous system. Insomnia is benefited by lesser altitudes, while chorea, hysteria, and most of the functional maladies, are likewise favoured by a sojourn at the sea-level, provided other meteorological conditions are good, such as equable temperature, heat, and the non-prevalence of atmospheric moisture. Melancholia and depressive diseases are helped by high winds with moderate heat, to aid in general bodily metabolism. In organic disease depending upon central or peripheral lesion, perverted function, as pain and sluggish circulation, will be helped by altitude ; a greater altitude being desirable for diseases of the central nervous system, a lesser altitude being the desideratum in the cases of peripheral diseases, as in neuritis and vaso-motor palsies, exemplified in Raynaud's disease, exophthalmic goitre, and allied affections.

DISCUSSION.

Dr. NEWTON : I have been greatly interested in this paper. I spent a few years myself on the plains and in the foot hills of the Rocky Mounta ins and know from experience that a great deal of what the doctor has said is true. These nervous patients, as a rule, bear the changes of climate better than you would expect, and yet at the same time, when a nervous patient undergoes a sudden change of climate, the result is necessarily more or less an unknown factor. Personally I have never been able to foretell what a certain climate would do for a nervous patient.

Dr. CAMPBELL : I think perhaps the circulation has much to do with the relief of many nervous troubles, and that the relief comes from the diminished barometric pressure, while the permanently good results come from the improved nutrition incident to life at an altitude so high, the sunshine, &c.

Dr. PHILLIPS : I understood Dr. Pearce to say that he considered reduced barometric pressure as favourable to increased metabolism. In this connection I recall some experiments reported by Professor Benecke, in which he endeavoured to find the rate at which a body lost heat. He took a closed flask filled with warm water and covered with cloth, and exposed it on the seashore, and noted the time the temperature required to fall a certain number of degrees He exposed similar flasks at several inland places and, if I remember correctly, one place was 6,000 ft. above the sea level, and he found in all his experiments that the water lost its temperature more rapidly at sea level than at the higher points. He came to the conclusion that inasmuch as rapid loss of heat must be met by rapid production, metabolism must therefore be more active at sea level.

Dr. PEARCE : I do not know whether these experiments would be exactly similar in human beings, but it seems to me the improvement in nervous patients going to higher altitudes is largely due to the effect upon the circulation, and this favours metabolism in a general way.

A REPORT OF THE LARGEST RECORDED ANEURYSM OF THE HEART, WITH SPECIMEN.

BY ROLAND G. CURTIN, M.D.
PHILADELPHIA.

CARDIAC aneurysms, although in themselves of little clinical importance, nevertheless, on-account of their rarity, are always interesting, and for that reason it is my desire to report the following case. I believe it to be unique, in that a careful search through medical literature has failed to reveal any instance in which the aneurysmal sac reached the tremendous proportions of this one.

Two years before the patient came under my charge, he was admitted to the Philadelphia Hospital with general dropsical symptoms. He was under my observation for two years. During this time, and one year before his death, Dr. Pepper decided that he had a left pleural effusion, and introduced an aspirating needle, drawing off 235 cc. of pure blood, which rapidly coagulated. The case was reported by Dr. Pepper as one of hemothorax. No unpleasant symptoms followed the operation.

When the patient came under my care the whole of the left anterior chest, nearly to the axilla and clavicle, was pulsating and heaving with each beat of the heart. To the left of the sternum, at the junction of the fourth and fifth ribs, there was a circumscribed, more markedly pulsating area. He had attacks of dyspnea on slight exertion, or when under excitement, for two years before death, associated with a cyanosed condition of the skin, particularly about the face. He was also dyspneic when the atmosphere was heavy.

PLATE I.

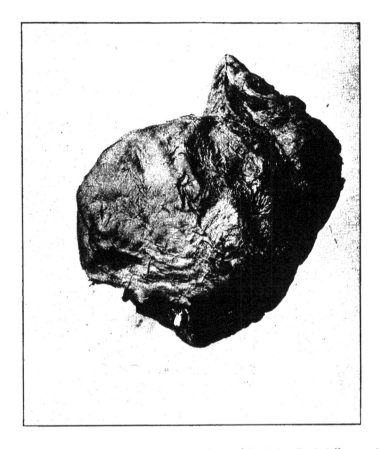

Posterior view of heart showing aneurysmal sac distended. Dotted line marks
boundary between left and right ventricles.

About two months before death, the anasarca, which had disappeared two years before, returned, with increased dyspnea. During the last two years of his life, his radial arteries had undergone rapid degenerative changes, so that at the time of his death these vessels were like a string of beads, from their atheromatous condition. During the last few months that he lived he became weaker and weaker, and death was looked for two days before it occurred. He died rather suddenly, apparently from apnea. At the time of death his face was greatly swollen.

Physical examination.—On inspection, a slow, outward wave towards the left was observed, which went far out beyond the left nipple, and high up near the left clavicle.

Palpation showed that this heaving, wavy impulse extended as far out as the midaxillary line, and at times beyond it. On percussion, the left side of the chest was found to be flat over its entire surface.

Auscultation showed an absence of all breath or voice sounds. On applying the ear to the chest to the left of the sternum at the fifth interspace, a long, rather soft, systolic murmur was heard, followed by a long, soft, whiffy sound, which corresponded in time with the diastole of the heart. The two sounds together occupied nearly the whole cardiac cycle.

Post-mortem examination.—The following notes were taken at the time of death, when the *post-mortem* examination was made :—

" The *left lung* was compressed to about one-third of the size of an ordinary fist, and pushed above the position of the root of the lung, where its apex should have been. The *right lung* was slightly compressed, as the heart encroached upon the right cavity of the chest. Here and there were emphysematous patches. The pleural cavities contained no effusions or adhesions, and were healthy.

" The *heart* itself was hypertrophied, particularly the left ventricle. The aortic valves were slightly thickened and stiff. The mitral valve and the pulmonary valves were healthy.

"Springing from the left ventricle was a very large aneurysmal sac, which was in close contact with the left side of the chest. The pericardium was thickened, and quite intimately adherent to the heart and the aneurysmal sac, but they could be separated by the occasional use of the knife. The mediastinal pleuræ were everywhere incorporated with the pericardium. Near the base of the heart, the pleura contained soft, yellow lymph, evidently the result of a recent inflammation.

"The aneurysmal sac formed the apex of the mass; its walls were about 0·3 cm. thick, and were composed of a dense, light, fibrous material, appearing to the naked eye to be made up of widely separated muscle-fibres, demonstrable after the pericardium was removed.

"When the sac was opened, it was found to contain a large amount of blood. In its lower part, and half way up its sides, it was coated with laminated clots, about 2 cm. in thickness. After the removal of the black, clotted blood, the cavity was filled with water. Upon weighing, its weight was found to be 2,850 grammes. On emptying the sac and re-weighing it, the weight was found to be 1,370 grammes less. As a cubic centimetre of water weighs a gramme, it will be seen that the cavity had a capacity of 1,370 cc., or nearly a litre and a-half (44 oz., or nearly 3 pts.).

"Two holes, communicating with the left ventricle, were discovered. They were about the size of a large quill. The apertures were about 1·25 cm. apart, and seemed to be located in a white substance, which was undergoing atheromatous change.

"The inside of the sac was here and there covered with plates of atheroma. In some places calcareous degeneration had taken place. Spicules of this material appeared in the incision, and at one place in the left side of the sac a hard plate gave forth a sharp click when struck with a knife.

PLATE II.

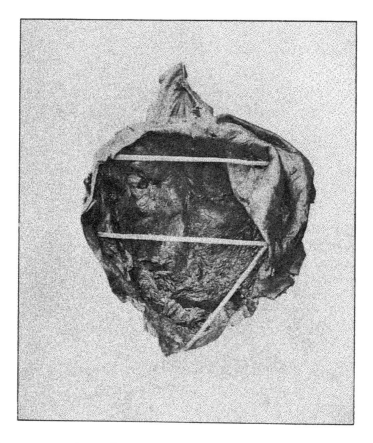

Shows aneurysmal sac laid open. Floor of sac formed by left ventricular wall 2·5 cm. thick. Capacity of sac 1,370 cc., length 15 cm., breadth 13·75 cm., depth 16·25 cm.

" The *liver* was contracted, indurated, and congested. Its edges were contracted and rounded. To the right of the transverse fissure was a white spot, depressed, and looking like a cicatrix, probably an old infarction.

" The *spleen* was small, blue, and firm.

" The *kidneys* were congested, slightly contracted, and a little granular. The capsule was quite firmly adherent. There was no erosion of the vertebræ."

Realising that the above notes, made many years ago, did not adequately describe the minute points of interest in this specimen, I asked Dr. David Riesman, an expert pathologist of Philadelphia, for a more systematic description of it, and he has most kindly furnished me with the following dictation:—

" *May* 26, 1901.—The specimen before us is that of a heart which has been kept in alcohol for nineteen years. The organ is very much enlarged toward the left side, on account of hypertrophy of the left ventricular wall, and the pressure of a large aneurysmal sac springing from the left ventricle.

" The *chamber of the left ventricle* is about normal in size, but its wall is greatly thickened; in the preserved specimen it measures more than 2·5 cm. in thickness.

" The *columnæ carneæ* are well marked, and the papillary muscles very thick and strong. The mitral valve, in its anterior leaflet, presents a small sclerotic patch; it is, however, perfectly pliable. The posterior leaflet is normal.

" The *tricuspid orifice* admits three fingers.

" The *aortic valve* presents nothing abnormal, except that on one leaflet, at its insertion into the aorta, there is a small, elevated ridge of atheroma on the ventricular surface.

" The *aorta* is of normal calibre, and has, scattered through it, a few calcified plates.

" The *coronary openings* are patulous, although one is rather small.

" In a somewhat funnel-shaped recess, situated between the two sets of papillary muscles of the posterior mitral leaflets, are two oval openings connecting the aneurysm with the ventricular cavity. One opening has its long axis transversely, and measures about 1 cm. in length, and 0·3 cm. in width; the second is of about the same dimensions as the first.

" The margins of both openings are smooth, and, so far as can be determined at the present time, have a glistening, fibroid appearance. This is particularly true of the inner opening. On the ventricular surface, these openings are separated by a bridge of tissue, 0·6 cm. wide, and 1 cm. long. On the aneurysmal surface the openings are large, somewhat funnel-shaped, and surrounded by fibrous tissue, slightly puckered.

" The outer opening is undermined, and communicates with the ventricle by a third perforation, opening about 0·8 cm. to the outer side of the median line, in a recess formed between the corresponding papillary muscles belonging to the anterior and posterior mitral leaflets. This opening on the ventricular surface is oval, with its long diameter vertical to the wall of the ventricle, and measures 1 by 0·3 cm. There are thus three openings on the ventricular surface, and two on the aneurysmal. They are all situated about 3·75 cm. from the auriculo-ventricular ring.

" The aneurysm itself is the size of a child's head, and springs from a point almost opposite the ventricular septum. It has thick, tough, fibrous walls, that can be separated into at least three layers.

" When not covered by clot, the internal surface is quite smooth and glistening. There are thick, laminated clots at the bottom of the sac, around its attachment to the ventricle, particularly at a point corresponding with the apex of the ventricle. The sac has been incised by a long, vertical cut, and shows no point of rupture. There are some signs of old adhesions on the external surface, especially at the base of the attachment of the sac to the wall of the heart. At its base, the sac measures 15 cm. vertically, and 13·75 cm. transversely, while from the ventricular wall externally, to the inner wall of the sac, the distance is 16·25 cm.

" To the outside of the openings is a crescentic, projecting ridge, forming a little niche about 2·5 cm. deep, and 5 cm. high. This ridge is continued below as a low elevation, for a distance of 5 cm., to a point 2·5 cm. below the openings.

" The *chamber of the right ventricle* is not enlarged. The wall is slightly thick, and measures about 1 cm. in diameter.

" The *right auricle* presents nothing abnormal.

" The *pulmonary* and *tricuspid valves* are normal.

" The *foramen ovale* is closed.

" The *left auricle* is normal.

" As the heart is now, it having been somewhat flattened in the jar, it would appear that the apex was in a large degree constituted by aneurysm."

There are three points of interest in this case :—

(1) So far as I am able to learn, it is the largest aneurysm of the heart that has ever been recorded.

(2) The patient lived for years, not only with greatly diminished breathing capacity, but also with a severe complicating cardiac condition.

(3) The removal of 235 cc. of blood, to accomplish which must have caused a break in the continuity of the aneurysmal walls, failed to produce any symptoms whatever.

REPORT OF A CASE OF INTERVENTRICULAR ANEURYSM OPENING INTO THE RIGHT VENTRICLE BY ULCERATIVE PROCESS; AND ANEURYSM OF THE ABDOMINAL AORTA; WITH AUTOPSY.

BY ROLAND G. CURTIN, M.D.

PHILADELPHIA.

History. January 9, 1885.—"M. D., aged 53, single; white; born in Ireland; came to America when 3 years old.

"*Family History.*—Mother and father died of old age. Has had three brothers and one sister. One brother died of typhoid fever, one was shot during the War of the Rebellion, and the third died of an unknown cause. The sister is alive and well.

"*Past Medical History.*—Has used whisky and beer to excess, and tobacco moderately, all his life. Has always had fairly good health. Had measles when a child, and chills and fever six years ago. Has never had rheumatism.

"In 1865 he had a primary sore, which made its appearance about nine days after exposure, and was followed by no secondary symptoms. Five years ago he had a severe fall from a horse. He first noticed palpitation of the heart and shortness of breath three years ago, but considered himself perfectly well, except for some precordial pain, until March, 1884. At that time he was seized with an attack in which he became very faint, fell down unconscious, and remained so for several minutes. On attempting to get up, some three hours later, he found himself still very weak. He did not have another attack until March, 1885. This attack lasted about an hour, with a period of unconsciousness of probably ten minutes. At this time he vomited, but on no occasion did he expectorate any blood.

" Since the date just mentioned, he had a number of attacks, which seemed to be becoming more frequent, although they were apparently not more severe than at first.

"*Physical Examination* shows that the precordia is prominent and bulging. There is a very apparent area of pulsation, 5 cm. in diameter, in the third interspace, between the mammary line and the left border of the sternum. The apex beat is visible within the nipple line, and extends over an area which would correspond to a circle with a diameter of 3·75 cm.

" Over the pulsating region, as above given, is heard a systolic murmur, most intense over and above the second costal cartilage, at a point midway between the nipple line and the left border of the sternum. Palpation shows that there is also present a marked thrill.

" The murmur is transmitted over the entire precordia, and into the great vessels of the neck. It is also heard in the left interscapular and axillary spaces, and at the angle of the scapula on the same side. Over its seat of maximum intensity, this murmur can be heard with the ear removed from the chest.

" The patient also complains of a sharp pain shooting through to the back, which, from the murmur also present here, probably has its origin in the abdominal aorta."

NOTE, NOVEMBER 20, 1885.

" The patient is now suffering from one of his attacks. He feels faint, and his whole body vibrates with each systole of the heart. The pulse is 136, gaseous, small, and feeble. He states that at the beginning and close of his attacks his eyesight fails, and his eyeballs become more prominent."

NOTE, DECEMBER 3, 1885.

"Posteriorly, the point where the murmur is heard with greatest intensity is on the left side, opposite to, and 5 cm. to the left of, the second dorsal vertebra. It is transmitted 5 cm. farther to the left, gradually growing fainter, but being still audible at the point of the shoulder. Anteriorly, the murmur is most intense in the second intercostal space, 2·5 cm. to the left of the sternum, where it may be heard with the ear 5 cm. from the chest.

"Associated with this murmur there is an area of dulness, over which may be felt a thrill, extending from 2·5 cm. below the clavicle to the lower border of the third rib, and from the right edge of the sternum to a point just in front of the anterior border of the left axilla. With the palm of the hand placed upon this area, the left arm extended, and used as a stethoscope, the murmur may be heard by another placing his ear at the left elbow joint."

AUTOPSY, MARCH 26, 1886.

All notes made at autopsy, and not directly bearing upon the physical signs, are omitted.

"Left thorax, prominent up to the upper border of the second rib, extending over the entire heart region. Pericardial sac bulging. Precordial space full, and entirely uncovered by lung. Thoracic aorta slightly dilated; there is a small, saccular dilatation above its origin anteriorly, capable of admitting a small chestnut. Inner surface roughened, with some calcified plates on the arch.

"*Heart.*—Left auricle much dilated; mitral orifice dilated, admitting more than three fingers. Valves slightly thickened.

"On opening the right ventricle, an aneurysm of the undefended portion of the interventricular septum is found bulging into the right ventricle, into which it opens through a small orifice, probably the result of an old ulceration. This aneurysm is large enough to contain a good-sized walnut.

"The right auricle is also dilated.

"The liver and kidneys show considerable passive congestion.

"The abdominal aorta is much thinned at its commencement, and throughout its entire length is the seat of extensive atheromatous changes. Extending from the diaphragm to the iliac arteries, is a fusiform aneurysm filled with old coagula, its lumen being occupied by recent clots. There is no erosion of the vertebræ."

A CASE OF ANEMIC NECROSIS IN THE WALLS OF THE LEFT VENTRICLE, ABOVE THE APEX OF THE HEART, ASSOCIATED WITH ANGINA PECTORIS AND LOCOMOTOR ATAXIA; WITH AUTOPSY.

BY ROLAND G. CURTIN, M.D.

PHILADELPHIA.

———

THE case is that of a practising physician, aged 54, who was working hard in a country practice. Fifteen or twenty years ago, Dr. D. Hayes Agnew said that a sore on his index finger was undoubtedly a chancre. No positive evidences of secondary or tertiary syphilis were observed. He had had mild symptoms of angina pectoris for the past three or four years, which gradually grew worse, until in October, 1899, he could scarcely walk, owing to the intense suffering. He had lightning and girdle pains, and was unable to walk in the dark, and in the daylight it was necessary for him to keep his eyes upon the ground.

At the time that I examined him with Dr. Stokes, there was no abnormal pulsation of the heart; no bruit, thrill, or murmur. Both pleural cavities contained fluid. After great suffering, he died about two weeks later.

In January, 1900, Dr. Stokes reported to me that soon after I saw the patient he grew much worse. He had oppression and increased dyspnea; a violent form of Cheyne-Stokes respiration set in; the lungs became congested, and the legs were paralysed. After lingering about six days, he died in great distress.

The autopsy showed effusion in both pleural cavities, and recent adhesions on the right side.   There was heptization of the middle lobe of the right lung, and part of the lower lobe of the left, and effusion and recent adhesions in the pericardium. The inner surface of the pericardium was quite rough.   The heart was large, weighing 468 grammes, with soft, flabby muscular walls.   An organised clot was found in the right auricle.   The coronary arteries were extremely rigid, and grated under the scalpel like plaster.   In the distribution of the anterior coronary artery, near the apex, a cavity of *anemic necrosis* was found, holding about 15 cc. of a chocolate-coloured, semi-fluid substance.

The specimen illustrates how an aneurysm could result by the rupture of such a cavity into the ventricle ; or should both walls give way, causing a communication between the ventricle and the pericardial sac, a complete rupture of the heart would naturally be the result.

REPORT OF A CASE OF SPONTANEOUS RUPTURE OF THE HEART.

BY ROLAND G. CURTIN, M.D.

PHILADELPHIA.

My reason for bringing this specimen before you is to illustrate a condition that might be produced by a weakening of the ventricular walls by disease, such as is shown in the case of myomalacia of the left ventricle, which I have just reported to you. The specimen was presented to me by Dr. J. S. Baer, of Camden, N. J. He obtained it from a patient whom he had under his care. The history was as follows:—

Mrs. —, aged 65.

The *Family History* contained no points bearing upon the case.

Previous History.—She had typhoid fever some thirty years ago, otherwise she had always been well, except for periodic attacks of severe pain in the hepatic region.

Present Condition.—When first called to see the woman, she was up and about the house, attending to her domestic duties. She was moderately jaundiced, with a temperature of 102 degrees F., and complaining of severe pain and soreness in the region of the liver. The doctor ordered her to bed at once, and placed her upon appropriate treatment. In about a week she was free from pain, and the jaundice was much lesss. Having had no fever for several days, she was considered convalescent. Contrary to instructions, however, she arose, walked about the house, and sat before an open window for some time. It was cold November weather. The next morning the doctor was sent for, and found her somewhat cyanosed, with rapid respiration and pulse, severe pain in the left axillary region, and slight cough. These symptoms continued for five days, when he was again sent for in haste, and found the woman in a state of collapse, with no radial pulse. A faint heart-beat could be heard over the left breast. The face was pinched, cold, and deeply cyanosed. There had been no nausea, vomiting, or straining, but dyspnea was very marked. The patient was very restless and delirious, and complained of feeling smothered. The above symptoms of collapse came on suddenly while the patient was in bed, but in spite of their severity, she lived for more than twenty-four hours before death occurred.

The *post-mortem* record shows that, upon opening the abdominal cavity, the gall bladder was found to contain 125 small gall-stones nearly equal in size. Both pleural cavities contained large quantities of serous fluid. Hepatization of the lower lobe of the left lung was present. The vessels of the pericardium were injected. Upon opening the pericardial sac, it was found to contain a good deal of dark, fluid blood. Upon turning up the heart, the left ventricle was found to be ruptured to the extent of from 2·5 to 3·75 cm. This rent was closed by a dark blood-clot.

This, then, is the history of the case; and in it we notice several interesting and unusual points :—

(1) The woman was but 65 years old, which is rather young for an accident of this character. When we discuss the causes, it will be seen why a more advanced age than this would render the occurrence more likely.

(2) Apparently she was asleep when the rupture occurred.

(3) A period of over twenty-four hours elapsed between the time when the rupture presumably took place and the time of death. There is, I believe, a case recorded in which the symptoms came on eleven days before death, but that is a very unusual case, and is cited in all the books as being remarkable.

The reason that this patient lived so long is probably because the rupture was small, and also because she was in a quiescent state; only a small quantity of blood was, therefore, allowed to escape slowly, and clot formation was thereby induced.

The autopsy notes say that this rupture was from 2·5 to 3·75 cm. long. It is now only about 2 cm. long on the outside, and inside it is much smaller than externally, but still large enough to admit the end of my finger. The shrinkage is probably due to the action of the preserving fluid used. The position of the rupture is on the posterior aspect of the outer wall of the left ventricle, which, as statistics show, is the most frequent seat of its occurrence. In Barth's series of 24 cases, every one occurred in the left ventricle. Meyer's table of 36 cases—all of which are recorded since 1870—shows that 25 were of the left ventricle, 7 of the right ventricle, and 4 of the right auricle.

Rupture of the heart is, as must be readily appreciated, a rare condition; and yet in talking to Dr. William S. Wadsworth, one of the coroner's physicians of Philadelphia, I asked him whether in his work he had discovered any cases, and he said that last spring he saw three in six months. He denied, however, that the records of the coroner's office would indicate that the condition is so common, and admitted that he had seen no other cases since he had been serving in his present capacity.

The causes of rupture of the heart may be stated in a few words; fibroid and fatty degeneration are the most common. These changes cause the muscle fibres to become tender, so that they may at any time give way under strain. Another not uncommon cause is occlusion of the coronary arteries, cutting off the blood supply, and interfering with the nutrition of the myocardium. In this way, too, the tissues are weakened, and rupture may be easily produced. Small abscesses occurring in the muscular structure may act in the same way.

It is exceedingly rare to have a rupture of the heart occur

in a person that is not exercising or straining. Generally, a person engaged in some usual or unusual muscular effort will suddenly fall and immediately die ; but, as we have seen, the rupture may occur some days before death takes place. In such cases, a positive diagnosis, although suspected, cannot be made, for, without an autopsy, it is not justifiable to say that the symptoms which might be produced by other well-known conditions were, in a given case, caused by rupture.

In the spring of 1899, Dr. Newton, of Montclair, New Jersey, presented a specimen at a meeting of the American Climatological Association held in New York City. It was taken from the body of a boy from 11 to 13 years of age. This boy was riding along on his bicycle, when he met another wheelman coming from the opposite direction. They made two or three attempts to avoid each other, but finally collided ; not, however, sufficiently hard to knock either rider from his wheel, and there was no rebounding. The boy dismounted, stood up for a moment, and then dropped dead. Dr. Newton made the autopsy, and found, in the middle of the ventricle, a small aperture, very like this one which I have shown you to-day. It looked as if a small piece had been torn up. There was no ulceration, fatty degeneration, or thickening of the wall ; and that the boy should have been killed by such an insignificant blow, seems very strange.

In the average college football match, there is not a participant who has not more force applied to his chest than this boy had ; and yet such an accident has never been known to occur on the football field. The most reasonable supposition is that the active exercise of bicycle riding had caused his heart to beat very fast, and that the handle-bar of his wheel struck his chest over the heart while the latter was in diastole.

The situation of the tear was, as in my case, in the wall of the left ventricle. Traumatic ruptures do not, however, occur in this locality with the same frequency as they do in spontaneous cases. Gamgee's figures on twenty-eight cases, in twenty-two of which the exact location of the lesion is specified, show that the right ventricle was ruptured in eight, the left in three, the left auricle in seven, and the right in four. Packard has reported a traumatic case which involved both auricles and the interauricular septum. From these figures it would appear that the left ventricle is the least liable to be affected in traumatic cases, while in spontaneous cases the left ventricle is almost invariably the one in which the rupture is to be found.

DISCUSSION.

Dr. ELSNER : In this connection I have an interesting experience to report. A man, aged 60, was suddenly seized with cardiac dyspnea and syncope. The pallor was alarming ; the pulse weak, thready, and rapid ; heart sounds distant, embryonic, almost inaudible. Stimulants restored the patient, but ten days later he died suddenly. The *post mortem* showed a degenerated heart-muscle with a rupture of the left ventricle—button-hole shaped. The first attack was shown to have been due to a partial rupture of the heart, the remnants of which were still visible in torn muscular fibres, holding a blood-clot which was held under the visceral pericardium. The coronary arteries, in fact the entire arterial system, were far advanced in sclerosis.

CAUSE OF DEATH IN ANEURYSMS OF THE THORACIC AORTA WHICH DO NOT RUPTURE. REPORT OF FIVE CASES.

BY HORACE D. ARNOLD.

BOSTON.

SUDDEN death from rupture of the sac of an aneurysm of the aorta is such a tragic event that it dominates our whole conception of the disease and the prognosis. Little is said in the text-books about the other ways in which these aneurysms may cause death, and even in some special works this topic receives scant attention. The prognosis is so generally considered to be fatal, that at the autopsy the discovery of the mere existence of an aneurysm is too often accepted as an adequate explanation of the death, without any careful investigation as to the way in which this result was brought about. The object of this paper is to show that the investigation of the cause of death in such cases is not without interest.

Owing to the frequency with which incomplete examinations have been made in cases of unruptured thoracic aneurysm, statistics based on such observations are far from satisfactory. The writer soon gave up as unprofitable the task of tabulating individual cases with reference to this point.

Hare and Holder* have collected from medical literature 953 cases of aneurysm of the arch of the aorta. This very valuable piece of work gives us better information on the point in question than any other collection of statistics that I have found. That it is not entirely satisfactory, is evidently due to the imperfection of the reports of cases on which it is based, and not to any lack of care in the collation of statistics.

Among their conclusions, these writers make the observation† "that in a large proportion of cases death did not ensue from rupture, but from pressure by the growth." In another place they say‡: "Death occurs as a result of aneurysm of the aorta, either from rupture of the aneurysmal sac, from pressure of the sac upon important nerves and blood-vessels, or from the secondary changes which take place in these tissues, and in other vital organs as a direct or indirect result of such pressure."

From various data in their article I have made the following tabulation of the number of cases in which it was stated that death occurred without rupture.

					Unruptured.	Per cent.
Ascending arch	...	..	...	570	... 93 =	16
Transverse arch	..	...	...	104	... 20 =	19
Descending arch	...	...	...	110	... 17 =	15
Unclassified	...	...	...	169	... 24 =	14
		Total		953	... 154 =	16

I have also made a tabulation of the cases in which rupture is definitely stated to have occurred.

					Ruptured.	Per cent.
Ascending arch	..	...	...	570	... 339 =	60
Transverse arch	...	...	...	104	... 39 =	38
Descending arch	...	...	...	110	... 72 =	66
Unclassified	...	...	...	169	... 74 =	44
		Total		953	... 524 =	55

Rupture of the aneurysmal sac caused death in 55 per cent. of this series, while in at least 16 per cent. of the cases death came without rupture. We are left uninformed of the cause of death in 29 per cent. It is useless to speculate as to what proportion of this 29 per cent. may have died without rupture, but we get from the following statistics a suggestion that it is not unreasonable to suppose that in a large majority of them rupture did not occur.

Browne,§ in a series of 173 cases, found that only 84, or

49 per cent. were due to rupture, a smaller percentage than that among the cases reported by Hare and Holder.

Sibson‖ made an analysis of 584 reported cases of aortic aneurysm, and of 296 museum specimens. Of the total number of 880 cases, 703 were instances of aneurysm of the thoracic aorta. Of these latter, 358 ruptured, or 51 per cent It is not explicitly stated that the other 49 per cent. did not rupture. However, in the two classes of aneurysm in which Sibson tabulated all the observations in detail (those of the sinuses of Valsalva, and those of the ascending arch), it is shown that with one or two exceptions, it was known that the balance of the cases did not rupture. If we may assume that the rest of the cases were divided with equal care, then we may assume that nearly 49 per cent. of these 703 cases did not rupture.

At first, with the prevalent ideas in mind about the frequency of rupture of a thoracic aneurysm, it is a little startling to learn that this is the cause of death in only about half of the cases. Yet this must be so, otherwise we cannot understand how in three large series of cases, reported by such able observers, the results arrived at independently should so nearly coincide.

				ases.		uptured.		Per cent.
Hare and Holder	...	...		953	...	524	=	55
Sibson	...	...	...	703	...	358	=	51
Browne	...	...	...	173	...	84	=	49
		Total		1,829	...	966	=	53

The inference seems almost as reliable, that nearly one half of the cases of aneurysm of the thoracic aorta die without rupture of the sac.

Turning now to the analysis of the 154 cases collected by Hare and Holder, of which it was stated that death was not due to rupture, I have made the following tabulation of the causes assigned for death by the various observers.

Obstruction to air passages								66.	
Dyspnœa						26			
Suffocation						10			
Pressure on trachea						27			
Pressure on bronchus						2			
Œdema of larynx						1			
Exhaustion							50		
Affections of lungs and pleura							28		
Apoplexy of lung						3			
Congestion of lungs						2			
Pneumonia from pressure						2			
Pneumonia						1			
Pleuro-pneumonia						1			
Abscess of lung						1			
Bronchitis						2			
Serous pleural effusion						14			
Pleurisy						2			
Péricardial affections							8		
Serous pericardial effusion						7			
Pericarditis						1			
Pressure on vena cava superior								1	
Collapse								1	
						Total	154		

It is clear at a glance, that this information is vague and unsatisfactory. The largest single item is death from exhaustion, comprising practically one-third of the cases. In too many of these cases, I fear, the reporter thoughtlessly said "exhaustion" without any special effort to see if there was a better explanation. Suffocation, credited with ten deaths, leaves the mind guessing as to the exact way in which it was caused. Pressure on the trachea, credited with twenty-seven deaths, is an adequate cause of death if the pressure is extreme; but moderate pressure does not necessarily cause death, though doubtless it may be one of the factors in producing that result. Dyspnea is fatal, not in itself, but from the condition of which it is a sympton. It may signify trouble in the respiratory organs, in the circulation, or irritation of certain parts of the nervous system. The twenty-six deaths caused by dyspnea might certainly be more carefully analysed. It is a noteworthy fact that any complication involving the heart is not once mentioned specifically as a cause of death in these cases, though recognised by all the leading authorities as holding an important place in this connection. Only one case is mentioned of pressure on the great vessels about the heart—another well-recognised factor in the fatal results. Undoubtedly more careful observation would have shown that many of the cases classed under the heads of exhaustion, dyspnea, suffocation, &c., were really deaths due to disturbance of the circulatory apparatus. It is not an exaggeration to say that many of these supposed explanations do not explain, and I think it is evident that there is need of a closer scrutiny of the fatal cases which do not rupture, and a more thoughtful consideration of the real cause of death.

Let us consider briefly some of the problems to be thought out in this connection. We may divide the cases into three classes.

(1) Cases in which an aneurysm of the arch of the aorta exists, but in which it is not the important factor in the fatal result.

(2) Cases in which death ensued from disease or disturbance of the circulatory system, not caused by direct pressure of the aneurysmal tumour.

(3) Cases in which death was due, directly or indirectly, to pressure of the aneurysmal tumour upon organs of vital importance.

Class 1 comprises those cases which die from some intercurrent disease, whose origin cannot properly be ascribed to the aneurysm. Diseases of other parts than the thoracic organs or circulatory apparatus need no special discussion, the aneurysm can be a factor only by diminishing the blood supply to important organs like the brain, or in so far as it may have affected the general health. Diseases of the thoracic organs may in some cases be so obviously due to other causes than the aneurysm that its existence is plainly an unimportant incident. On the other hand, it will not be easy in other cases to decide how far the aneurysm may have been a contributing factor in the causation of such disease. This is illustrated by the following case : —

CASE 1.—H. S., male ; white ; aged 51 ; stationary engineer. His father died of rheumatism and cardiac trouble ; otherwise the family history is unimportant. He had children's diseases. Later he had rheumatism at times for two years. This was some years before the present trouble. No history of syphilis could be obtained. Alcohol was not used to excess. When 20 years old, was thrown from a locomotive, and injured his back, so that he lost the use of his legs for one month. On December 31, 1897, he was assaulted by two men, strangled, and beaten until insensible. Whether the strangulation, together with the violence of his struggles, may have been the immediate cause of the giving way of the arterial wall, it is impossible to say. Certain it is that as a result he suffered from broken cardiac compensation. He was more or less sick for a number of months after this assault, and at the height of the sickness, in July, 1898, he had marked œdema of the lower extremities, ascites, a large amount of albumen in the urine, and a weak, dilated heart. The autopsy shows that this trouble could not have been due primarily to the kidneys, and also that there was an old endocarditis of moderate grade which had affected the mitral valve. It is highly probable that the violent struggle put a greater strain on the damaged heart than it could withstand; and it seems plausible that the same strain acting on a weakened arterial wall, should have been the starting point of the aneurysm. He had had two attacks of pneumonia, nine and seven years ago.

The more serious symptoms of his present trouble date from about April 1, 1901. For some time before that he had noticed dyspnea on slight exertion. He had also had a cough for about six months, with difficulty in raising phlegm. His first serious attack of dyspnea occurred on April 19. This attack resembled angina pectoris in the nature of its distress and anxious suffering. It also suggested to the attending physician emphysema, with an asthmatic attack. There was marked expiratory dyspnea, "rattling" breathing, and stridor. There was very little cough. It required four subcutaneous injections of morphia (each ¼ grain) for relief before the attack had subsided. On the night of April 25, after drinking a certain amount of liquor, while walking on the street, he "felt queer," rapidly choked up, lost consciousness, and did not recover consciousness until some hours later at the hospital.

At this time physical examination showed the pupils equal, with normal reaction. Pulse was regular, slow, of good volume and tension. The walls of the radial arteries were sclerotic. The right border of cardiac dulness was 3½ cm to right, and the left border 10½ cm. to left of the median line; upper border at the third rib. The apex was in the fifth interspace, 10 cm. to left of median line. The heart sounds were faint. No murmurs were detected. The lungs were negative except for a slight increase of voice sounds and tactile fremitus over the upper part of the right lung front and back. No signs of aneurysm were detected. He improved, and left the hospital April 27, at his own request.

On April 28 he had two attacks of dyspnea, similar to his first attack. On April 29 he had two attacks; on April 30 one attack. His next attack was on May 12. He had four attacks in the next two days, and the final attack began on the night of May 15.

He was brought to the hospital in a semi-conscious condition, due in part to morphia, which had been necessary to relieve his intense distress. For the same reason the pupils were contracted. The peculiar crowing respiration and brassy cough at once attracted attention, and suggested the possibility of aneurysm. A tracheal tug was found. Dulness in the second interspace extended 5 cm. to right of median line, but there was no impulse, thrill, or bruit detected. The right radial pulse was entirely obliterated; the left was regular, and of only fair strength and volume. The heart was the same as at previous examination, but weaker. Percussion showed fair pulmonary resonance throughout the chest. Auscultation showed exaggerated, crowing respiration, with many coarse bubbling and fine moist râles. He did not improve, the pulmonary œdema increased, and he died early next morning.

The autopsy showed a sacculated aneurysm of the transverse arch of the aorta and a dilatation of the ascending arch, chronic endocarditis of the mitral valve, hypertrophy and dilatation of the left ventricle, general chronic passive congestion, arterio-sclerosis, lobar pneumonia, acute congestion and œdema of lungs.

The heart muscle appeared of good quality, and showed no fatty changes microscopically. There was nothing noteworthy beyond a moderate thickening of the mitral valve and chordae tendinae, and moderate hypertrophy and dilatation of the left ventricle.

The aortic orifice measured 8 cm. in circumference; 1 cm. higher the aorta measured 9 cm., and 6 cm. beyond the valve it measured 11 cm. At 9 cm. from the valve a sacculated dilatation began, extending backwards and somewhat downwards and upwards from the transverse arch. The dilated aorta merged into the aneurysmal sac without a definitely marked border on the side toward the heart. The distal edge of the sac had a definite rounded border. At this latter point the aorta measured 6 cm. in circumference, and continued of this size to the diaphragm.

The opening from the aorta into the sac measured 4 to 5 cm. in diameter, and 14.5 cm. in circumference. The circumference about the sac and aorta was 15 cm. The measurement over the sac from proximal to distal border in the direction of the course of the aorta was 10 cm. The intima of aorta and the lining of the sac showed irregular thickened patches, but no calcification.

The posterior wall of the sac was in contact with the trachea just above its bifurcation. The wall of the sac was eroded at this point over an area 4 by 2 cm., and here the rough tracheal wall and the cartilaginous rings could be easily felt. The tracheal wall was somewhat thinned at this place. The trachea was somewhat flattened antero-posteriorly, but at the *post-mortem* examination there was no definite bulging of the aneurysm into the lumen of the trachea.

The cavity of the aneurysm contained fluid blood, except for a small amount of fresh red clot. The left pneumogastric nerve ran down the side of the sac anteriorly, but seemed perfectly free. The right pneumogastric nerve was not in direct relation to the sac.

The vessels to the neck arose from the anterior wall of the sac. The left carotid and subclavian arteries appeared normal. There was no opening to the innominate artery from the sac. Where the opening should be was a smooth, rounded thickening, with a very small depression. The smallest probe could not find a passage. On opening the innominate artery from its distal end, it appeared normal until within 1 cm. of the sac, when it suddenly narrowed, and was completely occluded by a firm, reddish-yellow thickening beneath the intima on one side. The arteries and veins of the right arm appeared normal and were filled with blood.

In the upper part of the lower lobe of the right lung was a fairly firm, reddish-grey area, involving about one-fourth of this lobe. On section of this area the tissue was rather dry and granular, and from the bronchi a slight amount of pus could be squeezed. Extending up from this area the root of the upper lobe was similarly involved by the pneumonic process. The middle lobe was not involved. The remaining portions of both lungs showed intense acute congestion and œdema. Death was evidently due to this congestion and œdema of the lungs, which in turn was caused probably by the toxines of the pneumonic inflammation. The stage of development of the pneumonia indicated that it was about the fourth or fifth day, which suggests that the series of attacks, beginning May 12, were induced by the pneumonic process.

What part did the aneurysm play in causing the death of this patient? It certainly was not the immediate cause, yet it

23

is hard to believe that it did not have an important contributing influence. In the first place, the recurrent attacks of extreme and prolonged dyspnea must have materially affected the general condition and strength of the patient. This reduced the resisting power of the system of an individual who was easily susceptible to pneumonic infection, as shown by the history of two previous attacks of pneumonia. It would seem probable, also, that the obstruction to the passage of air to the lungs might have induced changes in the lung tissue, rendering those tissues more susceptible to invasion by the pneumococcus. Finally, after the pneumonic process started, the frequent attacks of dyspnea from the pressure of the aneurysm on the trachea must have had a bad effect upon the patient's vitality in fighting the pneumonia. It is not clear how far the last attack of dyspnea was due to the aneurysm, and how far to the general acute congestion and œdema of the lungs. When he was examined at the hospital, pulmonary œdema was already well established, but he also had the crowing respiration and brassy cough of aneurysm.

In class 2, which includes cases of death from circulatory disturbance not caused by direct pressure on the blood-vessels, the chief doubt will arise in determining how far in cases associated with arterio-sclerosis death may have been caused by that disease, rather than by the aneurysm itself. Arterio-sclerosis may cause death independent of the aneurysm, either as a result of changes in the nutrition of vital organs, or by rupture of the diseased arteries, by the plugging of the arteries by thrombosis or embolism, or by its combined effect on the work and the nutrition of the heart. If death occur from embolism, its source may be the aneurysm itself, since coagulation of blood is favoured in the aneurysmal sac, and the danger of embolism is thus increased. Or again, the aneurysm may be an important factor in causing death by its effect upon the heart.

What effect may an aneurysm of the aorta have upon the

heart? It has been claimed by some that it causes hypertrophy of the heart. Calvert¶ has shown that this is not necessarily the case. His conclusion is based on statistics gathered by Dr. Oswald A. Browne, from the cases occurring in St. Bartholomew's Hospital in thirty years. Of 124 cases, 68 showed no hypertrophy; in 47 the hypertrophy could be satisfactorily explained by other causes, and in the remaining 9 hypertrophy could be explained as probably due to other causes. In arterio-sclerosis we have a very common cause of heart hypertrophy, so that in many cases the aneurysm and the heart hypertrophy are to be regarded as common results of the same cause, and not as one dependent upon the other. One form of aneurysm, however, certainly has a direct effect upon the heart. I refer to aneurysms situated close to the aortic valve, and involving a general dilatation of the aorta. If such an aneurysm enlarges enough, it will by its stretching cause dilatation of the aortic orifice, from which follows aortic regurgitation with its results. Case 2 belongs to this group.

CASE 2.—T. Y., a mulatto; male; aged 44; married; came to the Out-patient Department of the Boston City Hospital, February 18, 1899. His occupation was that of choreman. Family history is unimportant. He had syphilis twenty-five years before. He had used alcoholic drinks moderately.

His chief complaint was of pain and a feeling of pressure in the precordial region, increased by exertion. He had suffered from this about one week. His trouble, however, began at least a year before, at which time he began to have a severe boring pain in the back of the chest, together with dyspnea on exertion. At the time of examination he was not hoarse, but he had had several attacks of hoarseness in the last few days.

Physical examination showed a well-developed, fairly nourished man. Pupils equal and reacting normally. Inspection showed the pulsation of the carotid arteries more marked and jerky than normal. On the right side of the neck, just above the inner end of the clavicle, and also in the episternal notch, a marked pulsation was seen. Palpation showed that the pulsation in the episternal notch had a distinct lateral thrust from the right, indicating its origin from the innominate artery, and not from the arch of the aorta. A thrill was plainly felt just outside the sterno-mastoid muscle and above the clavicle. The right radial pulse was weaker than the left, but there was no perceptible difference in time. A slight, but distinct, tracheal tug was made out. The apex beat of the heart was felt in the sixth interspace in the left mammary line.

Percussion over the lungs was normal. Relative dulness of the heart extended to the left mammary line 4⅞ inches to left of median line, and on the right its border was 1 inch to right of median line. The area of dulness over the great vessels was increased in breadth. On the left, at the base of the heart, dulness extended 2 inches from the median line, diminishing to 1⅝ inches higher up. On the right the distance was 1 inch from the median line at the base of the heart, increasing to 1⅜ inches just below the clavicle. The line of dulness bounding the great vessels on the right, together with the abnormal pulsation beneath the inner end of the right clavicle, made the diagnosis of aneurysmal dilatation of the innominate artery practically certain. The breadth of the area of dulness over the vessels just at the base of the heart, with the tracheal tug and the associated aneurysm of the innominate artery, made it highly probable that an aneurysm existed in the ascending and transverse parts of the arch of the aorta. Physical examination gave no sign of the involvement of the descending arch.

Confirmation of the diagnosis was sought in an X-ray examination, which was very kindly made for me by Dr. F. H. Williams. The accompanying diagram shows the outline of the shadow cast by the heart and great vessels, as shown by the fluoroscope.

The point of special interest in the X-ray examination lies

in the shadow with a curved outline above the left base of the heart. This shadow extended upwards 3 inches from the base of the heart, and outward to the left 1¼ inches beyond the origin of the great vessels. Distinct expansile pulsation was seen in this shadow just following the systolic contraction of the ventricle. It evidently shows an aneurysm of the aorta

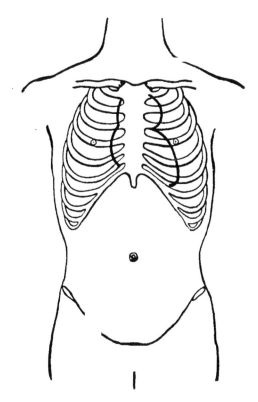

FIG. 1.—FLUOROSCOPIC EXAMINATION.   Fusiform aneurysm of ascending, transverse, and descending arch.

extending from the transverse arch to the descending arch. A distinct outline of the innominate aneurysm could not be obtained, perhaps owing to its relation to the shadow of the spine.

By the fluoroscopic examination we made certain the existence of an aneurysm of the arch of the aorta, whereas before we had great probability rather than certainty. We also learned that this aneurysm extended to the descending arch, of which fact the ordinary physical examination did not give even a clue, and we were able to outline the size of the heart more accurately than by percussion. In this instance the small, superficial aneurysm of the innominate artery was better demonstrated by the ordinary methods of examination than by the fluoroscope.

Auscultation of the lungs was normal. At the aortic area a systolic and a diastolic murmur were heard. The systolic murmur had its maximum intensity at the aortic area. It was transmitted upwards along the aorta, and could be heard faintly in the left carotid and subclavian arteries. Just at the inner end of the right clavicle the systolic murmur was markedly reinforced, and had an intensity even greater than at the aortic area (a condition which was interestingly explained by the *post-mortem* findings), and the murmur was quite loud in the right carotid and subclavian arteries. The diastolic murmur could not be heard in the left carotid or subclavian arteries, but was faintly audible in the corresponding vessels of the right side. Its maximum intensity was at and just above the aortic area. It was not carried downwards beyond the anatomical position of the aortic valve (the junction of the third left costal cartilage with the sternum), and at this point the second sound became distinct and somewhat accentuated. A slight systolic murmur was also heard at the apex, but was not transmitted far in any direction. It was not clear whether this was the aortic systolic murmur transmitted or not.

The diagnosis was aneurysm of the aorta, involving the ascending, transverse, and descending portions of the arch, aneurysm of the innominate artery, and regurgitation at the aortic valve. The patient was ordered to take iodide of potash, beginning with 10 grains three times daily, and he was specially cautioned against sudden or marked exertion.

On February 23, five days later, he returned. He felt

much better. The pain in the shoulders and upper chest was much less, but he still complained of the precordial pain. Physical examination was the same, except that the radial pulse was fuller, and apparently stronger. His condition was apparently improved. The dose of iodide of potash was increased to 15 grains.

This observation was made about 1 p.m. The patient was found not long afterwards on a doorstep, not far from the hospital. He looked sick and distressed, and was very weak. He told the person who found him that he had been at the hospital for treatment. This person assisted him to rise, but finding he was too weak to walk, left him and hurried to the hospital. An ambulance was sent at once. The patient was carried directly to the ward, and was seen at once by the house physician. He was in collapse, pale, and with no radial pulse. His mind was clear, and he told his name. He did not respond to stimulants, but grew steadily worse, and died in about ten minutes. This was about one hour after he was seen at the Out-patient Department. It was naturally supposed that the aneurysm had ruptured.

At the autopsy the following pathological conditions were found: Fusiform aneurysm of the aorta and of the innominate artery, general arterio-sclerosis, with calcification and atheroma, general chronic passive congestion, œdema of the lungs, healed tuberculosis of apex of left lung and of bronchial lymph nodes, chronic fibrous peritonitis, and chronic hydrocele.

The aneurysm had not ruptured. The heart was enlarged, somewhat distended with blood, and the right auricle was especially full and prominent, extending farther to the right than normally. The aneurysmal sac was not tensely distended, but rather relaxed. The aneurysm was of the fusiform type, involving the whole of the arch. There was also a fusiform aneurysm of the innominate artery, extending from its origin at the aorta to its bifurcaton.

The circumference of the aortic valve was 8·5 cm.; 6 cm.

above this the circumference of the aorta was 13¼ cm.; at the
innominate artery it was 13 cm.; at the left subclavian artery
10 cm.; and at the first intercostal branches 7 cm. The opening into the innominate artery had slightly thickened walls,
and measured 1·1 cm. in diameter. The artery gradually
increased in size as it ascended, until it reached a diameter of
2½ cm. From this point the enlargement gradually diminished to the division into the carotid and subclavian arteries,
which were normal in size. There was a marked general
arterio-sclerosis, with calcification and some atheroma, involving
the whole extent of the aorta.

The autopsy, then, thoroughly confirmed the diagnosis,
and showed that the extent of the aneurysm had been
accurately recognised. Moreover, the relative constriction of
the innominate artery as it branched off from the aorta, gave
an adequate explanation of the peculiar intensity of the systolic
murmur near the clavicle, namely, that a new murmur was here
created as the blood rushed through the narrow opening into
the larger space of the dilated innominate artery beyond.

Not only was death not due to rupture, but it was equally
evident that it was not due to any direct pressure of the
aneurysm. No organ of vital importance had been seriously
pressed upon, and the aneurysm at death was in a lax condition.

Death came from the cardiac complication. The existence
of aortic regurgitation had been recognised clinically by the
aortic diastolic murmur, the enlargement of the left ventricle
downwards and outwards, and the characteristic jerky pulsation
of the carotids. At the autopsy the aortic cusps were practically normal, but there was dilatation and slight hypertrophy
of the left ventricle, and the aortic orifice was somewhat
stretched, sharing in the dilatation of the aorta just above.
This is shown by comparing the measurements of this case
with the normal measurements (Mallory and Wright).**

			Normal.		Case 2.
Circumference of aortic orifice	...	...	7·7 to 8·0 cm.	...	8·5 cm.
,,	,, mitral orifice	...	10·4 ,, 10·9 ,,	...	10·0 ,,
,,	,, pulmonary orifice	...	8·9 ,, 9·2 ,,	...	8·0 ,,
,,	,, tricuspid orifice	...	12·0 ,, 12·7 ,,	...	12·0 ,,
,,	,, ascending aorta	...	7·4 ,,	...	8·5 to 13·25 cm.
,,	,, pulmonary artery	...	8·0 ,,	...	(?)
Thickness of left ventricular wall	...	·7 ,, 1·0 ,,	..	1·2 cm.
,,	,, right ventricular wall	...	·2 ,, ·3 ,,	...	·4 ,,

Here we find the measurements of all other orifices corresponding pretty closely to the minimum figures of the normal table, while we find the aortic orifice nearly 1 cm. larger than the minimum figure of the normal table.

The autopsy also showed a general chronic passive congestion of the organs. This suggests that the systolic murmur heard at the apex was due to mitral regurgitation. This regurgitation was secondary to the dilatation of the left ventricle, as the mitral curtains and chordæ tendinæ were normal. The œdema of the lungs, the distension of the cavities of the heart, and the clinical story of the rapid failure and death, all point to failure of the heart muscle as the immediate cause of death. Whether this in any way depended on nervous influence is a mere matter of surmise. The muscle seemed to be in good condition, and microscopical examination failed to find fatty degeneration in examining a fresh specimen. The coronary arteries were patent. We have, then, no anatomical explanation for the failure of the cardiac muscle, and we may rule out any serious interference with its nutrition due to arterio-sclerosis. We have to fall back on the well-known clinical fact that death is apt to ensue suddenly in aortic regurgitation—a fact for which we are not yet always ready to furnish a satisfactory explanation. We are apt to think of death from aortic regurgitation as more rapid than this, which lasted somewhere between one half and one hour. But Balfour†† has called attention to the fact that ingravescent asystole occurs in aortic regurgitation, and may even be much more prolonged than in this case.

Our story in this case would seem to be clear, and the sequence of events as follows: Syphilis, arterio-sclerosis of the aorta, fusiform aneurysm of the arch, resulting dilatation of the aortic orifice, aortic regurgitation, dilatation of the left ventricle, mitral regurgitation, general passive congestion, and death from asystole, accompanied by œdema of the lungs. The responsibility of the aneurysm for the death is indirect.

This case illustrates so well the view of fusiform aneurysms held by Sir Douglas Powell, that I will quote a few of his remarks on the subject. He says: ‡‡ " Clinically the phenomena characteristic of aneurysm are scarcely ever observed except in association with the sacculated form, the so-called 'fusiform aneurysm' being merged, as regards prognosis and treatment, in the class of heart disease with which they are most closely connected." " These general dilatations involve, for the most part, the first part of the aorta, and are associated with valvular lesions and secondary cardiac dilatations and hypertrophies; they give rise, with rare exceptions, to no pressure signs; they do not tend to cause death by rupture or by compression of vital parts, but rather through cardiac failure, angina, or syncope. The treatment is that appropriate to heart disease."

Class 3 includes by far the greatest number of cases. It is true that in the vast majority of cases of aneurysm of the aorta, that if death is not due to rupture, it is due, directly or indirectly, to pressure.

In its course from the left ventricle to the diaphragm, the thoracic aorta lies in close relation to many important structures. It is worth while in the study of the effects of pressure by the aneurysmal sac to briefly recapitulate those organs which may be affected.

The origin of the aorta is imbedded in the structures at the base of the heart. In front lie the conus arteriosus of the right ventricle, and the auricular appendage of the right auricle. The right auricle and the vena cava superior are in close contact on the right. Around the left the pulmonary artery winds from the front, while behind lie the left auricle and the right pulmonary artery.

Just above the heart the edges of both lungs separate the ascending arch of the aorta from the sternum in front. The pulmonary artery is on the left. Behind and below are the right branch of the pulmonary artery and the root of the right lung. On the right lies the vena cava superior and the right lung. It should be remembered that the pericardium extends up on the aorta from 1 to 1½ inches above the base of the heart.

The relations of the transverse arch are perhaps the most important of all. The ascending arch has a certain freedom of movement, and after it emerges from the structures at the base of the heart it may become considerably enlarged without serious results to surrounding organs; it displaces rather than compresses them. The transverse arch has much less freedom of movement; its relations to surrounding parts is closer, and these parts cannot readily be moved aside. Enlargement here causes compression rather than displacement. Symptoms of pressure, therefore, develop early in the process of enlargement.

The transverse arch passes backward and to the left in front of the trachea, and above the left bronchus. The bifurcation of the pulmonary artery is beneath the anterior part of this section of the aorta. Above lies the left innominate vein. Farther back than the trachea lie the œsophagus and thoracic duct. The relations of the nervous structures to this part of the aorta are important. The deep cardiac plexus lies behind the aorta, between it and the trachea, and above the bifurcation of the pulmonary artery. This is the main centre for the nerves distributed to the heart. The superficial cardiac plexus lies between the aorta and the right pulmonary artery. The left recurrent laryngeal nerve passes down in front of the aorta, passes backwards beneath it, and ascends behind it and in front of the trachea. In front also pass the left vagus and phrenic nerves. From the transverse arch are given off the innominate, the left carotid, and the left subclavian arteries.

The descending arch passes backwards and downwards to the left of the trachea, behind the root of the left lung, to the left anterior aspect of the dorsal vertebræ. As it passes downwards the œsophagus and thoracic duct lie on its right. The left pleura and lung lie to the left and anteriorly. The descending arch of the aorta and the thoracic aorta below are held firmly in place by the intercostal branches which are given off from the aorta.

We may now turn our attention to the ways in which pressure from an aneurysm upon the organs surrounding the aorta may contribute to a fatal result. It is clear that the results will depend partly upon the size of the aneurysm, and partly upon the vital importance of the organ or organs pressed upon. It is also manifest that the size of the aneurysm is of less importance than the place where the pressure is exerted. A striking case to illustrate this point is reported by Irvine.§§ It was a case of double aneurysm of the arch of the aorta. A relatively large aneurysm of the ascending arch caused very little trouble, whereas death came because a small aneurysm of the descending arch compressed the left bronchus, and induced extensive changes in the left lung.

Before considering the effect on individual structures, however, let us note that death may come from the gradual wearing out of the patient's strength without any extreme pressure on vital organs. When an aneurysm enlarges enough to press upon peripheral nerves, pain results. Pain may also be of the nature of " referred pain," as in cardiac disease. This may be of a severe anginous type, or a referred neuralgic pain. Pressure upon some of the nerves in close relation with the aorta causes irritation, and the impulse is carried by varying channels to the central nervous system, and gives rise to the " referred pains."

Such irritation may also cause dyspnea or cough, especially of a paroxysmal type. The suffering from the pain, the dyspnea and cough, and sleeplessness due to any of these factors, are the main cause of death in some cases. Such death comes from the gradual wearing down of the system. It may be properly called " death from exhaustion," and it is indirectly due to pressure of the aneurysm upon the nerves.

Pressure on the nerves may contribute to the death in other ways. Spasm of the glottis may result reflexly from irritation of the vagus nerve. And Gibson‖‖ says the same result " may possibly be an early symptom of interference with the motor nerve of the larynx," the recurrent laryngeal. To what extent pressure on the cardiac nerves or ganglia may exert an inhibitory or paralytic effect on the cardiac muscle, is not perfectly clear. It is mentioned by some writers, and it may be a possible explanation of some of the cases where the most careful *post-mortem* examination fails to reveal any adequate explanation. This subject needs further investigation, as does also the question of what effect pressure on the vagus may have on the condition of the lung.

In considering the effects of pressure on the heart and the great vessels, we may practically disregard the left ventricle and the aorta, for it is from the left ventricle and through the blood in the aorta, that the pressure is carried to the periphery of the aneurysmal sac. We cannot expect this pressure to be greater than its source, hence it cannot compress the left ventricle or aorta. An aneurysm arising at the root of the aorta may, however, by pressure distort the aortic or pulmonary valve. In either case we get regurgitation into the corresponding ventricle as the chief factor in causing cardiac failure and death. Compression or obliteration of the innominate or left carotid or left subclavian arteries may occur. This leads to impaired nutrition of the parts supplied by these arteries; but the collateral circulation is so good that a fatal result is hardly to be expected from this cause alone, unless all these were occluded together, of which occurrence I have found no reported case. The supply of blood to the brain is of course the most important item in considering obstruction of these arteries. Of the other branches of the general arterial system we need consider only the bronchial arteries—the nutrient arteries of the lung. Obliteration of one of these will cause gangrene of the part of the lung supplied by it with fatal termination. This is a less frequent occurrence than was at one time supposed, as the blood-vessels of the roots of the lung are so situated that they are generally protected by the resistance of the bronchi.

Returning to the heart, we have to consider pressure upon the auricles, the conus arteriosus of right ventricle, the pulmonary artery, and the pulmonary veins. In these cases we are dealing with obstruction of the circulation, essentially the same in its results as is found in valvular disease. Death may result in the same ways as from broken compensation. Pressure on the vena cava superior is by no means uncommon. We get venous stasis of the upper part of the chest, the head, and the upper extremities. Collateral circulation may lessen this by furnishing a channel to the vena cava inferior, by anastomosis with its branches, or to the vena azygos if the pressure be above the point of entrance of that vessel into the vena cava superior. Here, again, the brain is the important organ to consider, and death by coma from the obstructed venous circulation is reported. Œdema of the glottis has also been reported¶¶ as a cause of death from impeded venous circulation.

CASE 3 is an illustration of death caused by pressure interfering with the circulation. The point of application was the pulmonary artery.

O. D., male; white; aged 42; single; came to the Out-patient Department of the Boston City Hospital in the latter part of September, 1900. He was a painter by occupation. His father had died of heart disease, and his mother of cancer. He had diphtheria eleven years ago. Otherwise he had been in good health, except for a venereal disease about fifteen years ago, which was apparently syphilis. He had used alcoholic drinks to excess until quite recently, and used a good deal of tobacco.

His present illness began about one year ago. He began to get short of breath on exertion, and also had vertigo and palpitation. For some months he had had pain at times in the precordial region, radiating into the shoulders. Of late the pain had been worse and more frequent, and he complained of increasing dyspnea and weakness.

On physical examination the cardiac area of dulness was practically normal. At the base of the heart was to be heard a peculiar murmur. It was loud and harsh in quality. Its point of maximum intensity was to the left of the sternum at the second rib and first and second interspaces, at and just above the pulmonic area. In rhythm it began just after the first sound—that is, it was a somewhat late systolic murmur—and continued just a trifle after the second cardiac sound, yet it was clearly all one murmur, and not a systolic running into a diastolic murmur. There was also a loud, ringing, much accentuated second pulmonic sound, as exaggerated a second pulmonic sound as I have ever heard.

This peculiar combination was evidently due to something outside the heart itself. The peculiar late systolic murmur with this area of maximum intensity, and with the accentuated second pulmonic sound, are characteristic of a persistent ductus arteriosus. But it seemed highly improbable that such a case should live to this age, and without a longer history of cardiac trouble. The only other explanation which seemed at all likely was the existence of an aneurysm which compressed the pulmonary artery, and thus raised the tension in the pulmonary circulation. There was, however, no dulness, no pulsation, no tracheal tug, no hoarseness, no inequality of pupils, nor any other physical sign that I could find to confirm the suspicion of aneurysm of the arch of the aorta. I asked him to come again so that he could be examined with the X-ray, but he did not return. He got a chance to work, then attended another clinic, and finally returned for admission to the Boston City Hospital, December 7, 1900.

He was now much worse. He was weaker, had much more pain, more dyspnea, had been unable to do any work for three weeks, and had had orthopnea for two weeks. He had also become hoarse at times. He was pale, and had a slight cyanotic hue. The pulse was 80, regular, and of fair volume and strength. There was no perceptible difference in the two wrists. A distinct tracheal tug could now be felt.

There was now a slight bulging of the chest just to the left of the sternum, and from the second interspace nearly to the clavicle. A slight pulsation could be seen. On palpation, a distinct, coarse, rough thrill or grating sensaton could be felt over this bulging area. Percussion showed marked dulness over this area. On auscultation a rough, coarse, rumbling systolic murmur was heard, loudest over the bulging area, but transmitted to some distance in all directions. The second pulmonic sound was still somewhat accentuated, but was not as loud or clear cut as before. Moreover, it was followed by a diastolic murmur, with its maximum intensity in the pulmonic area, and transmitted downwards and diagonally across the sternum to the right, following the location of the right ventricle and not the left.

This murmur seemed to me to indicate pulmonary regurgitation. It was now perfectly evident that we had an aneurysm pressing front to the chest wall to the left of the sternum. This had in September been too small to be detected, but so situated as to press on the pulmonary artery, and greatly increase the resistance in the pulmonary circuit. This obstruction had now increased so much as to cause regurgitation through the pulmonary valve.

As a matter of interest, an X-ray examination was made in this case also. It showed the heart slightly enlarged to the left, but markedly enlarged to the right. Above the base of the heart was an abnormally broad shadow, extending especially to the left of the sternum, and very closely resembling the shadow of the aneurysm of the descending arch, as shown in fig. 1. The outline is shown in fig. 2.

In spite of rest in bed and other treatment, this patient gradually failed, and died December 17, 1900. Towards the

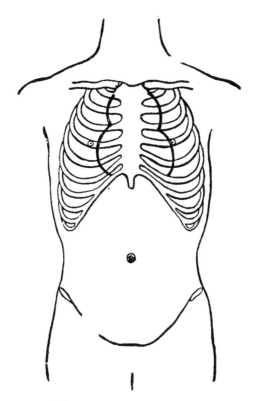

FIG. 2.—FLUOROSCOPIC EXAMINATION. Sacculated aneurysm of the ascending arch, growing forward and to the left, and compressing the pulmonary artery.

end the attacks of dyspnea were more frequent and severe. He had to be propped up in an upright sitting position for the last forty-eight hours of life. During the last few hours he developed pulmonary œdema, and his pulse gradually failed.

The autopsy showed a sacculated aneurysm of the aorta

24

compressing the pulmonary artery, hypertrophy, and dilatation of the right ventricle, hypostatic congestion of the lower lobes of the lung, and atelectasis of an area of left upper lobe of lung which was compressed by the aneurysm, chronic passive congestion of liver, spleen, intestines, and kidneys, fatty degeneration of the heart and kidneys.

On removing the sternum, the mediastinum presented a roughly spherical mass, about 10 cm. in diameter, projecting forwards and to the left. The mass is continuous with the heart and vessels of the base, and lies anterior and to the left of them. It projects 8·5 cm. to the left of the median line at about the level of the second rib. On dissection the mass is found to be an aneurysmal sac, 11 by 9 by 7·5 cm., which communicates with the aorta by an oval opening 2·75 by 2 cm. in diameter. This opening is situated in the anterior wall of the first portion of the aorta 3 mm. above the upper margin of the aortic cusps. The opening is on the left anterior aspect, above the junction of the anterior and the left posterior cusps of the valve. The edges of the opening are smooth and slightly raised (*see* fig. 3).

Inside the sac a rounded mass of firm, organised clot fills the cavity to within ½-cm. of the opening. This mass becomes firmly adherent to the inner wall of the aneurysmal sac at ½ to 1 cm. from the edge of the opening, except at the posterior side of the opening. Here a flattened pocket extends 3 cm. in depth between the rounded sac on the outside and the rounded mass of clot on the inside. The portion of this pocket farthest from the aortic opening is directly opposite the sinus of the right anterior cusp of the pulmonary valve. It is evident that this pocket is so situated as to have caught the greatest force of the blood current entering the sac, and this fact has prevented the formation of blood clot at this point. The cause of the peculiar murmur heard in this case was the eddying blood current in this pocket of the aneurysmal sac.

Elsewhere the whole aneurysmal sac is filled with firm clot.

An incision from the anterior surface of the tumour shows a firm, fibrinous, dark red, layered clot, everywhere adherent to the inside of the sac (*see* fig. 4). This aneurysm not only had not ruptured, but it presented that condition, filled with firm clot, which is called " cured."

The general direction of the growth of the aneurysm has been to the left and forward. It has also extended upward, as two-thirds of the mass is above the opening from the aorta. More important still is the growth of the tumour a short distance backward, crowding in between the aorta and the pulmonary artery, so that where the transverse arch should cross close above the pulmonary artery, it is separated from it by an aneurysmal mass 5 cm. in thickness. The arch of the aorta has been apparently pushed upward, backward, and to the right to accommodate this growth, but there has been little, if any, diminution of the lumen of the artery.

In the pulmonary artery, however, a different condition obtains. There has been a marked flattening from the encroachment of the tumour upon its lumen. The tumour presents as an irregular rounded mass, projecting downward and to the left into the pulmonary artery and the upper part of the right ventricle (*see* fig. 5). The right anterior cusp of the pulmonary valve is stretched taut over the rounded surface of the tumour. The tumour projects into the right ventricle just below this valve, and the distance over its rounded surface is 4 cm. from the right ventricular wall to the upper edge of the cusp, and from this point to the end of the projecting mass in the pulmonary artery is 7 cm. The tumour mass as felt from the right ventricle or pulmonary artery is firm everywhere except over the shallow pocket of the aneurysmal sac already mentioned. This sac lies behind the right anterior cusp of the pulmonary valve and part of the pulmonary artery just above it. Though yielding in the *post-mortem* specimen, it must have been firmly distended by the pressure of the aortic blood during life. The right anterior cusp of the valve must have lain flat over the surface, useless as far as its function was concerned.

The right ventricle was very much dilated, and the wall was hypertrophied to about four times its normal thickness. Death came from failure of the right ventricle, owing to the obstruction in the pulmonary artery, and the regurgitation through the crippled pulmonary valve.

Pressure on the trachea or the primary bronchi is a frequent cause of death in aneurysm of the aortic arch. This may act directly or indirectly. When it acts directly, death comes by suffocation, and the pressure is usually on the trachea just above its bifurcation. Death from this cause is rarely sudden, it is generally by slow asphyxiation, and the suffering is terrible. Sometimes the attack of asphyxiation is rather rapid in course, and unconsciousness ensues before there is much suffering, as in the following case.

CASE 4.—J. H., male; white; aged 39; married; labourer; entered the Boston City Hospital December 6, 1900. Family history was negative. He had had typhoid fever when young, and remembered no serious illness since then. At 22 he had gonorrhœa, and at 27 syphilis. Used alcohol moderately; tobacco to some extent.

His present illness began in August, 1900, four months before, when he began to have occasional spells of difficult breathing. He felt an attack coming on, would then sit down, and soon lost consciousness. If severe, the attack lasted about one to one and a half hours. The attacks were followed by great prostration. The attacks came on rather suddenly after exertion or excitement. He had one just before entrance to the hospital, another five days before, and another five weeks before that. The intervals between the attacks had been variable. In the attack, breathing was extremely difficult, and he got blue in the face.

In the intervals between attacks he had pain and discomfort in the precordia. There was some cough, but little expectoration. The voice had been husky since September.

Fig. 3.

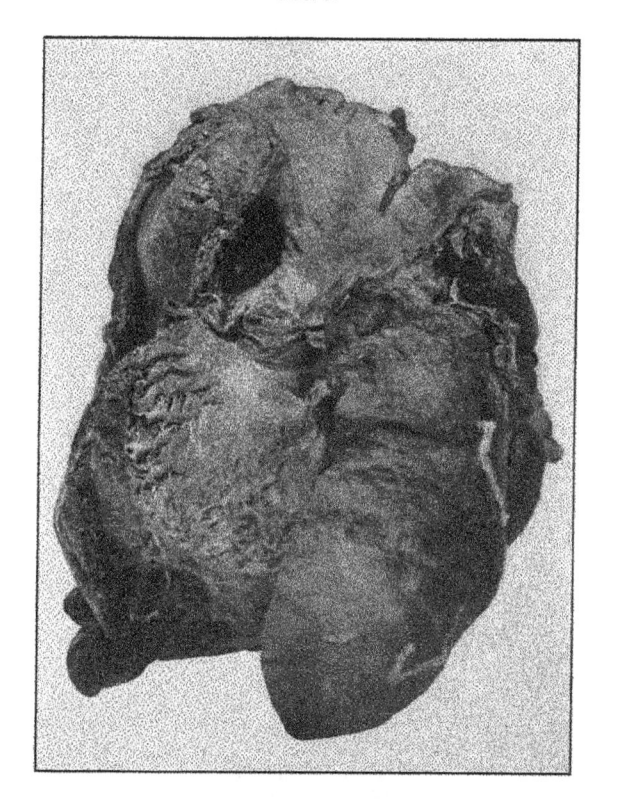

Interior of left ventricle and aorta, showing opening into aneurismal sac just above the cusps of the aortic valve.

FIG. 5.

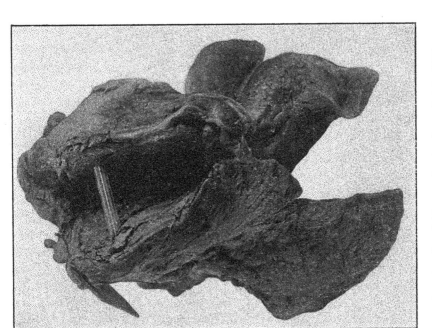

Interior of right ventricle and pulmonary artery. Cusp of pulmonary va stretched taut over bulging surface of aneurism.

Aneurismal sac laid open, showing layered clot within.

Physical examination showed the pupils equal, the left vocal cord immovable, and the radial pulses equal and of good volume and tension. Tracheal tug was present. There was no œdema. Examination of lungs was negative. Upper border of cardiac dulness was at the third rib. The right border was 1½ inches to right, and left border 5½ inches to left of median line. Apex beat was in the fifth interspace. A soft systolic murmur was heard at the base, loudest to the left of the sternum. The second pulmonic sound was accentuated. Physical examination was otherwise negative.

Up to January 21, 1901, a period of about six weeks, he had three attacks, all of them severe. The dyspnea was especially marked on expiration. He became cyanotic and lost consciousness. Nitroglycerine was employed subcutaneously and inhalation of oxygen. He recovered from these attacks, but was exhausted and weak for hours afterwards. The hoarseness had continued, but varied in degree. At times he had a metallic, barking cough. There was dyspnea on any marked exertion. He was able to be up and about the ward most of the time.

On February 9 he had an attack at night. On February 21 he had an attack while up and around the ward. Up to March 25 there were no more atttacks. He complained more of distress in the upper part of the chest, however, and his cough, dyspnea on exertion, ar⁴ hoarseness persisted. He was evidently losing ground. On March 25 he had a slight attack in the morning, and had another slight attack on March 27.

On April 3 he developed an inflammatory swelling on the left side of the neck. In a few days this showed fluctuation, and he was transferred to the surgical ward for operation, if necessary. It subsided under poulticing. While in the surgical ward he had another attack, April 18.

On April 23 he was returned to the medical ward. For the past month or two abnormal dulness had been found on level of first interspace. It had been increasing, and now measured 2¼ inches to right and 3¼ inches to left of median line. Slight pulsation could be seen and felt to the left of the sternum. There was no thrill. The systolic murmur was the same, and the second pulmonic sound was accentuated. An

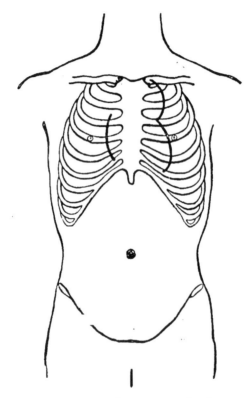

FIG. 6.—FLUOROSCOPIC EXAMINATION. Sacculated aneurysm of transverse arch, pressing on trachea.

X-ray examination had been made on December 21, 1900, and showed the following outline (fig. 6).

On May 3 he had an attack. On May 5 and 6 he had four attacks. On the night of May 7 he had an atttack, and died during the attack at 3 a.m.

The autopsy showed the following: Sacculated aneurysm of the transverse arch of aorta, and dilatation of the ascending arch, obstruction of trachea by pressure of aneurysm, distension of lungs, chronic healed tuberculosis of lung, arterio-sclerosis, and hypertrophy of heart.

The heart was somewhat enlarged, weighing 480 grammes, the principal change being in the left ventricle. The muscular tissue was firm and dark red, but showed some fatty degeneration on microscopical examination. The aorta is apparently dilated, and a mass about the size of a lemon lay below the clavicular notch, extending slightly into the left pleural cavity. This was a sacculated aneurysm of the transverse arch of the aorta, which had not ruptured.

The aortic orifice measured 8·5 cm. in circumference, and the ascending arch was somewhat dilated, measuring from 9 to 10·5 cm. in circumference. At a point 9·5 cm. from the aortic valve there is a rounded border forming part of the opening of an aneurysmal sac. This opening measured 8 by 9 cm. in diameter. This sac arose almost entirely from the posterior and inferior part of the transverse arch, while the innominate left carotid and subclavian arteries arose in front from the apparently normal aortic wall, and were practically normal. The sac was hemispherical in shape and the greatest circumference of it and the dilated aortic wall was 22 cm.

The aneurysm lay directly anterior to the trachea, just above its bifurcation. The trachea was flattened and curved back by the pressure, and its lumen was encroached upon from the anterior and left side by the bulging wall of the aneurysmal sac. Even with the sac empty the lumen of the trachea was only one-third of its normal size at this point.

The lungs were very much distended with air. When the sternum was removed, they did not collapse, but bulged forward, nearly covering the heart. On cutting the bronchi the lungs collapsed to less than one half their former size from the escape of air. There was an area of healed tuberculous tissue occupying about one-third of the right upper lobe. Elsewhere the lung tissue was normal. The bronchi were normal. The bronchial lymph nodes were normal.

It was clear that the distension of the lungs was due entirely to the pressure of the aneurysm on the trachea. The pressure of the distended sac must have been sufficient to entirely prevent the exit of air, and the patient died of suffocation. It is not difficult to understand how the air passed by this obstruction on inspiration, but could not escape again. With the descent of the diaphragm on inspiration, the heart and anterior part of the arch are drawn downwards. This drew the aneurysm away from the trachea enough to allow the entrance of air, but when this traction ceased at the end of inspiration, the pressure was at once resumed, and the aneurysm acted like a ball valve to prevent the exit of air. The resulting dyspnea caused more forcible inspiratory efforts, the entrance of more and more air which could not escape, and the extreme distension of the lungs resulted. With the complete distension of the lung no more air would enter, and respiration was brought to a standstill, and death ensued from suffocation.

Compression of one bronchus is not so likely to cause death by suffocation. It is rarely so sudden that the necessary supply of air cannot be obtained through the other lung. Death is more likely to come through secondary changes in the lung. How far these secondary changes may be the result of pressure upon the blood-vessels or nerves at the root of the lung has been a matter of dispute, and I do not think we are yet prepared to decide the question definitely. It is, however, certain that the mere mechanical occlusion of the bronchus may result in extensive and fatal changes in the lung tissue. This is due to the retention of secretions and the invasion of micro-organisms. Collapse and consolidation of lung tissue, a purulent bronchitis extending to the smaller divisions and then to the lung tissue, and causing multiple foci of suppuration and gangrene, are the manifestations of pulmonary disintegration which follow compression of the bronchus. Death in this case comes as an indirect result, not as the direct result of the pressure of the aneurysm. Irvine §§ has reported a case of this sort, and has called attention to the subject. Compression of one primary bronchus may, however, produce collapse and atelectasis of the corresponding lung, without further secondary results, as shown in case 5.

Pressure which results in a less complete obstruction of the trachea or bronchus, may contribute indirectly to death in another way. The pressure is enough to cause imperfect aeration of the lung, and an imperfect removal of secretions. The conditions are favourable for the establishment of bacterial infection, and thus the way is paved for a fatal result. Pulmonary tuberculosis may result, as pointed out by Stokes, or the patient may die from a more acute infective process, as in case 1.

Finally, in considering the effects of pressure on the pulmonary tissue, we must note the occurrence of cases where the aneurysm is so situated that it does not press on the main air passages, but upon the lung tissue itself. Here we get primarily a compression of the lung tissue, and may get secondary inflammatory processes in the tissues thus affected.

Pressure on the œsophagus may become so extreme as to prevent the passage of food and cause death by inanition.

In less degree it may be a more or less important factor in causing insufficient ingestion of food and imperfect nutrition, thus rendering the patient an easier victim to intercurrent disease of any kind. Compression of the thoracic duct may cause serious impairment of nutrition, with similar relations to the fatal termination, but this is extremely rare.

CASE 5 illustrates death by starvation from the pressure of aneurysm on the œsophagus.

J. A. F., female; aged 57; married; seamstress; had always enjoyed good health before the present illness. In the fall of 1893 she first noticed a pain in the lower left axillary region, which also shot into the back and up to the left shoulder. This continued at intervals, until the spring of 1895, when it was much improved by a course of iodide of potash treatment.

During the summer of 1895 she gained 9 lbs. in eleven weeks spent in the country.

In the fall of 1895 she began to have partial aphonia and difficulty in swallowing. After a time solids could not be swallowed at all but she could swallow liquids. In January, 1896, the pain in side and back returned with renewed vigour and reached around to the epigastrium. By the last of January a hacking cough had set in. Sibilant and sonorous râles were heard over both lungs. By March there was considerable expectoration, which was occasionally streaked with blood. By April dyspnea was caused by even slight exertion. She was very weak. She had been losing flesh since fall and was now greatly emaciated. Even liquids were now vomited or regurgitated, and nutritive enemata were resorted to after April 5. She failed gradually, and died quietly June 2, 1896. No new symptoms had developed and all the old ones had persisted.

During the latter part of her illness it was noted that the respiration was very faint on the right side of chest. Tuberculosis of the lung was thought of, but that diagnosis would hardly account for all the symptoms, and no tubercle bacilli could be found in the sputum. The probable diagnosis was thought to be a malignant tumour of the œsophagus. This would account for the obstruction of the œsophagus, the wasting and the pain, and by extension and pressure on the left recurrent laryngeal nerve and right bronchus, would account for the aphonia and diminished respiration of the right lung. This clinical diagnosis represented very closely the autopsy findings, except that the tumour was an aneurysm of the aorta instead of a malignant tumour of the œsophagus.

The autopsy showed a sacculated aneurysm of the thoracic aorta, atheroma of aorta, pressure of aneurysm on right primary bronchus and on œsophagus, atelectasis of right lung, bronchitis of left lung, and all other organs normal.

The aneurysm was a sacculated one, about 3½ inches in

diameter, arising from the upper part of the descending thoracic aorta. It had grown forwards and to the right, crowding in between the œsophagus behind and the air passages in front. The œsophagus was compressed flat against the vertebral column. The right primary bronchus was so completely occluded by the pressure toward the front, that the right lung had collapsed, and was in a state of atelectasis, but no inflammatory change had resulted. The fourth to sixth dorsal vertebræ (inclusive) were eroded on their right side from the pressure of the sac. The aneurysm was partly filled with lamellated clot. The thoracic duct could not be found. The anatomical relations of the aneurysm, the absence of other pathological cause, and the very extreme emaciation, showed that death came from starvation, of which the aneurysm was the immediate cause.

I wish to acknowledge my indebtedness to Drs. Withington, Williams, and Sears, of the staff of the Boston City Hospital, for permission to report the progress of cases 1, 3 and 4, while under their charge in the wards; to the Pathological Department of the Hospital for the excellent reports of autopsies; to Dr. H. C. Williams, of Boston, for the history of case 1; and to Drs. S. H. Ayer and W. H. Prescott, for the clinical history and autopsy report of case 5.

REFERENCES.

* Hare and Holder, *American Journal of Medical Sciences*, October, 1899.

† *Idem*, p. 410.

‡ *Idem*, p. 401.

§ Oswald A. Browne, "Aneurysms of the Aorta," London, 1897; statistics quoted by Gibson, "Diseases of the Heart and Aorta," 1898, p. 836.

‖ Sibson. "The Aorta and the Aneurysms of the Aorta," reprinted from *Medical Anatomy*, Fasciculus v., 1858.

¶ Calvert, *Brit. Med. Journ.*, 1899, vol. i., p. 84; statistics taken from Browne's observations.

** Mallory and Wright, "Pathological Technique," p. 36.

†† Balfour, "Clinical Lectures on Diseases of the Heart and Aorta," third edition, 1898, pp. 94, 318 ; also, "The Senile Heart," 1898, pp. 80, 139.

‡‡ Sir Douglas Powell, An Address on "The Diagnosis and Treatment of Aneurysm of Aorta," *Medical Society Transactions,* London, vol. xiii., 1890, p. 117.

§§ J. Pearson Irvine, *Transactions of the Pathological Society,* London, vol. xxviii., p. 63.

‖‖ Gibson, "Diseases of the Heart and Aorta," 1898, p. 846.

¶¶ Quincke, Ziemssen's Encyclopædia, Wm. Wood and Co., 1876, vol. vi., p. 426.

In addition to the works already referred to, valuable aid·has been derived from Stokes, "Diseases of the Heart and Aorta," 1855 ; Hayden, "Diseases of the Heart and Aorta," 1875 ; Broadbent, "Heart Disease," 1900.

DISCUSSION.

Dr. CURTIN: I am very much interested in Dr. Arnold's paper as I have studied aneurysms quite closely and have had unusual opportunities to observe a great many cases. I think, as the doctor has said, that we have a great aid in the diagnosis in the use of X-rays. Very recently I had a case complaining of persistent pain in the left side of the spinal column and an X-ray examination showed unmistakable indications of an aneurysm, which we had suspected, but could not diagnosticate because of the absence of all the physical signs. I have seen two or three cases that seemed to die of extreme weakness without any apparent cause for it, no pressure on the trachea, œsophagus, or any important structure, and no hæmorrhage. The majority of cases I have seen of thoracic trouble have died of rupture into the different cavities of the trunk. I have not been able to find the cause of death in some of these cases, and I have always thought that the patient was probably worn out by the suffering persisting for years.

Dr. ARNOLD : Dr. Curtin brings up a point that I have given more fully in that part of the paper which was not read, that you cannot in all cases assign a definite cause for death. The failure to do so, however, is sometimes due to the fact that the pathologist does not look carefully enough. He is too apt to accept the existence of the aneurysm as a sufficient explanation of death, the more so as the pathological evidence is not always marked and the right clue may be found only in the clinical aspect of the case. For example, in case 2, where death was due to aortic regurgitation the pathological changes indicating regurgitation were so slight that they did not in themselves attract attention. The knowledge that aortic regurgitation had been demonstrated clinically was responsible for a sufficiently thorough review of the pathological evidence and its proper interpretation. Only thus were we able to demonstrate the cause of death.

REMARKS ON STRYCHNINE

BY A. JACOBI, M.D., LL.D.

NEW YORK.

————

OF the fifteen pages of close print given by H. C. Wood[*] to the discussion of strychnine, there are only some brief sentences referring to the subject on which I intend to make a very few remarks.

On page 212 he says: "The full dose of strychnine produces a rise of the arterial pressure, which is enormously increased during the convulsion, after which there is a very pronounced fall in the arterial pressure." Page 213: "Our knowledge of the cardiac action of strychnine is still imperfect. Although Lahousse believes that in any dose strychnine depresses the intracardiac ganglia, it is probable that the small dose has a stimulating influence upon the heart." "In regard to the action of the alkaloid upon the vagi, there is much difference of statement by investigators." Page 214: "The fullest permissible doses stimulate very powerfully the respiratory centres, and also slightly increase blood pressure by stimulation of the vaso-motor centres, and probably also of the heart itself." Page 217: "Strychnine is an extremely serviceable remedy in the treatment of cardiac disease, with weakness of muscle. In mitral insufficiency we have seen it prolong life for years, after the failure of digitalis, and when before its administration

---

[*] "Therapeutics: its Principles and Practice," Eleventh Edition, 1900.

immediate death seemed inevitable. It should always be tried in cases of failing heart where digitalis disagrees, it not being possible at present to pick out those cases in which brilliant results are to be achieved by it. To be effective it must be given in rapidly ascending doses, the patient being kept, if necessary, for weeks and months on the verge of strychnine poisoning, with distinctly heightened reflexes and some muscular stiffness. Clinical experience shows that it has no cumulative action, but that the patient becomes accustomed to its use, so that a grain a day may finally be given without any serious effects."

The German literature does not favour strychnine. The latest text-books of Tappeiner (1899), Penzoldt (1900), the great cyclopædia of Liebreich (1894), and the pharmaco-therapeutics of Kobert (1897), contain but very few remarks. We learn that strychnine retards the pulse, and increases blood pressure by stimulating the centres of the vagus and the vaso-motors, but that it has no prominent therapeutic effect except occasionally in partial peripheral paralysis, in the psychical and nervous disorders of chronic alcoholism, in incontinence of the bladder, in amblyopia and amaurosis unattended with serious anatomical disorders, and in poisoning with chloroform or morphin. We are also told that a cumulative effect has sometimes been observed after many days, that poisoning has been observed after medicinal doses injected in diphtheritic paralysis, or administered during cardiac diseases, that now and then the secretion of urine is impeded, and that occasionally unexpected poisoning has taken place.

In the *Arztl. Sachverständ Zeit.*, of 1900 (August 1), for instance, Otto Jonas reported the case of a child, aged 2¼, that took two tablespoonfuls of "Fellow's syrup of the hypophosphites," which was advertised to contain some strychnine (0·001 in one teaspoonful), with poisonous effect.

In a similar manner the French literature disposes of strychnine and its cardiac effects with a few words. Even G.

M. Debove and Ch. Achard (*Manuel de thérap. med.*, vol. i., 1900, p. 444), have but little to say on the subject of strychnine in cardiac diseases. In their opinion, it is observed to be a general, and therefore a cardiac tonic, and to influence the myocardium particularly. It diminishes blood pressure, and retards the action of the heart, even in small doses (Lahousse); it paralyses the intracardiac motory centres, and in large doses, the terminal fibres of the pneumogastric. It is recommended in three daily doses of a half or of one milligramme, for valvular lesions in the period of compensation. Huchard combines it with spartein.

The English literature, for instance, J. Mitchell Bruce's "Principles of Treatment," 1899, treats the results of strychnine medication with more appreciation.

The daily practice of American physicians with whom I come in contact, and whose cases I read, gives no scanty recognition to strychnine in all sorts of diseases. I seldom meet a case of cardiac disorder, or of an anæmia, or of debility, no matter how caused, whether localised or general, or of collapse, in which strychnine has not been given long and extensively. Indeed, while formerly it was almost impossible to find such a case that was not attended with digitalis, strychnine is now considered the sheet anchor. Indeed, such dicta as that quoted from Wood, where he says that strychnine kept alive where digitalis had no effect, are quite capable of imbuing the profession with the belief in the identity of the two drugs. There is, however, no such identity.

When therapeutical measures are selected for cardiac diseases, we should not overlook the complex nature of the anatomy, the physiology, and the pathology of the organ. The muscle, the peri- and endocardium, the blood-vessels, or the innervation may be faulty. Part of the latter is controlled by centres located in the muscular substance. They are Bidder's and Remak's ganglia, which are connected by nervous plexuses. They are mostly found in the septum of the atria, and in the boundary between them and the ventricles.

Until a short time ago all the cardiac ganglia were believed to be motory organs. In a discussion, some years ago, before the Association of American Physicians, that opinion was upheld, and appeared to be sustained by a paper published in *Virchow's Arch.*, vol. lxxiv., written by Tutjanin, in 1878. But according to the researches of His and Romberg,[†] it seems to be proven that the ganglia come from the sympathetic plexus. Now the sympathetic ganglia were demonstrated by Onod[‡] to be derived from the spinal ganglia, which are exclusively sensitive. That is why the sympathetic and the cardiac ganglia should be sensitive only,[§] provided Onod's results are confirmed, which is demanded by the bewildering complexity of the anatomy and physiology of the sympathetic nerve in general.

Co-ordinate in importance with the ganglia, if they be motory at all, the pneumogastric nerve and branches of the sympathetic control the action of the heart. The cardiac branches of the former have mainly an inhibitory action, but contain accelerating fibres also; one of the upper cardiac branches is a depressor, which diminishes the tone of the blood-vessels and arterial blood pressure; its pericardial branches carry sensitive fibres. The sympathetic nerve is known to be sensitive, secretory, motory, vaso-motory, vaso-dilatatory, inhibitory, accelerating, and trophic. It sends accelerating branches from its cervical portion directly to the heart. There are many communicating branches between this and the cerebrospinal nerves. In this way the blood-vessels, the muscular layers of which are thus completely controlled, are influenced in the most various ways, which are seldom understood in an individual case. But there is one fact that is easily appreciated, viz., that in most cases it is utterly impossible to be quite certain of the correctness of our remedial indications in the diseases of an organ with such an inor-

---

† *Arbeiten aus d. Med. Klinik zu Leipzig.*
‡ *Arch. f. Mikrosk. Anat.*, 1886, vol. xxii.
§ A. Hoffmann, *Pathologie und Therapie der Herzneurosen*, 1901, p. 14.

dinately complex innervation Nor are these difficulties diminished or obviated by the heart muscle, for it is rarely diseased without some endocardial or (and) pericardial complication. The results of modern research tempt us often—indeed, should tempt us—to make the diagnosis of our forefathers, "carditis," more frequently than that of an isolated myocarditis, or endocarditis, or pericarditis.

Besides, the anatomical alterations of the myocardium vary considerably as to their etiology, nature, and seat. In regard to the latter, it should not be overlooked that the lesions of no disease are universal in the tissues of a whole organ. A pneumonia is local; a nephritis need not change all of the renal substance; an encephalitis is local. So a myocarditis is not, or need not be, universal; it is mostly focal; indeed, parts of the myocardium may be healthy, while others are diseased. That is why a drug that acts well on the healthy part of the muscle may not affect the abnormal portion, and *vice versâ*, and why the results of our medication may leave—do leave—much to be desired.

The character of myocardial changes may be inflammatory or merely degenerative. Inflammation may be acute or chronic, general, or interstitial. The latter is mostly chronic, and frequently toxic. The degeneration of the muscular tissue of the heart may consist of mere parenchymatous turbidity, or of granular degeneration, or may amount to segmentation and fragmentation (Hektoen, *American Journal*, 1897, November), which may have different causes, from very strong and irregular contractions to (more frequently) extended acute or chronic, primary or secondary textural changes, with results depending on the extent of the lesion.

Of the greatest importance to the practitioner, is the causation of myocardial anomalies which are usually chronic. Congenital smallness of the heart may lead to lipomatosis without secondary dilatation; that is what I have seen in a case of pernicious anæmia, which proved fatal to a woman, aged 34.

25

Insufficient nutrition, with secondary anæmia, injures mainly the muscular structure more than the interstitial connective fibres. Chronic disturbances of the circulation‖ disturb the nutrition of the heart by affecting its nutrient vessels. So does the obliteration of the pericardial cavity. Insufficient exercise in overworked school children, and persons with sedentary habits, though not so suddenly as overexertion, injures nutrition. Chronic changes of nutrition, for instance, the scrofulous tendency, and adiposity from whatever cause, have a similar effect. A certain number of myocardial alterations depend on nervous influences, which act either directly on the cardiac innervation, or influence the structure of the heart muscle by their effect on the cardiac circulation and nutrition.

The depressing effect of emotions causes distension, dilatation, or hypertrophy, by preventing the completion of systolic discharges, differently from what takes place during athletic sports. It is in these latter, particularly when the heart was not healthy previously, that temporary distension may become permanent. Indeed, fatigue alone renders the muscles more flaccid.

But many more structural changes of the myocardium are due to intoxications and infections. Alcohol, tobacco, syphilis, tuberculosis, and malaria, have long been known in that connection. The dangers of the acute and chronic myocardial changes that follow infectious diseases, have been studied these twenty years or less, since it became manifest that high temperatures alone were credited with more injurious consequences than they deserved. Typhoid fever, scarlatina, influenza, and diphtheria, particularly the latter, occupy the front rank as injurious influences. When their symptoms, principally arhythmia and extensive (mostly systolic) murmurs with (or without) accentuation of the second pulmonary sound, disappear within a few weeks, the prognosis as to complete

‖ Such as sclerosis of the coronary or universal atheromatosis or chronic nephritis.

recovery is good; it becomes doubtful when they remain a few months, and bad if after a year (good care being taken of the general health) the last symptoms are still persisting. The sudden deaths from heart failure, mainly during and after diphtheria, find their ready explanation partly in the muscular alterations, partly in the structural changes in the innervating fibres of their ganglionic centres.

I mentioned arhythmia of the heart as a prominent symptom. It has been attributed to a vast number of causes, to remember which taxes the memory unduly, unless we class them under two heads, the first of which is abnormal innervation (neuroses, and psychical diseases, cerebral affections, reflexes, poisoning with digitalis, coffee, tea, or alcohol); the second, a disease of the myocardium. All sorts of valvular affections have also been charged with having the same effect of causing arhythmia, but we should not forget that the murmurs which are believed to be valvular, are often myocardial, and that both stenoses and insufficiencies may depend on the condition of that small part of the myocardium in which the valves are inserted. Applications of ice, digitalis, or strychnine internally, or in other cases an opiate, will frequently diminish or remove a murmur that was erroneously attributed to the lesion of a valve. Myocardial arhythmia may be congenital; it is frequent in atheromatous and fatty degeneration, in acute or chronic inflammations, and in cases of pericardial adhesions. All the arhythmias observed in typhoid, variola and influenza, should be explained by the parenchymatous changes brought about by the microbic or toxic infection. These parenchymatous and the acute and chronic inflammations of the heart muscle have a characteristic peculiarity in this, that the lesions are not ubiquitous, or not equally disseminated. That is why the muscular contraction is not uniform, as, for instance, in the cases of fibroma of the heart muscle observed by Ebstein. The results may be irregularity or gallop rhythm, while in those cases in which the change is uniform, as in many forms of fatty degeneration, the result is either tachycardia or bradycardia.

Heidenhain and Knoll found also that arhythmia is observed when the heart is over-crowded with blood, and its force not commensurate with the resistance met with in the peripherous circulation. It is particularly in these cases, as in some of the conditions enumerated above, that cardiac stimulants such as digitalis and strychnine, seem to find their proper indications. In such cases we have to deal either with an incompetency of the whole myocardium, or with a local weakness, or fatigue depending on a local, perhaps not diagnosticable, alteration. Still, such instances are very perplexing, for it is exactly in them that the cardiac stimulants refuse to act, or become positively injurious.

Ethel Z., aged 10, was admitted to the "Jacobi Ward" of Roosevelt Hospital, February 21, 1901. Had diphtheria several years ago. Other history negative. Three weeks before admission child had an attack of pain in several joints, with fever; was in bed two weeks; out of bed since, but with dyspnea and some articular pains. Urine 1,026, trace of albumin, a few granular casts, no blood, no renal epithelia. Lungs, liver, and spleen negative. Apex beat in fifth space, outside of nipple line, cardiac dulness corresponding, and extending 1 cm. beyond the sternum about the second rib. Systolic mitral murmur quite loud. Second aortic and pulmonary sounds accentuated. Secona (mitral and tricuspid) sounds above the level of apex reduplicated; gallop rhythm. Took some salicylate of sodium, and was given strychnine, one-fiftieth grain, three times a day, February 26.

February 28.—Urine negative, no casts; gallop rhythm much more marked, and radial pulse slightly irregular. Strychnine was discontinued, and codeine one-quarter grain four times a day substituted.

March 4.—Systolic mitral murmur not changed; gallop rhythm less; it grew less from day to day, till March 9, when codeine was omitted and replaced by strychnine.

March 10.—Gallop rhythm more marked. Its intensity

grew until March 15, when strychnine was discontinued, and codeine resumed. After a week the second sound was no longer double, and the child, after having been out of bed, was discharged April 15.

Teresa de T., aged 9, was admitted March 7, 1901, with chorea minor. Had chorea five years previously, and never was quite free. Three months ago the twitching became worse. Urine negative, with the exception of a few pus cells. Lungs negative. Faint, soft systolic murmur at apex. Pulse very irregular and intermittent. Second sound over mitral and tricuspid duplicated; gallop rhythm. Appetite poor, but sleeps well, and feels comfortable when in bed. Liquor arsenitis potassii and, on account of deficient appetite and also the gallop rhythm, which was attributed to myocardial debility, strychnine nitrate, one-fiftieth grain three times a day were ordered.

March 10.—While continually in bed heart more irregular, gallop rhythm more marked. Strychnine stopped, and codeine, one-quarter grain four times a day, substituted.

March 14.—Pulse fairly regular, gallop rhythm much less.

March 18.—Pulse quite regular, and gallop rhythm almost disappeared. Strychnine was resumed and codeine omitted.

March 20.—While the condition of the child was improved, the pulse became slightly irregular again, and gallop rhythm returned. The experiment was not continued, strychnine omitted, and codeine resumed. Gallop rhythm became less within three days, and disappeared on March 31, when the patient was discharged.

In both these cases the temptation to consider the gallop rhythm as depending on general muscular weakness of the heart only was very great. If that diagnosis had been correct, strychnine would surely have been indicated. Failing utterly, it proved the incompleteness or the erroneousness of the diagnosis. Even if partly correct, the cases would prove the complex conditions of the cardiac lesions in many, perhaps most,

instances. It would also prove that the great pass-word " simplicity of prescription, only one drug at a time, no polypharmacy,
rely on nature," has its unscientific and ridiculous side. Muscle,
serous membrane, vagus, and sympathetic, may be affected at the
same time, or some of them at the same time. Rely on digitalis
alone? Yes, if you be sure you want nothing but the stimulation of the pneumogastric. On strychnine alone? Very
well, if you want a vaso-motor stimulus. Alcohol? If you
want to dilate blood-vessels, in conditions of spastic anæmia,
occasioned by fright, chill, or sepsis. Atropine? If you have
to combat the lowered number of cardiac contractions. Thus
I might go on teaching the necessity of combining medicines in
combined conditions.

Strychnine is eminently a vaso-motor remedy, which is indicated to correct defective distribution of the blood. It stimu-
lates the centre of the pneumogastric nerve, and thereby
contracts all the blood-vessels under its control, mainly those '
of the heart and of the abdominal cavity. These latter depend
on the action of the splanchnic nerve, the section or the
paralysis of which results in dilatation of the numberless
dilatable vessels of all the viscera. The vast amount of blood
thus stored in the abdominal cavity is withdrawn from the
aorta, the pressure of which is lowered (even much more than
in excessive aortic insufficiency), and from the brain. Pallor,
collapse, and syncope are the results.

Strychnine, through its stimulating influence on the centre of
the vagus, contracts the paralytic blood-vessels, and thus facili-
tates a new supply to the heart and brain.

The dose of a remedy required is by no means a stable one,
for the amount of blood appears to influence the action of a
drug in the living organism. Walker explains the resistance of
fish to the action of curare by their smaller amount of blood,
which has from one-fifty-third to one-ninety-third of their body
weight, while the proportion is in the dog from one-twelfth to
one-eighteenth, and in man, one-thirteenth to one-nineteenth,

the latter figures in the young, the former in the adult. It appears, therefore, that in fish the poison arrives at the periphery of the nerves more slowly than in the mammal. In accordance with this observation is that of Delaunay (*Comptes Rendus de l'Acad. des Sciences*, vol. xliii., p. 452), who found that when a frog was poisoned by strychnine after a depletion, its action was less marked than in a frog not so depleted. Of two frogs, that one which was better nourished was more sensitive to the action of a poison than that one which was emaciated by starving, and the right half of the body, which in frogs is more developed than the left, was more sensitive, more readily poisoned than the latter. It would consequently appear that like young infants, ill-fed, or emaciated, or slowly convalescent, or septic patients, or those in whom the nerves, for instance, in infectious fevers, have undergone organic deterioration, require larger doses of strychnine (also of other poisons, such as quinine, atropine, or nicotine) than the normal organism.

The newly-born is but little sensitive to strychnine. The spastic effect is obtained by $0 \cdot 415$ milligrammes of the nitrate in a kilogramme of the newly-born animal, $0 \cdot 347$ milligrammes of the animal when $2\frac{1}{2}$ days old, $0 \cdot 218$ milligrammes when $7\frac{1}{2}$ days old, $0 \cdot 210$ milligrammes when 10 days old (L. Lewin, *Die Nebenwirkungen d. Arzn.*, 3rd edition, 1899, p. 6).¶ This observation is fully in accordance with the fact (Soltmann) that reflex effects are but scantily obtained in the newly-born animal.

Still, in older children unexpected effects of strychnine have been observed. There are accidents on record after the subcutaneous use of strychnine in diphtheritic paralysis. Hyperæmia of and hemorrhage into the nervous centres, mainly the brain, seem to cause a great sensibility towards strychnine. I should judge that it is due to the diminished or paralysed inhibition

¶ F. A. Falck, *Arch. f. d. Phys.*, 1884, p. 525.

in the same way that patellar reflexes are exaggerated during cerebral diseases.

Some of the fatal terminations of strychnine treatment occurred in cardiac diseases. It is worth while to take notice of such facts, as long as the prevalent habit of prescribing strychnine is apt to run into the thoughtlessness of routine.

Strychnine is claimed as a vaso-motor stimulant. The centre of vaso-motor influences is located near the inhibitory, and also near the respiratory centres. The vaso-motor centre regulates blood pressure, and influences the contractions of the heart. They become more frequent during an increase, and more slow during a diminution of blood pressure. It appears evident that whatever drug influences blood pressure influences the heart. Blood pressure, however, does not depend on the heart, or the heart alone, but also to a great extent on the peripheral circulation, which is almost exclusively due to the action of voluntary and involuntary muscles. Their tone is influenced by their voluntary or involuntary action. Contractions of the voluntary muscles brought about or strengthened by strychnine, for instance, or by massage, or by electricity, increase general blood pressure by inciting arterial action and the force and number of the contractions of the heart. It is, indeed, in conditions of inactivity or insufficiency of the voluntary muscular system, no matter of what origin, with its incompetent effect on the general circulation, that strychnine finds one of its principal indications. That is why strychnine is not indicated in vascular neuroses, attended as they frequently are, with increased tendency to reflex action, no matter whether they are uncomplicated or form a part of general hysteria or neurasthenia, or are connected with organic nervous disorders. Some of these neuroses are dependent on or complicated with local endocarditis, or with general arteriosclerosis. In many the fundamental, in others the organic symptoms are predominant. To that general class belong the paroxysmal pulsation and dilatation of blood-vessels, mainly the aorta, the paroxysmal congestion of the face, the acute circumscribed œdema, the intermittent dropsy of the joints, Raynaud's disease, Weir Mitchell's erythromelalgia, Schultze's akroparæsthesia, and the intermittent limping (Erb's angiosclerotic, intermittent dysbasia).

THE HYGIENIC AND MECHANICAL TREATMENT OF HEART DISEASE.

BY BOARDMAN REED, M.D.

PHILADELPHIA, PA.

THE forms of heart disease particularly referred to in this paper are those involving autotoxic degenerative changes in the cardiac muscle, as well as those in which hypertrophy or dilatation has developed without any other cause discoverable than a faulty metabolism with or without an increase in the arterial tension. The chronic valvular affections caused by acute articular rheumatism and the various forms of chronic endocarditis and myocarditis which result from specific infection or from extraneous toxic agents, though less amenable to the methods of treatment now recommended, may yet usually derive benefit from them.

We all know that an increase in the arterial pressure adds to the work of the heart by increasing the resistance to be overcome, and many of us are also convinced that autointoxication plays an important *rôle* in arteriosclerosis, chronic myocarditis, &c., yet these etiologic facts do not always receive due consideration in the management of cardiac cases.

At the meeting of this Association held in Washington in the year 1894, a paper contributed by me, and kindly read in my absence by Dr. J. B. Walker, was entitled "The Ratio which Alimentation should bear to Oxygenation in Diseases of the Lungs." My observations up to that time had shown that not only in gastric and intestinal affections, but also in pulmonary disease, it is necessary to pay much attention to the diet and exercise, to see to it that the system is not burdened by an amount of food in excess of its powers to digest, oxidise, and assimilate. Recent personal experience has proved that in cardiac affections the same principle holds good. Indeed, in the case of an embarrassed heart, a disregard of sound dietetic rules can do far more harm than in tuberculosis.

In two ways at least the heart may be injured by the toxic products of imperfect digestion, as well as by suboxidation and other faults of metabolism: (1) Its muscles may be directly impaired by the circulating poisons, and at the same time be poorly nourished in common with all the other muscles by the blood previously impoverished from the same cause; and (2) its work may be much increased by the contraction of the arterioles resulting from the action of the alloxuric bodies and other products of imperfect metabolism.

It depends upon the particular fault in this process, and the nature of the resulting poisons in the circulation, whether on the one hand enfeeblement of the cardiac muscle and possible dilatation result, or on the other hand, primarily hypertrophy, with then dilatation as a later consequence. It would unduly prolong this paper to enter fully here upon a consideration of autointoxication and the most recent investigations concerning uric acid, the xanthin bases, &c. It is enough to cite the now admitted fact that certain of these products of nitrogenous katabolism present in excess in the blood, cause a contraction of the arterioles. Among the constituents of tea, coffee, and cocoa are active principles, which are very closely allied chemically to some of the highly toxic alloxuric bases, which the investigations of Rachford, Croftan, and others, show to be responsible for many of the harmful effects which Haig especially, has attributed to uric acid. These include the elevation of the arterial tension, and the causation of arteriosclerosis, Bright's Disease, &c. All these uratic products are of proteid derivation, and it follows, therefore, that a too predominantly nitrogenous diet, especially when made up largely of meat, and particularly the meat from those parts of animals' rich in nucleins, such as the pancreas, liver, kidneys, &c., must prove injurious to persons having a lithemic tendency.

According to the theory of Horbaczewsky, which is now pretty generally accepted, the alloxuric bases are produced by the katabolism of the nucleins of the body when there is deficient oxidation ; and Croftan in this country by recent brilliant experiments has demonstrated that xanthin and hypoxanthin can raise arterial tension, set up the characteristic changes of nephritis in the renal epithelium, and produce true cardiac hypertrophy.

The practical lesson to be drawn from these facts is, that for the prevention of threatened cardiac hypertrophy and the renal changes that so often accompany it, a suitable diet, not too nitrogenous in character, and an amount of careful moderate exercise in the open air, sufficient to oxidise fully the food taken, are indispensable. It should be still more important to regulate most carefully the diet and exercise in cases in which the heart and kidneys have already undergone pathologic changes from the irritation produced by the toxic products of an incomplete proteid katabolism. The uratic group of products of tissue metabolism has now been studied much more fully than the other leucomaines. Some of these katabolic products, while no less toxic than the xanthins, apparently act, to judge from clinical experience, in a different way, weakening the cardiac muscle and producing a rapid irregular pulse, with a tendency to degeneration or dilatation rather than hypertrophy of the heart. The following case, among many similar ones that have come under my observation, seems worth reporting : —

An unmarried lady, aged 25, came under my care in January, 1897, in a highly nervous excitable state, with marked general debility (almost entire inability to walk), and much indigestion. She had been previously robust, and very active, but had broken down rather suddenly without any ascertainable cause. In the previous treatment of her atttack of what seemed to be nervous prostration, champagne had at times been freely administered to keep her up. Her pulse was very feeble, and somewhat irregular, though no actual enlargement of the heart could then be made out, and there were no signs of valvular disease. Her stomach was a little dilated, and the gastric juice deficient in HCL. There was also constipation. The urine was variable; sometimes an excess of uric acid and urates, and at other times a deficiency of all the solids, but never any albumen or sugar. It was not my custom then, as it now is, to examine the urine of every patient for either indican or the aromatic sulphates, or both, as well as for the total acidity, and examinations for these were not then made in this case. What would otherwise be a long story, being much condensed, this patient was treated *secundum artem* for nervous prostration with gastric and cardiac complications. She had a rest cure, was allowed a very nourishing though careful diet, which probably included, however, more meat than was best for her, took various cardiac tonics at times during a period of several months, and had the benefit meanwhile of the invigorating climate of Atlantic City, spending much time in a wheeled chair on the Boardwalk there. Her nerve tone and stomach improved markedly, but her heart grew worse if anything, the pulse becoming at last more rapid and irregular under moderate doses of digitalis and strophanthus carefully alternated, than without them. The Schott movements against resistance (*Widerstandgymnastik*) were tried in a desultory way, but I had then had little experience with the method. By my advice, in July, 1897, the patient was sent to Nauheim, Germany, and after the special treatment there, returned with her heart considerably stronger, though still irregular. I did not see much of her after this until the spring of 1898, when I was summoned to the country residence of the family in North-eastern Pennsylvania. Her pulse was then rapid, weak, and irregular, and the heart slightly enlarged. She was also by spells much depressed mentally. Her urine showed at times a large excess of uric acid, and occasionally oxalic acid crystals. In the following June the patient with her mother and brother went again to Nauheim, and I accompanied the party. Another course of the baths and special movement benefited her, the heart returning to within normal limits and becoming stronger, without, however, losing the irregularity. I think now that the gain would have been greater if we had allowed her less nitrogenous food, and paid more attention to the renal excretion, as all along she was manifestly lithemic. Since her return to this country, in the autumn of 1898, though residing at a distance from Philadelphia, she has followed out a line of treatment laid down by me. This has included a diet from which sugar and alcoholic stimulants have been wholly excluded, while acids, fresh yeast bread, coffee, tea, and chocolate, and meat taken from the glandular organs of animals, were avoided so far as possible, and other kinds of flesh food allowed once a day only. She has taken very little medicine, except occasionally small doses of calomel, with a laxative as required, and a very free use of the milder alkaline waters. She has been required to practice the Schott movements daily, and to spend most of her time in fair weather out of doors in light exercise, such as walking or driving, and when tired of these, has sat out in the open air, well wrapped up, of course, in the colder weather.

When I saw her last, in the summer of 1900, her pulse was fairly good, and much more regular than formerly. She had not only retained the improvement made at Nauheim, but had acquired a decided additional gain in health. She wrote me in April of this year that she felt well, and had done much walking in the open air nearly every day all the winter.

It seems probable that many of us have occasionally overlooked the real etiology in these cases of heart disease from lithemia and other forms of autointoxication, and in treatment have relied too largely upon drug remedies of the digitalis group, which by further contracting the arterioles, aggravate the difficulty.

The treatment of lithemia, when recognised, is now fairly well understood, and need not be further enlarged upon here, except to urge the great importance of massage, and an abundance of out-door air, as well as a strict regulation of the diet. When the gastric or intestinal digestion is primarily more at fault than the metabolism, treatment, of course, must be directed accordingly, and the modern exact methods of investigating the secretory and motor functions of the stomach should not be neglected. It is equally unnecessary to discuss at length in this connection the Nauheim baths and special gymnastics, since numerous books have been devoted to them. It is highly important, however, to emphasise the fact that the artificial carbonated baths, to be had in this country, are useful, and that the ordinary hot sea water or salt water baths can be made effective, if employed cautiously, to dilate the blood-vessels of the skin and external muscles, with an ample period of rest following each bath, and the conjoint use of massage and exceedingly mild exercises between.

The great point to remember in this kind of treatment is, that both the baths and exercises are designed to lessen the labour of the heart by dilating the vessels, and need to be so managed as never to fatigue that organ. The pulse should be closely watched during each bath, never being allowed to be accelerated, and the gymnastic movements should be so controlled (as they always can be) that the pulse shall be slowed rather than quickened by them.

Oertel's carefully graduated system of hill climbing is based upon a similar principle, though it is not adapted to advanced cases.

To sum up: (1) Cardiac disease is often due to auto-intoxication, especially to poisoning by the alloxuric bases. (2) Cure or amelioration in such cases requires at first, in addition to appropriate diet, not too nitrogenous, the utmost

practicable rest of the crippled organ.   This cardiac rest may
be further promoted by very gentle exercises, which dilate the
capillaries without taxing the heart.   (3) The Nauheim method
of treatment spares the heart by dilating the too contracted
arterioles in two ways: (*a*) By stimulating the peripheral circulation through carbonated saline baths; and (*b*) by massage
and forms of exercise (*Widerstandgymnastik*) so mild as not
to quicken the pulse.

A CASE OF MALIGNANT ULCERATIVE MITRAL VALVULITIS.

BY W. DUFFIELD ROBINSON, M.D., AND JUDSON DALAND, M.D.
PHILADELPHIA.

THE patient from whom this heart was removed was a male, aged 68; married. He was always most temperate in food and drink, and of most hygienic life habits. Until the age of 46 he had always enjoyed good health, and there was no history of rheumatism, typhoid fever, malaria, pneumonia, nor intestinal disease, and at no time was he confined to bed because of illness. At the age of 45 he was extremely exhausted by running for a train. At or about the age of 46 he complained of headaches, which were looked upon as congestive by his physician. In April of this year he suffered an attack of fever, which confined him to the house for three weeks, and after which he did not fully regain his strength until late in the winter. At first the fever was looked upon as typhoid, and later was diagnosed as simple continued fever.

A few months after this attack of fever he complained of numbness, with partial loss of power of the left side, which was diagnosed as slight hemiplegia, due to apoplexy or embolism. Several months elapsed before he regained full control over the side affected.

At the age of 58 he had a severe attack of diarrhœa, which lasted several weeks.

Previous to this time he had successfully passed several

26

Life Insurance examinations, but the following year he was rejected because of the discovery of a heart murmur.

In December, 1899, after having been thoroughly exhausted by a long journey, he took a long drive in the cold while attending a funeral in New England, and became thoroughly chilled. He was greatly prostrated upon his arrival in Philadelphia, and at this time placed himself under the care of Dr. W. Duffield Robinson, who then noticed the characteristic signs of nervous enfeeblement, similar to those observed in collapse following shock. His colour was pale, and speech slow and irregular, but the symptoms present did not direct attention to any special organ. The cardiac murmur presented the same character it had some years previously, *i.e.*, low pitch and blowing quality. The urine when examined gave negative results.

Within a week there was a slight rise in temperature in the late afternoon. His feebleness was so great that he was compelled to rest in bed. Repeated careful physical examinations during the first three weeks of his illness failed to demonstrate the existence of any disease. Typhoid fever was suspected, more especially as an epidemic prevailed at that time, but no symptom of this disease could be discovered, other than the continued fever, and the Widal test was negative. His temperature curve showed an increase of 0·50 at the end of each week, as compared with the previous week, and gradually the number of hours he had fever each day increased until there was continued fever. The morning temperature averaged 99·4 degrees, and the evening temperature 102 degrees during the tenth week. Gradually the temperature rose to 102 degrees in the morning, and to 105 degrees in the evening.

During his entire illness no cardiac symptoms were present, and although he was frequently questioned, he related none of the subjective symptoms of disease of this organ. There was no dyspnea nor nausea ; the appetite was fair, and the body weight was fairly well preserved. He frequently complained of a distressing, burning sensation of the skin of the limbs during the last six weeks of his life, but no abnormality could be detected by inspection.

Owing to the presence of an enlarged prostate, cystitis developed, and catheterisation became necessary during the last ten years of his life.

There was no sweating, diarrhœa, constipation, delirium, disease of the lungs, nor bronchial tubes, and the spleen was not enlarged. Although his body weight was maintained, he gradually grew more feeble, and was practically helpless, and could only whisper a few words. There were no bedsores.

A slight albuminuria appeared six weeks before death, probably due in large part to cystitis. A few hyaline casts were discovered.

The high temperature was unassociated with any of the ordinary symptoms. The burning of the skin of the legs was oftentimes so marked that he sought relief by keeping them uncovered, and by the application of very hot or very cold fomentations.

His pulse rate followed the rise in temperature, and during the interval of fever his pulse would oftentimes beat 140 per minute. During the last ten days of his illness nothing of importance was observable, excepting progressive, extreme asthenia.

This case was also carefully studied by Drs. J. M. DaCosta and Horatio C. Wood.

The mitral regurgitant murmur was faint, and oftentimes inaudible. The diagnosis of ulcerative endocarditis was concurred in by all who saw him.

Two examinations of the blood were made by Dr. Daland, one about ten weeks before death, which showed 80 per cent. of red blood corpuscles, and an equal percentage of hæmoglobin. At the time of the second examination, about two weeks before his death, the red blood cells had been reduced to 58 per cent., and the hæmoglobin to 45 per cent. At the time of the first examination the approximate number of leucocytes per cubic millimetre was 60,000, and at the time of the second examination a count of the leucocytes showed 40,400 per cubic millimetre. The red blood cells were practically normal in appearance, excepting that at the time of the second examination they seemed a trifle pale.

Four analyses were made; two about ten weeks before death, and two about two weeks before death. The first two specimens showed a specific gravity of 1018 and 1020; the reaction was faintly acid, and both showed a faint trace of indican and a slight excess of urates and phosphates, but no albumin, sugar, nor acetone. Microscopically, these specimens showed many red blood cells; a moderate number of leucocytes, pus.cells, uric acid crystals, urates and phosphates, and occasional hyaline casts. The last two specimens examined showed a specific gravity of 1009 and 1010; the reaction was intensely acid; albumin was present in the evening specimen to the extent of ½ bulk, and in the morning specimen ¼ bulk; there was an excess of phosphates, but no sugar, indican, nor acetone. Microscopic examination showed every field full of leucocytes and pus cells, and a few short, broad hyaline tube casts. He died from asthenia on April 15, 1900.

The autopsy was performed the following day, and with the exception of the heart, nothing of importance was observed.

Examination of the brain was not permitted.

The heart showed a moderate enlargement, more especially of the left side, which enlargement was chiefly due to a thickening of the left ventricular wall. Upon examination this muscle showed evidences of fatty degeneration. The left ventricular cavity was only slightly dilated. The columnæ carneæ had the appearance of slight hypertrophy. Many of the chordeæ tendineæ attached to the mitral leaflets showed attenuation, and some were ruptured, and those that were inserted in the free edge of the posterior leaflets of the mitral valves were remarkably thickened and fibroid. The entire leaflet was greatly thickened, and all over the surface was observed small, granular, hard fibroid deposits. This roughening was particularly conspicuous upon the auricular surface. The anterior leaflet of the mitral valve showed similar changes, but to a less extent. Viewing the surface of the interior leaflet from the auricular side, plainly can be seen numerous large and small, flat, fresh vegetations, whereas the coarsely granular, fibroid projections upon the same portion of the posterior leaflet were whitish in colour, hard in consistency, and were evidently the result of a former inflammation. A careful study of the mitral valve and its relation to the mitral orifice, makes plain the origin of the faint systolic murmur already described. The anatomical conditions present were such as to produce a pre-systolic murmur, but in all probability the weak cardiac systole was unable to propel the blood with sufficient velocity to produce this murmur. The aortic leaflets were competent, but were thickened. The coronary orifice was unusually large and patulous. The aorta was moderately atheromatous. The right ventricle presented nothing unusual, but it was plainly apparent that the hypertrophied intraventricular septum encroached especially upon this cavity. The pulmonary and tricuspid valves and orifices presented no abnormality. There was a considerable deposit of fat over the surface of the heart, more especially the right ventricle and apex region. The superficial veins were all enlarged and distended with blood. The pericardium was normal.

It is not at all improbable that the attack of fever at the age of 46 was rheumatic in character, and was accompanied by endocarditis, and that the hemiplegia, which occurred a few months later, was embolic in origin. A mitral systolic murmur was known to exist for fourteen years before death.

The exhaustive journey in December, 1899, followed by thorough chilling, probably induced a recurring attack of endocarditis, which engrafted itself upon the already diseased mitral valve. The excessive asthenia, both physical and mental, was probably due to extremely weak circulation, secondary to the mitral disease. It is interesting to note the entire absence of œdema.

The prolonged fever, which was first observed about four and a half months before death, was due to ulcerative endocarditis, affecting more particularly the anterior leaflet of the mitral valve. This is interesting as showing that malignant ulcerative endocarditis may occur in an old man, without well-defined cause, accompanied by profound asthenia as practically the only symptom, and the only physical sign was an intermittent, soft blowing, almost inaudible, apex systolic murmur in association with an extremely feeble cardiac first sound. The occurrence of leucocytosis adds another example of this sign in ulcerative endocarditis.

DISCUSSION.

Dr. CURTIN: The cause is a very remarkable one and the changes around the mitral valve are much more marked than is usual in cases of this kind. It seems that there is an atheromatous change there as well as an inflammatory one.

Dr. BALDWIN: This case calls to my mind one in which the diagnosis of miliary tuberculosis was made by mistake. The patient was a young physician of good physique who had the opinion of the best consultants, and the concensus of opinion was that he had better take the benefit of the doubt and go to Saranac. The fluoroscope shewed a shading at both bases and the heart was enlarged, but no murmurs existed and the cardiac enlargement could not be made out on percussion. The cardiac disease developed markedly in a few weeks and he returned home to die within about six months.

Dr. FISK : At the last meeting of the Association I mentioned a case of diphtheria with endocarditis. The first symptom apparent was a valvular murmur. The heart symptoms appeared before there was any evidence of a membrane.

I have in mind two other cases of acute endocarditis that seemed to be greatly relieved by the administration of salycilate of sodium, and in its administration I believe we should endeavour to get the drug derived from the willow.

Dr. ARNOLD : It seems to me this case illustrates the well-known fact that cases of malignant ulcerative endocarditis are extremely difficult to diagnosticate. The physicians are to be congratulated upon making the diagnosis as they did. It is also interesting as showing how such an extensive disease may exist without anything more marked in the way of physical signs. I would like to ask if examination of the myocardium showed anything definite.

Dr. ROBINSON : No, sir, nothing, even when examined microscopically.

Dr. NEWTON : That is an interesting point, as I understand these cases usually involve the myocardium and we are told that most of our cases get along all right until the myocardium is involved.

INDEX.

Lightning Source UK Ltd.
Milton Keynes UK
UKHW020019160219
337399UK00010B/704/P